Genetics and Genomics
of Neurobehavioral Disorders

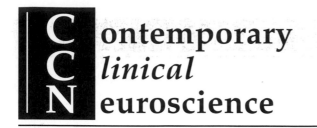

Contemporary Clinical Neuroscience

Series Editors:
Ralph Lydic and
Helen A. Baghdoyan

Contemporary Clinical Neuroscience

Genetics and Genomics of Neurobehavioral Disorders

Edited by

Gene S. Fisch

*Department of Epidemiology and Public Health
and the Child Study Center
Yale University School of Medicine
New Haven, CT*

Humana Press 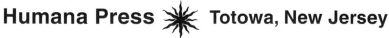 Totowa, New Jersey

Library of Congress Cataloging-in-Publication Data

Genetics and genomics of neurobehavioral disorders / edited by Gene S. Fisch.
   p. cm. -- (Contemporary clinical neuroscience)
  Includes bibliographical references and index.
  ISBN 1-58829-045-X (alk. paper); 1-59259-353-4 (e-book)
   1. Neurobehavioral disorders--Genetic aspects. I. Fisch, Gene S. II. Series.
 RC455.4.G4 G493 2003
 616.8'0442--dc21

                2002068944

Preface

Although it seems clichéd to say so, we live in a time of great discovery. With the remarkable advances in molecular genetics and genomics, and the Human Genome Project essentially completed, the feasibility of establishing meaningful genotype–phenotype correlations for complex human neurobehavioral disorders is within our reach.

In recent years, molecular geneticists have cloned, among others, genes producing Huntington's disease, spinal cerebellar ataxia, myotonic dystrophy, the fragile X syndrome (FXS), FRAXE (the "other" fragile X disorder), α-thalassemia mental retardation (ATR-X syndrome), neurofibromatosis types 1 and 2, tuberous sclerosis 1 and 2, and Rett syndrome. Researchers have also identified many of the genes in regions containing microdeletions that are associated with other neurobehavioral disorders, e.g., Prader–Willi/Angelman syndromes, Williams syndrome, and velo-cardio-facial syndrome (del22q11). Other genes associated with nonsyndromal X-linked mental retardation (MRX) have also been identified.

At the phenotypic end of these disorders, the development, refinement, and standardization of psychometric, clinical, and neuropsychological instruments have led to greater precision in the quantitative assessment and evaluation of cognition deficits and behavioral dysfunction. Among other neuroimaging techniques, functional magnetic resonance imaging (fMRI) now permits noninvasive access to brain function during the performance of various cognitive tasks. The development of animal models to emulate cognitive–behavioral features associated with many human genetic mutations, e.g., α-calcium-calmodulin kinase II, FXS, and Rett syndrome, also permit us to examine neurobiological and neurophysiological functions, as well as neuroanatomical structures that could not have been previously investigated.

The time has come to weave the various molecular genetic, genomic, neurophysiological, and neurobehavioral threads together into a cohesive fabric of human genes, brain, and behavior. The goal of *Genetics and Genomics of Neurobehavioral Disorders* is to provide the reader with a clear and comprehensive account of how genetic abnormalities, neurobiology, and neuropsychology work in concert to manifest cognitive–behavioral dysfunction.

To achieve our objective, we have divided *Genetics and Genomics of Neurobehavioral Disorders* into four distinct parts. In the first we present an introduction and overview of neurobehavioral disorders. Chapter 1 introduces neurobehavioral disorders from an historical prospective. Chapter 2 considers the neuroanatomical aspects of neurogenetic disorders, and Chapter 3 examines animal model strategies to investigate cognitive–behavioral deficits. The fourth chapter discusses the utility of examining behavioral phenotypes to investigate the pathway between genes and behavior.

The second part of the text is devoted to autosomal disorders that produce neurobehavioral dysfunction. Chapter 5 explores the genetics and pleiotropic phenotype of neurofibromatosis type 1. Chapter 6 is devoted to the cognitive–behavioral phenotype in Prader–Willi syndrome and Angelman syndrome and the genes in the deleted region that seem to affect specific functions in PWS/AS. The seventh chapter examines tuberous sclerosis 1 and 2 and genes recently discovered that cause these disorders. Chapter 8 investigates the behavioral phenotype in del22q11 (velo-cardio-facial syndrome), the psychopathology associated with the disorder, and the genes known to be deleted from the region. In Chapter 9, Williams–Beuren syndrome and genes in the deleted region on chromosome 7 known to be associated with the disorder are presented. The chapter on myotonic dystrophy (Chapter 10) describes the phenotype and the difficulties in teasing out the psychopathology associated with the disorder from what may be produced by the mutation itself.

The third and fourth parts consider X-linked disorders in which syndromal and nonsyndromal forms of XLMR are present. First, the nonsyndromal forms of X-linked mental retardation are presented in Chapters 11 and 12. Chapter 11 is a comprehensive examination of all known genes that produce syndromal and nonsyndromal XLMR (three of which are discussed in Part IV). Chapter 12 is the first comprehensive account of the genotype and phenotype in FRAXE, the "other" fragile X mutation. In Part IV the final three chapters are devoted to the three major syndromal forms of XLMR. In Chapter 13, α-thalassemia mental retardation (ATR-X) syndrome is described and both gene and gene function are reported. Chapter 14 is a comprehensive account of the fragile X syndrome and the fragile X mutation. Chapter 15 discusses Rett syndrome, an X-linked disorder primarily affecting females.

The editor and authors thank Martine Borghgraef, Edward Cook, Stewart Einfeld, Jean-Pierre Fryns, Miriam Grosof, Keith Johnson, Samantha Knight, Hans-Pieter Lipp, James MacPherson, Barbara Pober, Charles Schwartz, Roger Stevenson, and Flora Vaccarino for reviewing the chapters, and for their many comments and suggestions.

Gene S. Fisch

Contents

PART III. X-LINKED NONSYNDROMAL DISORDERS AND NEUROBEHAVIORAL DYSFUNCTION

PART IV. X-LINKED SYNDROMAL DISORDERS AND NEUROBEHAVIORAL DYSFUNCTION

Contributors

MÒNICA BAYÉS, PhD • *Departament de Ciències Experimentals i de la Salut (Genetics), Universitat Pompeu Fabra, Barcelona, Spain*

SUZANNE B. CASSIDY, MD • *Director, Division of Human Genetics, Department of Pediatrics, University of California at Irvine, Orange, CA*

JAMEL CHELLY, MD • *Institut Cochin, Laboratoire de Génétique et de Physiopathologie des Retards Mentaux, Paris, France*

RUI M. COSTA, PhD • *Departments of Neurobiology, Psychiatry, and Psychology, and Brain Research Institute, University of California Los Angeles, Los Angeles, CA*

JOANNA DRAGICH, BS • *Department of Human Genetics, University of California Los Angeles School of Medicine, Los Angeles, CA*

ELISABETH M. DYKENS, PhD • *Neuropsychiatric Institute, University of California Los Angeles, Los Angeles, CA*

YPE ELGERSMA, PhD • *Departments of Neurobiology, Psychiatry, and Psychology, and Brain Research Institute, University of California Los Angeles, Los Angeles, CA*

GENE S. FISCH, PhD • *Senior Research Scientist, Division of Biostatistics, Department of Epidemiology and Public Health, and the Child Study Center, Yale University School of Medicine, New Haven, CT*

JONATHAN FLINT, MD • *Wellcome Trust Centre for Human Genetics, University of Oxford, Oxford, UK*

ALBERT M. GALABURDA, MD • *Emily Fisher Landau Professor of Neurology and Neuroscience, Harvard Medical School, Beth Israel Deaconess Medical Center, Boston, MA*

JOZEF GÉCZ, PhD • *Department of Cytogenetics and Molecular Genetics, Women's and Children's Hospital; Department of Paediatrics, Adelaide University, Adelaide, SA, Australia*

RICHARD J. GIBBONS, DPhil, FRCP • *MRC Molecular Haematology Unit, Weatherall Institute of Molecular Medicine, University of Oxford, John Radcliffe Hospital, Oxford, UK*

BEN C. J. HAMEL, MD • *Department of Human Genetics, University Medical Centre Nijmegen, Nijmegen, The Netherlands*

MARK C. HIRST, DPhil • *Molecular Genetics Section, Department of Biological Sciences, The Open University, Milton Keynes, England*

LUIS A. PÉREZ JURADO, MD, PhD • *Departament de Ciències Experimentals i de la Salut (Genetics), Universitat Pompeu Fabra, Barcelona, Spain*

JULIA C. LEWIS, MRCPsych • *Institute of Medical Genetics, University of Wales College of Medicine, Cardiff, UK*

KIERAN C. MURPHY, MMedSci, PhD, MRCPI, MRCPsych • *Department of Psychiatry, Royal College of Surgeons in Ireland; Education and Research Centre, Beaumont Hospital, Dublin, Ireland*

KATHRYN NORTH, MD, FRACP • *Department of Paediatrics, University of Sydney; Head, Neurogenetics Research Unit, Deputy Head, Institute of Neuromuscular Research, The Children's Hospital at Westmead, Westmead, Sydney, NSW, Australia*

ALAN K. PERCY, MD • *Departments of Pediatrics, Neurology, and Neurobiology, University of Alabama at Birmingham School of Medicine, Birmingham, AL*

NANCY RATNER, PhD • *Department of Cell Biology, Neurobiology, and Anatomy, University of Cincinnati College of Medicine, Cincinnati, OH*

JULIAN R. SAMPSON, DM • *Institute of Medical Genetics, University of Wales College of Medicine, Cardiff, UK*

N. CAROLYN SCHANEN, MD, PhD • *Head of Human Genetics Research, Nemours Research Programs, Alfred I. duPont Hospital for Children, Wilmington, DE*

J. ERIC SCHMITT, MD • *Stanford Psychiatry Neuroimaging Laboratory, Stanford University School of Medicine, Stanford, CA*

ALCINO J. SILVA, PhD • *Departments of Neurobiology, Psychiatry, and Psychology, and Brain Research Institute, University of California Los Angeles, Los Angeles, CA*

JEAN STEYAERT, MD • *Department of Clinical Genetics, University of Maastricht, Maastricht, The Netherlands; Department of Child Psychiatry, University of Leuven, Belgium*

TAKAHITO WADA, PhD • *MRC Molecular Haematology Unit, Weatherall Institute of Molecular Medicine, John Radcliffe Hospital, Oxford, UK*

I

INTRODUCTION AND OVERVIEW

1

THE GENETICS AND GENOMICS OF NEUROBEHAVIORAL DISORDERS

Historical Introduction and Overview

Gene S. Fisch

1. INTRODUCTION

Broadly speaking, the genetics and genomics of neurobehavioral disorders examine the causal relationship between genetic mutations on the one hand, and impaired development, particularly cognitive–behavioral development, on the other, and the neurobiological and neurophysiological functions that are disrupted in between. Although genetics and genomics form the biological bases of behavior, we do not assume that the biological components are the sole or necessarily the most important contributors to cognitive–behavioral development. During the past century, research by experimental psychologists have clearly demonstrated the extent to which environmental stimuli and the context in which they are presented are salient factors in behavioral growth and development, language, learning, and memory. Humans develop along many psychological dimensions behaviorally, but this text focuses on known genetic anomalies and the cognitive–behavioral deficits that result in difficulties in learning and memory, problem-solving, language, and other associated limitations in psychomotor development. That is not to say no other aspects of behavior may be affected. Various forms of psychopathology may develop concomitantly with many neurodevelopmental genetic abnormalities. Children with the fragile X mutation manifest mild to severe mental retardation, but are also frequently hyperactive, inattentive, and impulsive. Children and adolescents with velo–

From: *Contemporary Clinical Neuroscience:*
Genetics and Genomics of Neurobehavioral Disorders
Edited by: G. S. Fisch © Humana Press Inc., Totowa, NJ

cardio–facial syndrome develop mild cognitive deficits but an unusually high proportion manifest schizophrenia.

2. COGNITIVE FUNCTION, INTELLIGENCE, AND GENETICS

2.1. Cognitive Ability and Intelligence

Any discussion of cognitive–behavioral impairment should begin with a description of cognitive–behavioral ability, and that involves the definition of intelligence. Recounting the famous remark by E.G. Boring, Jensen *(1)* stated that the operational definition of intelligence is what intelligence tests measure. Jensen continued, saying that problems arose only when more was attributed to intelligence than what was measured. Unfortunately, there is more than one point of view regarding the definition of intelligence, and that has been at issue for more than a century. In 1921, the editors of the *Journal of Educational Psychology* convened a symposium on intelligence and its measurement. Fourteen experts (among them, Edward L. Thorndike and Lewis Terman) provided nearly as many definitions, the central theme of which, according to Sternberg *(2)* was the ability of an individual to adapt to the environment. Sixty five years later, Sternberg and Detterman *(3)* convened a second symposium consisting of 24 experts who reiterated the earlier idea of adaptation. On the other hand, Sattler *(4)* highlighted 10 definitions provided by psychologists dating from Binet and Simon *(5)* through Sternberg *(6)* and, although many agreed that adaptation to the environment was a core component, not all included it as part of their definition. Some definitions emphasize the ability to learn. For example, Spearman *(7)* said that intelligence was "a special case ... of educing either relations or correlates." Others define intelligence as the ability to think abstractly. For example, Wechsler *(8)* defined intelligence as "the global capacity ... to act purposefully, to think rationally ..." More recently, Baroff and Olley *(9)* argued that intelligence is composed of three factors: practical problem solving, verbal ability, and social intelligence. However, Snyderman and Rothman *(10)* who asked more than 1000 experts in psychology, in fields related to psychology, and in genetics to define intelligence, found that these authorities nearly unanimously agreed otherwise. Experts said the three major components of intelligence were problem-solving ability, abstract reasoning, and the capacity to acquire knowledge.

2.1.1. A Brief Historical Survey of the Concept of Intelligence

The difficulty in defining intelligence has not been confined to 20th century psychology. Historically, the earliest conceptualizations of intelligence likely predate the notions espoused by Plato and the Socratic philosophers of the 5th century BC which involve the structure of mental processes. Plato argued that all knowledge was inborn and teaching merely extracted that which was already known. Aristotle, one of Plato's students, held a somewhat different point of view. According to Aristotle, humans, unlike other animals, had three internal senses or mental faculties with which to interpret the externally sensed universe: common sense, memory, and imagination *(11)*.

As with its definition, localization of intellectual function has also proved problematic. In the 11th century, Abu Ibn Sina, the great Muslim physician also known as Avicenna, contended that there were three faculties of function in the body, one of which, the nervous faculty, was centered in the brain *(12)*. Ibn Sina, an adherent of Aristotle's philosophy, updated the Aristotelian point of view, contending that the internal senses could be located in various brain regions. By the 15th century, physicians had extended Sina's model by adding a fourth internal sense, estimation. However, within the next 100 years, Vesalius, who actually dissected the human body, showed that these notions of brain localization were incorrect. Nonetheless, the idea of localization of brain function and its relationship to intelligence would resurface in the early part of the 19th century.

In the late 18th–early 19th century, Franz Gall revived the notion of brain function previously held by the post-Aristotlean physicians. Specifically, Gall argued that all mental activities proceeded from the brain, that brain was the organ for the mind and, like Avicenna before him, that individual mental faculties resided in different parts of the brain. Those portions of brain that were well developed would be larger than those that had evolved less favorably. Physionomically, these regions would emerge as bumps and depressions on the skull. Gall's theory of mind, brain and behavior—phrenology—was the first to argue that cranial prominence, which could be observed and measured, varied in size according to the magnitude of the cortical region beneath it. The size of the cortical region was, in turn, related to some innate mental faculty manifested at the behavioral level. Later in the 19th century, physiologists such as Flourens and Hughlings Jackson would find the Gallian notion of localization of brain function without merit. However, phrenology and craniometry flourished in the early to mid-19th century, particularly in anthropology and genetics, lending credence to some of the most egregious forms of racism and sexism Western society would encounter.

Craniometry was applied to collateral areas of research, specifically anthropology, by way of the physician and surgeon, Paul Broca, who founded the Anthropological Society of Paris in 1859 *(13)*. Broca was the first to observe that patients with speech dysfunctions exhibited brain damage in similar regions of the left frontal lobe. Although he rejected phrenology, Broca's researches provided support for the notion that a language faculty resided in part of the brain. He also believed that brain size was related to intellect. Unfortunately, his beliefs about brain function would also provide a scientific foundation for racism and sexism. Broca stated that "In general, the brain is larger ... in men than in women, in eminent men than in men of mediocre talent, in superior races than in inferior races" *(13)*. Ironically, Gall's brain weighed only 1198 grams, much smaller in size than that of the average European (1300–1400 g). Indeed, many of the anthropometric measures used to establish intellectual, racial or gender superiority, especially brain volume, were found to be flawed or even fraudulent *(13)*.

2.2. Heredity and the Assessment of Intelligence

In addition to the discord created by a lack of agreement on the definition of intelligence, there is the matter of how one measures a nonphysical attribute. Craniometry had been one quantitative inferential approach, but its popularity had waned toward the end of the 19th century. Another, more sustainable approach was developed by Francis Galton. Galton, Charles Darwin's nephew, was keenly interested in quantitation and measurement, particularly as related to human features. In *Hereditary Genius*, Galton acknowledged the extent to which the Belgian statistician, Quetelet, influenced his own interests in statistics and measurement *(14)*. Quetelet, in addition to his contributions to economics, applied Gauss' Theory of Errors to account for the variability and frequency distribution of adults' heights. Galton also investigated human attributes such as beauty, moral quality, socioeconomic status, ethnicity, the anthropometric measurements from craniometry and sensory processes (e.g., reaction time), and how these features could be related to intelligence *(4,13,15)*. Galton adapted Quetelet's application of the normal distribution of errors to his own concept of mental ability and intelligence *(14)*, the consequences of which continue to affect present day psychometrics, as well as researchers' efforts to estimate the prevalence of individuals with mental retardation (MR). It should be noted that the assumption of a Gaussian or normal distribution of frequencies as an appropriate model of psychological characteristics has never been satisfactorily demonstrated *(15)*.

As a result of his seminal efforts in statistics, psychological measurement, and genetics, Galton engendered several important principles for the formal development of psychometrics and the rise of IQ testing. Galton was first to introduce the twin concepts of general mental ability and specific aptitude. These two "factors" of intelligence would eventually find favor in the early 20th century work of Charles Spearman. Like his predecessor, Spearman's "monarchic" (a single or unitary) theory of intelligence posited that mental processes could be subsumed principally under a common factor, *g*, and secondarily under factors specific to individual processes, *s*. Spearman contended that *g* represented mental energy used by the entire cortex and possibly the nervous system as well *(16)*.

Spearman's *(17)* application of factor analysis to develop a two-factor theory of intelligence laid the foundations for later, more complex factor-analytic approaches. Thorndike *(18)* postulated that intelligence was formed by clusters of abilities connected to one another. Thurstone *(19)* devised a method of factor analysis showing that intelligence was composed of many factors. Guilford *(20)* devised a three-dimensional structure organizing intellect. Other quantitative psychologists conceived of intelligence as composed of two major components: fluid (nonverbal) and crystallized (culture-specific) abilities *(21,22)*. Later, Gustaffson *(23)* would add a third factor to this two-factor model, visualization. A more complete survey of factor-analytic theories of intelligence can be found in Sattler *(4)*.

At about the time Spearman was developing his two-factor theory, Alfred Binet had begun to test intelligence in French schoolchildren. Earlier, Binet had studied the relationship between craniometry and intelligence and found it wanting *(13)*. Binet, along with his collaborator, Theodore Simon, were commissioned by the French educational system to devise a means by which to differentiate generally educable children from those who required special means. Accordingly, Binet and Simon set about collecting many different types of test items *(24)*. Some items were related to vocabulary, some related to visual discriminations, some related to memory, some related to quantitative skills, that would satisfy four essential features that continue to form a basis for psychometric testing: (1) that items measure ability related to intellect; (2) that items be ordered by degree of difficulty; (3) that items be age-related; and (4) that items be standardized *(25)*.

Interestingly, despite the many differences in conceptualization, IQ tests based on any of the aforementioned factor-analytic approaches produce remarkably similar results. The age range of the WISC-R overlaps the WPPSI from 6 to 6 1/2 years, and the Full Scale IQ scores from each test generated by a sample of 6-year-olds are highly correlated ($r = .82$). Median correlations between the WISC-R Full scale and the K-ABC Mental Processing Composite are also high ($r = .70$; *4*). Composite IQ scores from the WISC-R and Stanford–Binet (4th Edition) are also highly correlated ($r = .69$ to $r = .83$), particularly among learning disabled and mentally retarded children *(26)*. This is likely due to the many high positive correlations obtained from the various subtests that constitute specific factors, whether they are verbal or nonverbal, abstract/visual, quantitative, or associated with visual or auditory features of short-term memory.

The notion of a single score to represent intelligence, the intelligence quotient or IQ score, was generated by Lewis Terman *(27)*. Terman was concerned about Binet's use of the term "mental age" and its relationship to chronological age in the testing procedure. Binet used mental age (MA) as the point at which a student could no longer produce correct responses, given the child's chronological age (CA). Terman, however, argued that calculating the difference between, for example, a 6-year-old child performing at the level of a 3-year-old is strikingly different from a 12-year-old performing at the 9-year-old level. Terman adapted the term "mental quotient" from Stern *(28)*, contending that "this value expresses not the difference, but the ratio of mental to chronological age, and thus is partially independent of the absolute magnitude of chronological age" (cf. *4*). Terman called his ratio, MA ÷ CA, the "intelligence quotient" or, as it has come to be known, IQ, and composite intelligence test scores typically have been referred to as IQ ever since.

2.3. Mental Retardation and Intelligence

2.3.1. A Brief History

The earliest references to MR date back more than 3500 years, but systematic evaluation and training of individuals with MR is a relatively recent phenomenon, and associated with the post-Renaissance Age of Enlightenment of the late 18th, early 19th century (cf. *12*) for a comprehensive historical review). Historically, individuals with MR were not treated well by the societies into which they were born. One means of inferring the manner in which individuals with MR were treated is to examine the Termanology used to describe them. The term "idiot" is derived from the Greek and was reserved for individuals unable to participate in the public forum, whereas "imbecile" is derived from the Latin and refers to a small stick indicative of frailty *(29)*. It has been asserted that both the Greeks and Romans practiced infanticide as a means of dealing with babies born with physical and/or developmental disabilities *(12)*.

The earliest attempts to train individuals with MR have been attributed to Jean M.G. Itard and his efforts to educate a 12-year-old boy named Victor of Aveyron, a putatively feral child *(30–33)*. Itard, who believed that Victor's psychosocial development had been stunted, began an intensive program to civilize him. Although his successes were limited, Itard was able to train Victor to recognize letters of the alphabet, develop a small receptive language, to name several objects, and make fine motor discriminations *(30)*.

Edouard Seguin, a former student of Itard, went on to develop his own "physiological treatment" to stimulate the nervous system so that a child with mental deficits could develop physically and intellectually. Every child was evaluated individually, and training exercises were based on the strengths and weaknesses observed in each, not unlike the extensive regimens employed currently by applied behavior analysts. Johann Guggenbühl, a physician contemporaneous with Sequin and who established a facility in Abendberg, Switzerland, primarily treated children with cretinism. He claimed to cure them of their MR, but when his facility was examined by outside experts, the treatments were found ineffective. Until then, Guggenbühl enjoyed a brief notoriety, and Samuel G. Howe, who visited him, returned to Massachusetts to establish an experimental program based on his teachings for individuals with MR *(32)*. Seguin's greater effect in the United States was due in part to his emigration to New York in 1852. Earlier, Horace Mann had met Seguin in Paris, as did Hervey Wilbur and James Richard, all of whom went on to establish special education programs for the mentally retarded in the United States *(34)*. In 1876, Seguin, Wilbur and Richard, along with several others, established the first professional association for individuals with MR.

Often, individuals with MR were conflated by the general public with persons suffering from mental health disorders. This resulted partly from the fact that individuals with MR were protected by the so-called Lunacy Acts passed in England centuries earlier *(35)*. Recent surveys suggest, however, that individuals with MR are at increased risk for developing maladaptive behavior and other forms of psychopathology *(36)*. This may account for some of the early findings by Goddard *(37)* in which the Kallikak family was described as prone to certain forms of criminal and maladaptive behavior; or other studies in which alcoholism and/or criminal activity were segregating *(30,38,39)*.

2.4. Genetics and Intelligence

The link between genetics and intelligence was first clearly articulated by Galton *(14)*, who later coined the term "eugenics" and reiterated "the practicability of supplanting inefficient human stock by better strains" *(40)*. Galton also referred to his study of twins and the "vast preponderating effect of nature over nurture" *(40)*. Statistical models for heritability estimates were subsequently devised by Fisher *(41)* and are at the core of ongoing nature–nurture debates, that is, the extent to which heredity and environment affect cognitive ability as reflected in the IQ score. Sattler *(4)* notes that differences in the percent of variance in IQ score accounted for by genetics ranges from 30% to 50%. However, Goldstein and Reynolds *(42)* state the range is much broader, that heritability of IQ can be as small as 20% or as large as 80%, depending on the model employed.

The heritability (and stability) of IQ is central to psychometric testing, although Binet not only questioned the utility of a single IQ score, but also declined to make use of it as a measure of inborn ability *(13)*. Also, although some prominent geneticists and statisticians continued to propose more and complex statistical models of inherited intelligence *(43,44)*, others would find fault with their respective methodologies *(45,46)* or data *(15,46,47)*. Currently, the statistical models and data used to support the heritability of intelligence are, at best, controversial.

The concept of MR as represented by the lower tail of a frequency distribution of IQ scores is derived from a statistical formulation used in quantitative psychology and the presumed normal distribution of individual abilities. Developmental psychologists were saddled with the psychometric point of view until Piaget, who had worked with Binet, left to develop his own qualitative developmental psychology. Binet and Simon were concerned about how to evaluate correct responses; but Piaget, who was dissatisfied with this formulation, became interested in the types of incorrect responses children made and how remarkably similar those errors were at specific ages. Piaget conceived of human development as unfolding through several consecutive stages, that children pass through the same stages in the same sequence, and have similar intellectual structures *(48)*. Piaget's theories of child development would later be taken up by Zigler *(49,50)* and his colleagues who would also differentiate familial MR from organic MR.

2.5. Genetics and Mental Retardation

Organic forms of MR were first identified clinically in the mid 19th century by J. Langdon Down *(12)*. Down, along with other physicians of his time, for example, William Ireland, P.M. Duncan, and W. Millard, were seeking to classify MR according to its severity, phenotype, and possible etiology. Down's text, *The Mental Affections of Children and Youth* (1887), proposed three types of MR: congenital, accidental, and developmental *(51)*. The etiology of those categorized as congenital MR were primarily genetic in origin and classified according to ethnic features: Negroid, Mongoloid, and so on. It has been argued that, as a self-described liberal, Down's ethnic classification was not intentionally racist *(12)*. However, Down stated that many individuals with congenital MR exhibited anatomical features lacking in their parents but associated with the "lower races." Given the tenor of his time and the extent to which anthropometry was used to assess intelligence, one would be hard-pressed not to consider his remarks as at least tainted with racism. As an example: "The boy's aspect is such that it is difficult to realize that he is the child of Europeans, but so frequently are these characters presented, that there can be no doubt that these ethnic features are the result of degeneration" *(13)*. Although the genotype for this disorder, trisomy 21, was identified in 1959, the term mongolism persisted until only recently, when it was renamed Down syndrome.

The putative role heredity played in MR was widely believed by many who studied individuals with developmental disorders. Many physicians reasoned that alcoholism was caused by hereditary factors *(48)*. Others attributed criminality to heredity, as in the case of the"Jukes" family *(52,53)*. The "Kallikak" family *(37)* was also frequently cited. It should be noted, however, that Gould *(13)* discovered the photographs used to depict the disordered features of several members of the Kallikak family, including that of Deborah Kallikak, had been retouched around the eyes and mouth to give them a more insidious appearance.

Although identification of many genetic causes of MR would have to await the cytogenetic and molecular genetic revolutions of the mid-to-late 20th century, many causes and clinical forms of the disorder were recognized by the mid-to-late 19th, and early part of the 20th century. In the 19th century, for example, neurofibromatosis type 1 (NF1) was first described by von Recklinghausen in 1863; tuberous sclerosis was reported by Bourneville in 1880; and cretinism was associated with hypothyroidism by Curling in 1860 and Fagge in 1870. In the early middle part of the 20th century, microcephaly associated with dysmorphic craniofacial features was identified by Cornelia de Lange in 1933; phenylketonuria (PKU) was observed by Fölling in 1934; gonadal dysgenesis recognized by Turner in 1938; and trisomy 21 (Down's syndrome) discovered cytogenetically by Lejeune and his colleagues in 1959 (cf. *12*).

3. THE DEFINITION OF MENTAL RETARDATION

Eventually, Down's conceptualization of congenital MR would become more restricted to identifiable genotypes, whereas his notion of developmental MR would expand to incorporate familial forms. As mentioned earlier, Zigler and his colleagues also differentiated between familial MR (also referred to as cultural–familial MR) and organic MR *(49,50)*. His two-group approach to MR has its roots in Down and Ireland's classificatory schemas. Zigler defined individuals with organic MR as those who sustain organic damage from inborn or prenatal causes or postnatal trauma, whereas those with no known organic etiology would be categorized as cultural–familial

MR *(50)*. The cultural–familial form of MR is also distinguished from organic causes by the greater severity and syndromal nature of the latter. Earlier, Dingman and Tarjan noted an excess in the frequency of individuals with MR based on the normal distribution of IQ scores in the general population and two standard deviations below the mean as the criterion for MR (IQ scores <70), and proposed a two-group approach to MR also *(54)*. U.S. census data have been used to estimate the prevalence of MR, and that proportion has varied from 0.5% to 3% of the general population *(12)*. The 3% estimate is typically adopted by other researchers (e.g., *55*) and used to justify the two-group approach. However, Reed and Reed *(56)* examined subsequent generations of families of persons institutionalized with MR. Of the 289 probands whose IQ scores were below 70 and who showed no signs of organicity, 20% of their children were also MR, much higher than expected if only cultural–familial factors were involved. Their data suggest that the two groups are not necessarily distinct from one another, an argument made recently by *(57)*.

As research into the causes of MR has expanded and advocates for those with MR have become more vocal, the definition of MR has also evolved. Unfortunately, the current definition does not take into account the possible differences between cultural–familial and organic MR, nor its overlap, although earlier versions of the Diagnostic and Statistics Manual (DSM) provided subcategories for organic causes *(58)*. The Association for the Advancement of Mental Retardation (AAMR) proposed that a diagnosis of MR can be given if

1. An individual's intellectual functioning is approx 70–75 or below.
2. There are significant disabilities in two or more adaptive skill areas.
3. The age at onset is below 18 years.

The AAMR definition of MR is essentially that of the American Psychiatric Association's DSM-IV diagnostic criteria *(59)*:

1. Significant subaverage intellectual functioning: an IQ of approx 70 or below on an individually administered IQ test (for infants, a clinical judgment of significantly subaverage intellectual functioning).
2. Concurrent deficits or impairments in present adaptive functioning in at least two of the following: communication, self-care, home living, social/interpersonal skills, use of community resources, self-direction, functional academic skills, work, leisure, health, and safety.
3. Onset before 18 years.

Although the current definition of MR does not differentiate between the organic and cultural–familial forms, it does oblige the diagnostician to employ both a psychometric instrument to test cognitive ability and a means by which to evaluate adaptive behavior. Other, neuropsychological measures have also been recommended to obtain a more comprehensive profile of strengths and weaknesses *(60)*.

3.1. Genetics and Mental Retardation: The One and the Many

Despite differences in etiology between cultural–familial and organic MR, defining MR in this fashion compels researchers to think about MR as a single disorder with degrees of severity based upon IQ score: mild (55–69), moderate (40–54), severe (25–39), and profound (<25). Using his two-group approach to MR, Zigler *(49,50)* demonstrated that children with cultural–familial MR performed as well as mental age equivalent children without MR on a broad array of Piagetian tasks *(61)*. However, children with cultural–familial MR perform less well on tasks involving learning and memory *(62)*. On the other hand, children with organic MR do not perform as well on Piagetian tasks as do mental age equivalent children without MR *(61)*.

There not only are differences between children with cultural–familial MR and those with organic MR, but among the different genetic disorders that produce cognitive impairment as well. Hodapp et al. *(63)* found that individuals with fragile X syndrome (FXS) exhibit sequential processing deficits on the K-ABC, while individuals with Down syndrome (DS) do not. Children with Williams syndrome (WS) seem to show remarkable expressive language skills given their typical level of MR *(64)*, although other researchers have found similar cognitive–behavioral profiles between children with WS and age-matched children with FXS, despite the obvious phenotypic differences between the two genetic disorders *(65)*.

Differences between groups of individuals with different genetic disorders manifest themselves both cross-sectionally and longitudinally. It has been shown that IQ scores among children and adolescents with DS decline as these individuals age *(66–67)*. More recently, other researchers have found that both IQ and adaptive behavior scores in children and adolescents with FXS also exhibit longitudinal decreases *(68,69)*. However, IQ scores do not show longitudinal declines among individuals with other genetic disorders. For example, children and adolescents with Prader–Willi syndrome show no significant differences between test and retest IQ scores *(70)*, nor are there longitudinal changes in IQ scores in children with FRAXE, a nonsyndromal X-linked disorder *(71,72)*. These results strongly suggest that each genetic disorder should be examined comprehensively and individually at the cognitive–behavioral level employing as many of the same assessment tools in each case for comparative purposes *(60)*.

There are types of cognitive impairment that exist at the edges of MR, other than those described. Some cognitive impairment has been described as "borderline MR" in which IQ scores range from 70 to 79 *(4)*. Other forms of dysfunction exhibit markers for syndromes that tend to form a cluster of clinical behaviors—hyperactivity, distractability, impulsivity, and learning performance below expected levels of achievement. Originally, these symptoms were designated minimal brain dysfunction (MBD) but most recently have been cast under the general heading of learning disabilities (LD).

LD was defined by the federal government as part of the law (PL 94-142) passed by the U.S. Congress in 1975, and corresponds to a significant discrepancy between "ability" (as measured by psychometric testing) and "achievement" (as measured by accomplishment in school). Since the definition of a significant discrepancy between these two measures varies from one school district to another, prevalence estimates can range from 1% to 30% *(73)*. According to one recent survey *(74)*, as many as 50% of all children requiring special education were classified as LD. Interestingly, many school districts will label a child as LD instead of MR because of the stigma attached to MR. To date, there is no single psychometric instrument developed to evaluate LD. Indeed, the factor-analytic approach of psychometric testing used to evaluate individuals with LD or organic MR may also be of limited utility, especially for those who are most severely affected with MR.

Early studies of MBD suggested, but were unable to demonstrate, genetic factors associated with dysfunction *(75,76)*. More recently, however, as the syndromes have become more clearly delineated phenotypically and genotypically, genetic causes for LD have been found. For example, among individuals with NF1, 40–60% exhibit some form of LD *(77)*. Besides NF1, evidence for a genetic basis for LD has been obtained from concordance studies of monozygotic and dizygotic twins, which strongly suggest a genetic factor or factors related to reading disabilities *(78)*. Linkage analysis has also provided statistical support for a gene or genes producing dyslexia on chromosome 15 *(79)*, and developmental dyslexia on chromosomes 6 and 15 *(80)*.

3.2. Organic Bases for Cognitive Impairment

Cultural–familial MR notwithstanding, a large proportion of the general population is affected by genetic disorders that produce some form of cognitive–behavioral dysfunction. Broman et al. *(81)* estimated that neurobiological disorders caused about 0.5% of the incidence of MR in the population. However, Fisch *(82)* noted that the proportion cited by Broman et al. excluded many currently known genetic disorders, for example, the fragile X mutation, Williams syndrome, velo–cardio–facial syndrome, as well as the many nonsyndromal XLMR types. The prevalence of these disorders combined is probably about 0.3%. As result of the advances made in molecular genetics in the past 20 years, the number of genes identified as producing cognitive–behavioral disorders is increasing at an exponential rate. One might then expect that organic causes of MR or LD may well exceed 1% of the general population.

4. GENETICS AND GENOMICS OF NEUROBEHAVIORAL DISORDERS

To date, molecular geneticists have cloned many genes causing MR or LD: fragile X syndrome, FRAXE, myotonic dystrophy, α-thalassemia mental retardation (ATR-X syndrome), Rett syndrome, neurofibromatosis types 1 and 2, tuberous sclerosis 1 and 2, and other syndromal forms of XLMR. Researchers have also identified genes in regions containing microdeletions that are associated with other neurobehavioral disorders such as Prader–Willi syndrome/Angelman syndrome, Williams syndrome, and del22q11. Other genes related to nonsyndromal XLMR have also been discovered.

At the behavioral end of the genotype–phenotype spectrum, the development, refinement, and standardization of psychometric, clinical, and neuropsychometric instruments has led to greater precision and quantitative assessment of cognitive–behavioral phenotypes identified with neurobehavioral disorders. Functional magnetic resonance imaging (fMRI) now permits noninvasive access to brain function during the performance of a variety of cognitive and memory tasks. The development of transgenic strategies in rodent models to emulate cognitive–behavioral features of human genetic mutations, for example, α-calcium–calmodulin kinase II, the fragile X mutation, neurofibromatosis type 1, has permitted scientists to examine neuroanatomical, neurobiological, and neurophysiological, functions that could not be investigated previously.

Given standardized instruments by which to assess the multidimensionality of behavior, molecular techniques by which deTermane the genetic causes of MR and LD, the development of mouse models to emulate cognitive impairment, and the knowledge of brain function obtained from many areas of investigation in neuroscience, researchers are now in a position to examine and provide a comprehensive analysis of many of the outstanding issues related to genetic and genomic etiologies of cognitive–behavioral dysfunction and their respective neurobiological and neurophysiological roles. Scientists are at a point where it is possible to weave the various molecular–genetic, genomic, neurobiological, neurophysiological, and neurobehavioral threads together into a cohesive fabric of genes, brain, and behavior in ways about which previous generations of scientists could only dream.

REFERENCES

1. Jensen AR. How much can we boost IQ and scholastic achievement? Harvard Educ Rev 1969,33:1–123.
2. Sternberg RJ. The search for criteria: why study the evolution of intelligence? In Sternberg RJ, Kaufman JC, eds. The evolution of intelligence. Mahwah, NJ: Lawrence Erlbaum, 2002;1–25.
3. Sternberg RJ, Detterman DK. What is Intelligence? Norwood, NJ: Ablex, 1986.
4. Sattler JM. Assessment of children, 3rd ed. San Diego, CA: Sattler, 1988:37–59, 61–83, 646–61.
5. Binet A, Simon T. The development of intelligence in children. Baltimore: Williams & Wilkins, 1916.
6. Sternberg RJ. Intelligence applied: understanding and increasing your intellectual skills. San Diego: Harcourt, Brace, Jovanovich, 1986.
7. Spearman C. The nature of intelligence and the principles of cognition. London: Macmillan, 1923;300.
8. Wechsler D. The measurement and appraisal of adult intelligence, 4th ed. Baltimore: Williams & Wilkins, 1958;7.
9. Baroff GS, Olley JG. Mental retardation: nature, cause and management, 3rd ed. Philadelphia: Brunner/Mazel, 1999:2–46.
10. Snyderman M, Rothman S. Survey of expert opinion on intelligence and aptitude testing. Am Psychol 1987;42:137–144.
11. Leahey TH. A history of psychology: main currents in psychological thought, 2nd ed. Englewood Cliffs, NJ: Prentice-Hall, 1987;34–57.
12. Scheerenberger RC. A history of mental retardation. Baltimore: Brookes, 1983;1–23, 51–87, 91–135.
13. Gould SJ. The mismeasure of man. New York: WW Norton, 1981;73–107, 135, 146–233.
14. Galton F. Hereditary genius. New York: D. Appleton,1884.
15. Evans B, Waites B. IQ and mental testing: an unnatural science and its social history. London: Macmillan, 1981;33–61, 145–178.
16. Spearman C. The abilities of man. New York: Macmillan, 1927.
17. Spearman C. The theory of two factors. Psychol Rev 1914;21:105 ff.
18. Thorndike EL. Human nature and the social order. New York: Macmillan.
19. Thurstone LL. Primary mental abilities. Psychometric monographs. Chicago: University of Chicago Press, 1938.
20. Guilford JP. The structure of intellect. Psychol Bull 53:267–93.
21. Catell RB. Theory of fluid and crystalized intelligence: a critical experiment. J Educ Psychol 1963;51:1–22.
22. Horn JL. Organization of abilities and the development of intelligence. Psychol Rev 1968;75:242–59.
23. Gustafsson JE. A unifying model for the structure of intellectual abilities. Intelligence 1984;8:179–203.

24. Binet A, Simon T. Méthodes nouvelles pour le diagnostic du niveau intéllectuel des anormaux. Ann Psychol 1905;11:191–244.
25. Styles I. The study of intelligence—the interplay between theory and measurement. In Anderson M, ed. The development of intelligence. Sussex, UK: Psychology Press 1999;19–42.
26. Thorndike RL, Hagen EP, Sattler JM. Technical manual, Stanford-Binet 4th Edition. Chicago: Riverside, 1986.
27. Terman L. The measurement of intelligence. Boston: Houghton Mifflin, 1916.
28. Stern W. The psychological methods of testing intelligence. Baltimore: Warwick & York, 1914.
29. Smith GF. Clinical aspects of genetics in mental retardation. In Allen RM, Cortazzo AD, Toister RP, eds. The role of genetics in mental retardation. Coral Gables, FL: University of Miami Press, 1970;25–48.
30. Penrose LS. Mental defect. New York: Farrar & Rinehart, 1934;1–13, 45–52, 53–84, 85–95.
31. Kanner L. Itard, Seguin, Howe—three pioneers in the education of retarded children. Am J Ment Defic 1960;65:2–10.
32. Kanner L. Medicine in the history of mental retardation: 1800–1965. Am J Ment Defic 1967;72:165–70.
33. Doll EE. Trends and problems in the education of the mentally retarded: 1800–1940. Am J Ment Defic 1967;72:175–83.
34. Talbot M. Édouard Seguin. Am J Ment Defic 1967;72:184–89.
35. Herd H. The diagnosis of mental deficiency. London: Hodder and Stoughton, 1930;3–11.
36. Bregman JD. Current developments in the understanding of mental retardation Part II: Psychopathology. J Am Acad Child Adolesc Psychiatry 1991;30:861–72.
37. Goddard HH. The Kallikak family, a study in the heredity of feeblemindedness. New York: Macmillan, 1912.
38. Goddard HH. Feeblemindedness: its causes and consequences. New York: MacMillan, 1914.
39. Town CT. Familial feeblemindedness: a study of one hundred forty-one families. Buffalo: Foster & Stewart, 1939.
40. Galton F. Inquiries into the human faculty and its development. London: JM Dent & Co, 1883;217.
41. Fisher RA. The correlation between relatives on the supposition on Mendelian inheritance. Trans Roy Soc Edinburgh 1918;52:399–433.
42. Goldstein S, Reynolds CR, eds. Handbook of neurodevelopmental and genetic disorders in children. New York: Guilford Press, 1999;3–8, 101–53.
43. Jinks JL, Fulker DW. Comparison of the biometrical, genetical, MAVA, and classical approaches to the analysis of human behavior. Psychol Bull 1970;73:311–49.
44. Rao DC, Morton NE, Yee S. Resolution of cultural and biological inheritance by path analysis. Am J Hum Genet 1976;28:228–42.
45. Lewontin RC. Genetic aspects of intelligence. Ann Rev Genet 1975;9:387–405.
46. Goldberger, AS. The nonresolution of IQ inheritance by path analysis [letter]. Am J Hum Genet 1978;30:442–5.

47. Kamin L. The science and politics of IQ. Hillsdale, NJ: Lawrence Erlbaum, 1974.
48. Inhelder B, Piaget J. The growth of logical thinking from childhood to adolescence. New York: Basic Books, 1958.
49. Zigler E. Familial mental retardation: a continuing dilemma. Science 1967;155:292–8.
50. Zigler E. Developmental versus difference theories of retardation and the problem of motivation. Am J Ment Defic 1969;73:536–56.
51. Down, J. Mental affections of children and youth. London, J & A Churchill, 1887.
52. Dugdale R. The Jukes: a study of crime, pauperism, disease, and heredity. New York: GP Putnam, 1877; reprinted by Arno Press, 1970.
53. Estabrook A. The Jukes in 1915. Washington, DC: Carnegie Institute of Washington, 1916.
54. Dingman HF, Tarjan G. Mental retardation and the normal distribution curve. Am J Ment Defic 1960;64:991–4.
55. Stevenson RE, Schwartz CE, Schroer RJ. X-linked mental retardation. New York: Oxford University Press, 2000;23–67.
56. Reed EW, Reed SC. Mental retardation: a family study. Philadelphia: WB Saunders, 1965;1–18.
57. Burack JA, Hodapp RM, Zigler E. Issues in the classification of mental retardation: differentiating among the organic etiologies. J Child Psychol Psychiatry 1988;29:765–79.
58. American Psychiatric Association. Diagnostic and Statistical Manual of Mental Disorders, 2nd ed. Washington, DC: American Psychiatric Association, 1968.
59. American Psychiatric Association. Diagnostic and Statistical Manual of Mental Disorders, 4th ed. Washington, DC: American Psychiatric Association, 1994.
60. Fisch GS. Psychological assessment on XLMR: a proposal for setting international standards. Genet Counsel 2000;11:85–101.
61. Weisz J, Yeates K, Zigler E. Piagetian evidence and the developmental-difference controversy. In Zigler E, Balla D, eds. Mental retardation: the developmental-difference controversy. Hillsdale, NJ: Lawrence Erlbaum, 1982.
62. Weiss B, Weisz J, Bromfield R. Performance of retarded and nonretarded persons on information-processing tasks: further tests of the similar structure hypothesis. Psychol Bull 1986;100:157–75.
63. Hodapp RM, Leckman JF, Dykens EM, Sparrow SS, Zelinsky DG, Ort SI. K-ABC profiles in children with fragile X syndrome, Down syndrome, and nonspecific mental retardation. Am J Ment Retard 1992;97:39–46.
64. Bellugi U, Wang P, Jernigan T. Williams syndrome: an unusual neurocognitive profile. In Broman SH, Grafman J, eds. Atypical cognitive deficits in developmental disorders. Hillsdale, NJ: Lawrence Erlbaum, 1994;23–56.
65. Fisch GS, Carpenter N, Howard-Peebles PN, Tarleton J, Holden JJA, Simensen RJ. Longitudinal changes in cognitive ability and adaptive behavior in children and adolescents with fragile X or Williams syndrome. Paper presented at the 10th International Workshop on Fragile X and XLMR, September 19–22, 2001, Frascati, Italy.
66. Carr J. Longitudinal research in Down syndrome. In Bray NW, ed. International review of research in mental retardation. San Diego: Academic Press, 1992;18:197–223.

67. Wishart JG. The development of learning difficulties in children with Down syndrome. J Intell Disab Res 1993;37:389–403.
68. Fisch GS, Simensen R, Tarleton J, et al. Longitudinal study of cognitive abilities and adaptive behavior levels in fragile X males: a prospective multicenter analysis. Am J Med Genet 1996;64:356–61.
69. Fisch GS, Carpenter N, Holden JJ, et al. Longitudinal changes in cognitive and adaptive behavior in fragile X females: a prospective multicenter analysis. Am J Med Genet 1999;83:308–12.
70. Dykens EM, Hodapp RM, Walsh K, Nash LJ. Profiles, correlates and trajectories of intelligence in Prader–Willi syndrome. J Acad Child Adolesc Psychiatry 1992;31:1125–30.
71. Abrams MT, Doheny KF, Mazzocco MMM, et al. Cognitive, behavioral, and neuroanatomical assessment of two unrelated male children expressing *FRAXE*. Am J Med Genet (Neuropsychiatr Genet) 1997;74:73–81.
72. Fisch GS, Carpenter NJ, Simensen R, Smits APT, van Roosmalen T, Hamel BCJ. Longitudinal changes in cognitive–behavioral levels in three children with *FRAXE*. Am J Med Genet 1999;84:291–2.
73. Ingalls S, Goldstein S. Learning disabilities. In Goldstein S, Reynolds CR, eds. Handbook of neurodevelopmental and genetic disorders in children. New York: Guilford Press, 1999;101–53.
74. Lerner JW. Learning disabilities: theories, diagnosis, and teaching strategies, 6th ed. Boston: Houghton Mifflin, 1993.
75. Omenn GS. Genetic approaches to the syndrome of minimal brain dysfunction. In: de la Cruz FF, Fox BH, Roberts RH, eds. Minimal brain dysfunction. Ann NY Acad Sci 1973;205:212–22.
76. Vandenberg SG. Possible hereditary factors in minimal brain dysfunction. In: de la Cruz FF, Fox BH, Roberts RH, eds. Minimal brain dysfunction. Ann NY Acad Sci 1973;205:223–30.
77. North KN, Riccardi V, Samango-Sprouse C, et al. Cognitive function and academic performance in neurofibromatosis 1: Consensus statement from the NF1 cognitive disorders task force. Neurology 1997;48:1121–7.
78. LaBuda MC, DeFries JC. Genetic etiology of reading disability: evidence from a twin study. In: Pavlidis GT, ed. Perspectives in dyslexia: Vol. 1. Neurology, neuropsychology, and genetics. New York: Wiley, 1990;47–76.
79. Smith SD, Kimberling WJ, Pennington BF, Lubs HA. Specific reading disability: Identification of an inherited form through linkage analysis. Science 1983;219:1345–7.
80. Grigorenko EL, Wood FB, Meyer MS, Hart LA, Speed WC, Shuster A, Pauls DL. Susceptibility loci for distinct components of developmental dyslexia on chromosomes 6 and 15. Am J Hum Genet 1997;60:27–39.
81. Broman S, Nichols PL, Shaughnessy P, Kennedy W. Retardation in young children: a developmental study of cognitive deficit. Hillsdale, NJ: Lawrence Erlbaum, 1987;1–12, 24–37.
82. Fisch GS. Psychology genetics. Am J Med Genet (Semin Med Genet), 2000;97:109–11.

2

Neuroanatomical Considerations Specific to the Study of Neurogenetics

Albert M. Galaburda and J. Eric Schmitt

1. INTRODUCTION

There is a great need to understand the fundamental bases of complex behaviors such as language, memory, attention, music, emotion and affect, mathematical thinking, executive functions, visual cognition and mental imagery, and consciousness. These behaviors arise from intricate, developmental, and on-line interactions between genes and environment, having their ultimate effects at the molecular level. This understanding is difficult to achieve, as the interrelationships between genes and environmental factors that control the serial and parallel molecular events that build, adapt, and maintain the extremely complex neural structures that support these behaviors are great. The ultimate promise of neurogenetics research is the understanding of at least part of the molecular basis of behavior, which has to do with the influence of hard-wired genetic factors. As before in the history of this field, the study of disorders, in this case genetic disorders, is a reasonable start.

Identification of the genes and downstream events that lead to mental retardation and affective disorders will doubtlessly be invaluable in the diagnosis, treatment, and even prevention of human genetic disorders, with the desirable added effect of shedding light on the normal biology of behavior and cognition. There is a dearth of information about the participation of specific brain regions—and combinations thereof—in complex behaviors, which provides the opportunity for linking genes to behavior via the study of the brain. Thus, the brain represents the halfway point between genes and behaviors, and the first challenge is to understand how the brain is built from the functions of genes and their interactions with the early environment. At the same time, it is increasingly possible to link brain and behav-

From: *Contemporary Clinical Neuroscience:*
Genetics and Genomics of Neurobehavioral Disorders
Edited by: G. S. Fisch © Humana Press Inc., Totowa, NJ

ior, the other half of the trajectory. In addition to the traditional analysis of effects of focal brain injury, this is accomplished by using techniques of modern cognitive neuroscience, including structural imaging as well as activating and mapping techniques, which permit a more complete picture of the participation of the neural components involved in behavior. These, coupled with advances in cellular, molecular, and systems neurobiology using whole animal and tissue models, optimistically helps to round off the knowledge necessary for going from genes, through brain, to behavior.

Decades of research have revealed that the interaction between gene and brain can be quite complex and nonlinear. Furthermore, the effect of (aneuploidy) haploinsufficiency for even a single gene can have dramatic and widespread effects on brain structure and function. Neuroanatomical differences associated with neurobehavioral disorders resulting from genetic abnormalities encompass virtually every morphologic anomaly imaginable, from the microcephaly of Down syndrome, through the specific neuronal migration anomalies associated with the 7p13.3 deletion associated with the Miller–Dieker malformation, to the relatively targeted striatal atrophy of Huntington's disease. It cannot be assumed that a smaller brain is bad or a larger brain size (or portion thereof) is advantageous, as normal variation and some pathological conditions demonstrate. The writer Anatole France, for instance, seems to have had a small brain. Conversely, the fragile X syndrome is associated with increased brain volume in the presence of significant behavioral anomalies. Further, the possible mechanisms by which a gene may exert its influence on the brain are numerous. For example, a gene may produce a protein with a direct role in synaptic transmission during on-line execution of behavior, may be required for building a specific structure during neural development at a critical time point, or may be a transcription factor responsible for the expression of other genes. Thus, a single change in the molecular structure of a gene could, in principle, produce myriad downstream neuroanatomical effects that, at first glance, have no apparent relationship to one another.

Equally daunting is interpreting the relationship between neuromorphology and behavior. Most studies investigating the neural substrates of behavior show that even a "simple" cognitive function or emotion can be immensely complex in its degree and pattern of brain involvement when compared to elementary sensory and motor processes. Further, unlike those neurologic diseases in which the symptoms are motoric or sensory, cognitive behavior often involves more widespread brain loci with significant individual variability. For example, it is not uncommon to find a brain lesion that produces cognitive loss in one patient and a different loss or nothing at all in another. Conversely, it is not uncommon to see similar behavioral profiles in two patients with different brain lesions. Thus, determining how and which of several behaviors is linked to a specific lobe, convolution, or cytoarchitectonic region can be problematic. Then there is the effect of learning and the environment, which modify the effects of lesion and change the expression of genes. A given language, for instance, because of its peculiar phonological properties, may be more or less resistant to the effects of genes that cause dyslexia, or may modify the details in aphasia-producing brain lesions. Or, a longer experience with formal education may modulate the time of clinical onset of Alzheimer's disease in a given patient.

Despite intellectual and methodological obstacles toward understanding the genetic impact on brain and behavior, the advent of modern neuroscience has brought impressive advances to the field of neurobiology. Improvements in cellular and molecular methods, such as patch clamping, high-resolution microscopy, hybridization, and cloning, have provided the well established fields of histology and cellular and molecular neuroscience with new tools to elaborate on their discoveries. The ongoing characterization of genetic sequences has allowed construction of probes that react with brain tissue with increasingly greater specificity, as well as construction of mouse models for genetic disease. In addition, the invention of positron emission tomography (PET) and structural and functional magnetic resonance imaging (MRI and fMRI) have allowed the in vivo investigation of brain structure and function in cognitive and behavioral disorders, including neurodevelopmental disorders, in addition to increasing our knowledge of normal brain function.

This chapter is an attempt to explore several neuroanatomical considerations specific to the examination of neurodevelopmental disorders. We describe herein several approaches toward a common goal: the discovery of the connections between gene, brain, and mind. In our presentation, we review some of the current advances in the field, discuss advantages and disadvantages of each approach, and try to provoke new thinking about how to proceed in this area of research.

2. NEUROGENETIC SYNDROMES

Genetic syndromes with well defined etiologies provide an excellent opportunity for examining the contributions of genetics to behavior and brain development. Unlike most psychiatric conditions, the behaviors associated with known syndromes can be traced to a reasonably uniform etiology. Often, the behavioral phenotype of a neurogenetic syndrome is the result of a microdeletion of a very small number of genes that is fairly consistent from one affected individual to the next; or, in some cases, can be traced to a single gene mutation. Although the most straightforward single-gene syndromes can result in complex and extensive neuroanatomical anomalies, research on neurogenetic conditions represents one of the most direct ways for looking at human gene–brain–behavior relationships. The following syndromes provide examples of the diversity of genetic mechanisms, behavioral phenotypes, and neuromorphology found within this field.

2.1. Down Syndrome

As a result of its relatively high prevalence and distinct cranio-facial features, Down syndrome (DS) is perhaps the most widely recognized genetic syndrome *(1)*. DS is almost always caused by a complete trisomy of chromosome 21 that results from a non-disjunction event, usually with a maternal origin *(2)*. Occurring once in approx 800 live births, DS is the most common genetic cause of mental retardation. In addition to low IQ scores, problems related to memory, language, speech, and motor coordination are frequently reported *(3–6)*.There is now a renewed interest in DS because persons with this condition are at an increased risk for developing Alzheimer-like dementia beginning at a young age.

Geneticists have been able to estimate that chromosome 21 contains only 225 genes *(7)*. However, the genes that are involved in the cognitive phenotype have not yet been identified; multiple genes may be involved. DS has a distinct neuroanatomical phenotype. Postmortem studies indicate that microcephaly and brachycephaly are common in DS *(8)*. MRI studies suggest disproportionate volume reductions in the cerebellum, beyond the decrease in general intracranial volume *(9)*. When examining neuroanatomical differences in greater detail, specific reductions are found in the frontal and temporal lobes *(10)*. Hand measurements (rather than computer or automated measurements) have found significant reductions in the superior temporal sulcus and hippocampus *(11,12)*. Preservations in subcortical tissue and parietal–occipital tissue also are seen *(13,14)*.

The neuroanatomical profile of DS appears to conform to its behavioral phenotype. Selective decreases in frontal lobe volumes have been associated with the characteristic mental retardation seen in DS affecting executive functions. Temporal lobe and hippocampal reductions can be linked to deficits in language and memory. Decreases in the cerebellum are seen to underlie the motor control problems and hypotonia typical of DS. In contrast, the relative preservation of parietal–occipital tissue may be related to the relative sparing of visual–spatial ability in this condition. In addition, preservations in subcortical tissue conform to embryological results in DS that indicate that brain abnormalities in DS do not begin until the third trimester of pregnancy, after the formation of subcortical structures has already taken place *(8)*.

Interestingly, histological investigations reveal that even before the end of the second decade of life persons with DS commonly have neuropathological features that are similar to those of Alzheimer disease. Young subjects with DS often display amyloid(A)-β42-containing neuritic plaques typical of much older patients with Alzheimer disease *(15,16)*. A postmortem study of 100 subjects with DS found that 56% had amyloid plaques or plaques and neurofibrillary tangles; all subjects older than 30 years showed evidence of amyloid plaques *(17)*. Subjects with DS overexpress amyloid β protein as early as 21 gestational wk of age *(18)*. DS subjects typically exhibit progressive mental deterioration in the third and fourth decades of life, and there is good reason to believe that, as in Alzheimer disease, the dementia in DS is in part caused by excessive amyloid β protein deposition in the brain. However, in DS, unlike Alzheimer disease, this excess reflects the presence of the extra copy of the amyloid precursor protein gene on chromosome 21.

Investigations in DS introduce several issues that are commonly encountered in neurogenetics research. First, because the exact genes responsible for the syndrome are not yet known, the molecular mechanisms responsible for cellular and ultimately brain abnormalities remain a mystery, which makes interpretation of abnormal morphology difficult. Part of the behavioral phenotype may reflect abnormal brain structure formation, and part of it may result from subsequent changes in the brain because of additional acquired damage. Second, because the neurobehavioral phenotype of DS encompasses several cognitive and behavioral domains, and its neuroanatomical profile includes significant differences in several regions, linking a specific behavioral feature (i.e., language difficulty) to the morphology of a single neuroanatomical structure (i.e., temporal lobe) can be quite challenging. There is the problem typical of all developmental disorders, whether genetic or acquired, by which normal organization of function, for instance, cerebral laterality, cannot necessarily be invoked, as the developing brain is apt to change markedly in response to a change in one of its components. As a result, standard localization of function may be bypassed. The challenge in DS remains trying to identify genes that alter the development of the brain, genes that modify maintenance of brain structure throughout life, and genes affecting the formation of other organs, the malfunction of which could affect brain integrity. Each change in structure thus obtained and combinations of changes need to be studied in terms of effects on behavior.

2.2. Williams Syndrome

Williams syndrome (WMS) is a rare (1/20,000 live births) and fascinating neurogenetic condition that typically results from an unequal recombination during meiosis prior to conception *(19,20)*. The consequences of this event are that persons with WMS have only one copy of approx 20 genes in the 7q11.23 region of chromosome 7. The resulting phenotype presents a broad spectrum of unique physical and behavioral characteristics. The physical features of WMS include distinct craniofacial features, hypercalcemia in infancy, widely spaced teeth, strabismus, and narrowing of the vasculature, particularly supravalvular aortic stenosis (SVAS) *(21)*.

However, what is perhaps most interesting in WMS is a truly unusual profile of behavioral features *(22)*. The cognitive hallmark of WMS is a dissociation between a seemingly relatively preserved linguistic ability and profoundly impaired visual–spatial ability. In addition, a preserved social drive, and oddly, an enthusiasm for and love of music characterize WMS. Increased anxiety and attentional problems also are common in this condition *(20,23)*.

As with DS, research into the underlying neuroanatomical features of WMS reveals patterns of alteration concordant with our current understanding of functional neuroanatomy and the behavioral phenotype of WMS. Although both autopsy and MRI studies have shown that the overall brain size of persons with WMS is substantially decreased relative to typically developing controls, certain regions are relatively spared *(24–26)*. As expected from the observation of preserved language and musical abilities in this condition, the temporal lobe, specifically the superior temporal gyrus (STG), is relatively preserved in volume. In addition, the cerebellum is preserved in volume, and, on average, is of similar size compared to typically developing individuals *(25–27)*. Given recent studies implicating the cerebellum in higher cognitive and social abilities *(28,29)*, disproportionately increased cerebellum may be related to the hypersociability seen in this condition. In contrast, regions of the brain that play a large role in visual–spatial ability (i.e., parietal and occipital lobes) are disproportionately decreased compared to expectations based on total cranial volume.

More detailed investigations of WMS also have been performed on a few autopsy specimens, which allows for a much higher resolution of cortical anatomy than that permitted by MRI studies *(24,30)*. Gross examination of the WMS brain shows that there is an overall decrease in brain weight, with parietal and occipital hypoplasia common. Other than focal changes suggestive of immaturity of development, no consistent differences were found in the cytoarchitectonic organization of the cerebral cortex of subjects with

WMS. Motor and sensory association areas are easily identifiable by architectonic features typical of these areas. However, at the histological level, changes are seen in cell packing density and cell size suggesting abnormal neuronal development and connectivity.

The shape of the WMS brain also is unique. Overall, the brains of subjects with WMS are dolichocephalic and have some anomalous gyral patterns. The most consistent gross anatomic observation is a foreshortening of the dorsal central sulcus *(24)* Unlike most typical brains in which the central sulcus extends fully to the interhemispheric fissure, in WMS the central sulcus usually terminates prematurely on the dorsal, but not ventral end. The second common shape difference is a bilateral forshortening of the parieto–occipital region, effectively a curtailment in the superior–inferior dimension posteriorly in the telencephalon.

Gross morphological differences observed in autopsy specimens have been supported by several recent structural MRI studies that confirmed in larger samples autopsy findings of abnormal central sulcus morphology, posterior curtailment, and anomalous gyri *(31–33)*. Observations made on necessarily small numbers of autopsy specimens direct attention to specific brain areas that can be assessed in large numbers of living subjects. MRI provides highly automated, in vivo evidence with sample sizes that provide more statistical power that can commonly be obtained in autopsy studies. Conversely, observations made using MRI can lead to more detailed studies in autopsy specimens at the architectonic and histological levels. We have found that this cross-level combination of histology, gross anatomical observation, and MRI analyses is a productive strategy for furthering neurogenetics research.

Despite the relatively small size of the WMS deletion region, several genes have likely roles in brain development or synaptic functioning. For example, the gene *STX1A* encodes for *syntaxin1A*, a member of a gene family that has role in neurotransmitter release *(34)*. A second gene, *LIM-kinase1*, has been shown to play a role in growth cone formation and axon guidance *(35,36)*, which may partially underlie the abnormal white matter volume demonstrated by MRI in WMS. Hemizygosity for *LIM-kinase1* has been correlated with visual–spatial impairment for both subjects with WMS and subjects with microdeletions of only the elastin *(ELN)* and *LIM-kinase* genes *(37)*. Another gene in the WMS critical region, *FZD9* (formerly known as *FZD3*, the human homologue of *Drosophila's* frizzled gene), is expressed strongly in adult brains and appears to play a key role in global brain development *(38)*. *FZD9* is a putative receptor for the *Wnt* gene family, which encode for secreted signaling glycoproteins and are known to be involved in controlling early cell development, tissue differentiation, segmentation, and dorsal–ventral polarity *(39)*.

Neuroanatomical studies on WMS suffer from many of the same methodological limitations that are seen in DS research. Specifically, the broad array of neuroanatomical differences seen in WMS make interpretation of relationships to genetics and behavior difficult. Fortunately, there are many fewer genes in the critical WMS deletion region than in DS (about 20 compared to >200), although several of these have prominent roles in brain development. In addition, as with other developmental disorders of known genetic origin, WMS is a rare condition that can lead to difficulties in gathering statistically powerful results, particularly for studies requiring tissue samples. Finally, as with other mental retardation syndromes and developmental disorders affecting emotional behavior, the noisy and relatively stressful environment of the MRI lab can be a barrier to research.

Study of the WMS neuroanatomical phenotype also raises the question of how to interpret relative involvement in neurodevelopmental conditions. For example, although the STG is relatively preserved in WMS, can it be assumed that this volume preservation is related to the relative preservations in language in this condition? First, there is a strikingly phrenological quality to this form of reasoning, whereby volume of brain tissue is assumed to be causally related to quality of performance. Second, this argument assumes that the superior temporal gyrus in WMS serves the same function as in normal individuals. Third, regional measurements may assume a greater degree of functional localization than is evident from contemporary studies using activation approaches, such as functional MRI and PET. On the other hand, focal measurements provide clues for focusing other types of studies, and it is only through convergent evidence derived from various methodologies that a clearer picture of structure–function relationships begins to emerge.

2.3. Fragile X Syndrome

In the field of neurogenetic conditions, fragile X syndrome (FXS) is somewhat unique in that the primary genetic cause of the disease has been traced to the inactivation of a single gene. Affecting approx 1/4000–6000 live births, FXS is the most common form of inherited mental retardation resulting from a known gene *(40)*. The physical characteristics include macroorchidism, large ears, and a long face *(41)*. A distinct neurobehavioral phenotype, which differs between males and females, is present. Males with FXS are typically quite affected, with mild to severe mental retardation and learning disability. Deficits are present in short-term memory speech and language, and stereotypic behaviors also are typical *(42–44)*. In addition, boys with FXS often have autistic features such as social withdrawal and gaze aversion *(42–45)*. Although females heterozygous for FXS generally have a similar phenotype compared to males with the disorder, their problems are typically less severe and more variable *(46–49)*.

FXS is one of the recently characterized family of genetic disorders caused by trinucleotide repeat expansions. In FXS, the expansion of a (CGG)*n* trinucleotide sequence ultimately produces methylation in the first exon of the 5' end of the *FMR1* gene, which in turn inactivates gene expression through transcriptional silencing *(50)*. Although the function of FMRP, the protein product of *FMR1*, is not yet understood, its structure suggests that it binds to RNA and can enter the nuclear envelope and therefore may possibly regulate mRNA transcription *(51)*.

Postmortem studies on brain structure in FXS have been instrumental in understanding how a genetic defect in *FMR1* leads to cognitive and behavioral problems. Interestingly, gross morphological examinations report macrocephaly and increased brain weight in FXS *(52)*, which is unusual in genetic conditions. *In situ* hybridization studies for *FMR1*-mRNA and immunohistochemistry and Western blot studies for FMRP have localized the regions within the body that typically express the *FMR1* gene. Not surprisingly, *FMR1* is expressed in brain tissue during normal human development. *FMR1*-mRNA is highly expressed in fetal CNS tissue at 8–9 mo of gestation, particularly in the telencephalon *(53)*. As development continues, there is evidence that expression of *FMR1*-mRNA becomes more specific. Abitbol et al. found that at 25 mo of age, *FMR1* mRNA is most strongly expressed in deep structures (hippocampus, putamen, diencephalon), ventricular and subventricular areas, the neocortical plate, and the cerebellum. Similarly, monoclonal antibodies to FMRP bind strongly to adult brain tissue *(54)*. In cerebellar tissue, Purkinje cells were most reactive. Cerebral tissue showed FMRP expression most prominently in the cytoplasm and proximal regions of dendrites and axons.

Histological studies of the brain have consistently shown abnormalities of neuron structure in FXS. Specifically, the dendritic spines in brains of persons with FXS are longer and thinner when compared to the "mushroom shape" of mature spines seen in typically developing individuals *(52,55–58)*. Long, thin spines in FXS resemble the immature spines of healthy controls and indicates that FMRP may play a role in synaptic development. This hypothesis is supported by observations that dendritic spines are more densely packed in FXS, which suggests a failure of natural synaptic pruning during dendrite formation *(56)*. A recent study found that FMRP interacts with two other proteins, CYFIP1 and CYFIP2 *(59)*. Although the precise functions of these proteins are not yet known, recent studies have shown that CYFIP1 interacts with other proteins (members of the Rho family of GTPases) that have roles in the dynamic reorganization of the actin cytoskeleton *(60)*. They also play a role in the formation and maintenance of dendritic spines *(61)*. Thus CYFIP1 may be the important link between FMRP and the observed neuromorphological changes seen in FXS.

Imaging studies have allowed a new perspective on the global effects of the fragile X mutation. In addition to macrocephaly, MRI samples had the statistical power to detect morphological differences in localized regions of the brain. The hippocampus, in particular, has been shown to be larger in FXS *(62,63)*. Two studies that specifically examined the posterior fossa found decreases in the size of the posterior vermis in both males and females (particularly lobules 6 and 7) compared to normally developing controls and persons with nonspecific mental retardation *(64–66)*. Conversely, relative increases were seen in the caudate nucleus, thalamus, and lateral ventricular volumes *(67)*.

How these anatomic changes relate to the genetic, molecular, and behavioral characteristics of FXS is still unclear. Mostofsky et al. have found significant correlations between the size of the posterior vermis and verbal (Partial regression coefficient $[pr^2] = 0.150$; $p < 0.01$) and performance ($pr^2 = 0.099$; $p < 0.05$) IQ in 37 females with FXS *(66)*. Two functional imaging studies provide additional evidence of the neural substrates of the FXS behavioral phenotype. During tests of visual–spatial working memory, Kwon et al. found that whereas 15 typically developing female control subjects had increased activation in the inferior and middle frontal gyrus and superior parietal and supramarginal gyrus as task difficulty increased, 10 subjects with FXS did not *(68)*. Subjects with FXS also performed worse than controls during the more difficult tests of working memory. Further, Menon et al. found significant correlation between both FMRP expression and activation ratio (fraction of cells with the *FMR1* gene active) and activation bilaterally in the middle frontal gyrus (right $r = 0.71$, $p = 0.022$; left $r = 0.81$, $p = 0.004$), right inferior frontal gyrus ($r = 0.69$, $p = 0.027$), and the right supramarginal gyrus ($r = 0.7$, $p = 0.024$) *(69)*.

Because of excellent research on genetic, molecular, neuroanatomical, neurophysiological, and behavioral levels, FXS is a prime example demonstrating the promise of neurogenetic investigation. FXS, however, presents several difficulties and mysteries of its own. Unlike DS and WMS in which extra or missing genes usually appear within the genome *de novo*, the genetic mechanism that primarily causes FXS (CGG trinucleotide repeat expansion) is not clear cut. Inactivation of *FMR1* generally occurs when the number of (CGG)n repeats exceeds 200; however, typically developing individuals have approx 5–50 repeats. As the number of repeats increases, so too does the probability of transcriptional silencing. When an individual has 50–200 repeats they are considered to have a premutation. Most studies agree that the premutation is not associated with cognitive and psychiatric problems, but there is some evidence that large premutations may indeed have an abnormal effect *(70)*. Thus, the existence of a premutation, particularly com bined with the sex-linked nature of FXS and its differential effect on males and females, changes a relatively "ideal" single-gene disorder into a more challenging family of conditions.

2.4. *FMR1 Knockout Mouse:* Example of Animal Models in Neurogenetics

The *FMR1* knockout mouse was generated to study FXS under highly controlled experimental conditions and is an excellent example of the power of this type of research. The *FMR1* gene shares 97% homology between mice and humans *(71)*, and this loss-of-function mouse model has become a valuable tool for understanding the *FMR1* mutation. Since its creation in 1994 *(72)*, studies have shown that the *FMR1* knockout mouse has similar neuropathological findings and physical anomalies when compared to persons with FXS. Like males with FXS, male knockout mice have enlarged testes, learning deficits, and hyperactivity *(72)*. Differences in learning, as assessed by a water maze task, seem to be relatively mild in these mice *(73,74)*. Fisch et al., 1999 studied the *FMR1* knockout mouse for learning capacity. In an operant conditioning paradigm, older and naive mice could learn to discriminate visual from auditory stimuli, even when the task was quite difficult, raising questions about this mutant mouse's suitability as a cognitive–genetic model. In addition, recent studies have demonstrated that the *FMR1* knockout mouse has an increased likelihood for audiogenic seizures and startle responses to loud noises when compared to wild-type mice *(75,76)*. Given that persons with FXS have increased sensitivity to sensory stimuli (which may be associated to autistic-like behavior) *(71,77)*, audiogenic seizures in the *FMR1* knockout mouse may be related to abnormal auditory processing.

Equally intriguing are investigations into the neuropathology of the *FMR1* knockout mouse. As in FXS, dendritic spine abnormalities have been reported *(78,79)*. Specifically, these mice have significantly longer, more immature dendritic spines than wild-type control mice. There is also some evidence of increased spine density in the *FMR1* knockout. These findings suggest that *FMR1* is necessary for normal pruning and development of dendritic spines, and is yet another similarity between FXS and the murine FMR1 model.

Thus far, abnormal dendritic morphology is the only confirmed neuroanatomical feature of the *FMR1* knockout mouse. Although the learning deficits in this mutant mouse would suggest that *FMR1* plays a role in long-term potentiation (LTP), no differences compared to control mice were found when hippocampal slices were stimulated electrically *(80,81)*. This finding is in contrast to experiments using other types of knockout mice that also perform poorly in water mazes but do show differences in LTP when compared to control mice *(82,83)*.

Although experiments using the *FMR1* knockout mouse provide a wealth of new data on the nature of FXS, several limitations are also apparent. First, the mechanism of *FMR1* inactivation differs between it's the mouse model and its human counterpart; whereas FXS typically results from a CGG trinucleotide expansion, the *FMR1* knockout mouse was created using homologous recombination *(72)*. Second, the *FMR1* gene homologue in mice is not identical to *FMR1*, raising the possibility that it may have a different function. However, two studies provide evidence that the murine homologue has a similar role as *FMR1*. A study using antibodies against human FMRP found that binding occurred with a high specificity for mouse neurons *(84)*. Glial cells were not labeled. The second study used a yeast-artificial chromosome (YAC) containing the human *FMR1* gene in an attempt to "rescue" *FMR1* knockout mice from the affected phenotype *(85)*. Interestingly, the presence of human FMRP in the mouse was able to prevent some alterations in physical development and produced anxiety reduction, although other behavioral problems arose as a result of *FMR1* overexpression.

From the neuroanatomical and behavioral perspectives, the *FMR1* knockout mouse raises several questions. Despite striking similarities with the fragile X phenotype at the cellular level, no global structural changes have been observed in the mouse *(86)*. This is a matter of concern given the relatively robust findings of macrocephaly in FXS, as well as the findings in the hippocampus, posterior fossa, and thalamus. Similarly, the FMR1 mouse model is unlikely to explain some of the typically human aspects of higher cognition affected in FXS, such as language and social communication problems.

3. CONCLUSION

The study of genetic contributions to cognitive and behavioral disorders is having some success and is likely to proceed at a quick pace increasing research interactions among clinicians, psychologists, and neuroscientists.

It is likely that correlations will be discovered between genetic defects and specific anomalies in brain structure and behavior. What is likely to be more problematic will be the quick unraveling of the relationships between normal gene function and normal behavior. Complete understanding of intervening structure and development of the brain, as well as the myriad environmental influences, are likely to make this job a slow one over the next decades.

REFERENCES

1. Bishop J, Huether CA, Torfs C, Lorey F, Deddens J. Epidemiologic study of Down syndrome in a racially diverse California population, 1989-1991. Am J Epidemiol 1997;145:134–47.
2. Antonarakis SE. Parental origin of the extra chromosome in trisomy 21 as indicated by analysis of DNA polymorphisms. Down Syndrome Collaborative Group. N Engl J Med 1991;324:872–6.
3. Carlesimo GA, Marotta L, Vicari S. Long-term memory in mental retardation: evidence for a specific impairment in subjects with Down's syndrome. Neuropsychologia 1997;35:71–9.
4. Wang PP, Bellugi U. Evidence from two genetic syndromes for a dissociation between verbal and visual-spatial short-term memory. J Clin Exp Neuropsychol 1994;16:317–22.
5. Jarrold C, Baddeley AD, Hewes AK. Genetically dissociated components of working memory: evidence from Down's and Williams syndrome. Neuropsychologia 1999;37:637–51.
6. Silverstein AB, Legutki G, Friedman SL, Takayama DL. Performance of Down syndrome individuals on the Stanford–Binet Intelligence Scale. Am J Ment Defic 1982;86:548–51.
7. Capone GT. Down syndrome: advances in molecular biology and the neurosciences. J Dev Behav Pediatr 2001;22:40–59.
8. Schmidt-Sidor B, Wisniewski KE, Shepard TH, Sersen EA. Brain growth in Down syndrome subjects 15 to 22 weeks of gestational age and birth to 60 months. Clin Neuropathol 1990;9:181–90.
9. Aylward EH, Habbak R, Warren AC, et al. Cerebellar volume in adults with Down syndrome. Arch Neurol 1997; 54:209–12.
10. Jernigan TL, Bellugi U, Sowell E, Doherty S, Hesselink JR. Cerebral morphologic distinctions between Williams and Down syndromes. Arch Neurol 1993;50:186–91.
11. Becker L, Mito T, Takashima S, Onodera K. Growth and development of the brain in Down syndrome. Prog Clin Biol Res 1991;373:133–52.
12. Wisniewski KE. Down syndrome children often have brain with maturation delay, retardation of growth, and cortical dysgenesis. Am J Med Genet Suppl 1990;7:274–81.
13. Pinter JD, Eliez S, Schmitt JE, Capone JD, Reiss AL. Neuroanatomy of Down syndrome: a high-resolution MRI study. Am J Psychiatry 2001;158:1659–65.
14. Aylward EH, Li Q, Habbak QR, et al. Basal ganglia volume in adults with Down syndrome. Psychiatry Res 1997;74:73–82.

15. Mann DM, Yates PO, Marcyniuk B. Some morphometric observations on the cerebral cortex and hippocampus in presenile Alzheimer's disease, senile dementia of Alzheimer type and Down's syndrome in middle age. J Neurol Sci 1985;69:139–59.
16. Glenner GG, Wong CW. Alzheimer's disease and Down's syndrome: sharing of a unique cerebrovascular amyloid fibril protein. Biochem Biophys Res Commun 1984;122:1131–5.
17. Wisniewski KE, Wisniewski HM, Wen GY. Occurrence of neuropathological changes and dementia of Alzheimer's disease in Down's syndrome. Ann Neurol 1985;17:278–82.
18. Teller JK, Russo C, DeBusk LM, et al. Presence of soluble amyloid beta-peptide precedes amyloid plaque formation in Down's syndrome. Nat Med 1996;2:93–5.
19. Korenberg JR, Chen XN, Hirota H, et al. VI. Genome structure and cognitive map of Williams syndrome. J Cogn Neurosci 2000;12:89–107.
20. Morris CA, Demsey SA, Leonard CO, Dilts C, Blackburn BL. Natural history of Williams syndrome: physical characteristics. J Pediatr 1988;113:318–26.
21. Kaplan P, Wang PP, Francke U. Williams (Williams Beuren) syndrome: a distinct neurobehavioral disorder. J Child Neurol 2001;16:177–90.
22. Bellugi U, Lichtenberger L, Jones W, Lai Z, St George M. I. The neurocognitive profile of Williams Syndrome: a complex pattern of strengths and weaknesses. J Cogn Neurosci 2000;12:7–29.
23. Einfeld SL, Tonge BJ, Rees VW. Longitudinal course of behavioral and emotional problems in Williams syndrome. Am J Ment Retard 2001;106:73–81.
24. Galaburda AM, Bellugi U. V. Multi-level analysis of cortical neuroanatomy in Williams syndrome. J Cogn Neurosci 2000;12:74–88.
25. Reiss AL, Eliez S, Schmitt JE, et al. IV. Neuroanatomy of Williams syndrome: a high-resolution MRI study. J Cogn Neurosci 2000;12:65–73.
26. Jernigan TL, Bellugi U. Anomalous brain morphology on magnetic resonance images in Williams syndrome and Down syndrome. Arch Neurol 1990; 47:529–33.
27. Wang PP, Hesselink JR, Jernigan TL, Doherty S, Bellugi U. Specific neurobehavioral profile of Williams' syndrome is associated with neocerebellar hemispheric preservation. Neurology 1992;42:1999–2002.
28. Schmahmann JD, Sherman JC. Cerebellar cognitive affective syndrome. Int Rev Neurobiol 1997;41:433–40.
29. Schmahmann JD. An emerging concept. The cerebellar contribution to higher function. Arch Neurol 1991;48:1178–87.
30. Galaburda AM, Wang PP, Bellugi U, Rossen M. Cytoarchitectonic anomalies in a genetically based disorder: Williams syndrome. NeuroReport 1994;5:753–7.
31. Schmitt JE, Eliez S, Bellugi U, Reiss AL. Analysis of cerebral shape in Williams syndrome. Arch Neurol 2001;58:283–7.
32. Schmitt JE, Watts K, Eliez S, Galaburda AM, Bellugi U, Reiss AL. Increased gyrification: evidence using 3D MRI methods in Williams syndrome. Dev Med Child Neurol 2002;44:292–5.

33. Galaburda AM, Schmitt JE, Bellugi U, Eliez S, Reiss AL. Dorsal forebrain anomaly in Williams syndrome. Arch Neurol 2001;58:1865–9.
34. Botta A, Sangiuolo F, Calza L, et al. Expression analysis and protein localization of the human HPC- 1/syntaxin 1A, a gene deleted in Williams syndrome. Genomics 1999;62:525–8.
35. Arber S, Barbayannis FA, Hanser H, et al. Regulation of actin dynamics through phosphorylation of cofilin by LIM-kinase. Nature 1998;393:805–9.
36. Yang N, Higuchi O, Ohashi K, et al. Cofilin phosphorylation by LIM-kinase 1 and its role in Rac-mediated actin reorganization. Nature 1998;393:809–12.
37. Frangiskakis JM, Ewart AK, Morris CA, et al. LIM-kinase1 hemizygosity implicated in impaired visuospatial constructive cognition. Cell 1996;86: 59–69.
38. Wang YK, Samos CH, Peoples R, Perez-Jurado LA, Nusse R, Francke U. A novel human homologue of the *Drosophila* frizzled wnt receptor gene binds wingless protein and is in the Williams syndrome deletion at 7q11.23. Hum Mol Genet 1997;6:465–72.
39. Cadigan KM, Nusse R. Wnt signaling: a common theme in animal development. Genes Dev 1997;11:3286–305.
40. Kooy RF, Oostra BA, Willems PJ. The fragile X syndrome and other fragile site disorders. Results Probl Cell Differ 1998;21:1–46.
41. Hagerman RJ, Cronister A. Fragile X syndrome: diagnosis, treatment, and research. Baltimore: Johns Hopkins University Press, 1996.
42. Cohen IL, Fisch GS, Sudhalter V, et al. Social gaze, social avoidance, and repetitive behavior in fragile X males: a controlled study. Am J Ment Retard 1988;92:436–46.
43. Kemper MB, Hagerman RJ, Altshul-Stark D. Cognitive profiles of boys with the fragile X syndrome. Am J Med Genet 1988;30:191–200.
44. Sudhalter V, Cohen IL, Silverman W, Wolf-Schein EG. Conversational analyses of males with fragile X, Down syndrome, and autism: comparison of the emergence of deviant language. Am J Ment Retard 1990;94:431–41.
45. Reiss AL, Freund L. Behavioral phenotype of fragile X syndrome: DSM-III-R autistic behavior in male children. Am J Med Genet 1992;43:35–46.
46. Miezejeski CM, Jenkins EC, Hill AL, Wisniewski K, French JH, Brown WT. A profile of cognitive deficit in females from fragile X families. Neuropsychologia 1986;24:405–9.
47. Reiss AL, Freund L, Abrams MT, Boehm C, Kazazian H. Neurobehavioral effects of the fragile X premutation in adult women: a controlled study. Am J Hum Genet 1993;52:884–94.
48. Freund LS, Reiss AL, Abrams MT. Psychiatric disorders associated with fragile X in the young female. Pediatrics 1993;91:321–9.
49. Prouty LA, Rogers RC, Stevenson RE, et al. Fragile X syndrome: growth, development, and intellectual function. Am J Med Genet 1988;30:123–42.
50. Oberle I, Rousseau F, Heitz D, et al. Instability of a 550-base pair DNA segment and abnormal methylation in fragile X syndrome. Science 1991; 252:1097–102.

51. Tamanini F, Bontekoe C, Bakker CE, et al. Different targets for the fragile X-related proteins revealed by their distinct nuclear localizations. Hum Mol Genet 1999;8:863–9.
52. Sabaratnam M. Pathological and neuropathological findings in two males with fragile-X syndrome. J Intell Disab Res 2000;44:81–5.
53. Abitbol M, Menini C, Delezoide AL, Rhyner T, Vekemans M, Mallet J. Nucleus basalis magnocellularis and hippocampus are the major sites of FMR-1 expression in the human fetal brain. Nat Genet 1993;4:147–53.
54. Devys D, Lutz Y, Rouyer N, Bellocq JP, Mandel JL. The FMR-1 protein is cytoplasmic, most abundant in neurons and appears normal in carriers of a fragile X premutation. Nat Genet 1993;4:335–40.
55. Irwin SA, Galvez R, Greenough WT. Dendritic spine structural anomalies in fragile-X mental retardation syndrome. Cereb Cortex 2000;10:1038–44.
56. Irwin SA, Patel B, Idupulapati M, et al. Abnormal dendritic spine characteristics in the temporal and visual cortices of patients with fragile-X syndrome: a quantitative examination. Am J Med Genet 2001;98:161–7.
57. Rudelli RD, Brown WT, Wisniewski K, et al. Adult fragile X syndrome. Clinico-neuropathologic findings. Acta Neuropathol 1985;67:289–95.
58. Wisniewski KE, Segan SM, Miezejeski CM, Sersen EA, Rudelli RD. The Fra(X) syndrome: neurological, electrophysiological, and neuropathological abnormalities. Am J Med Genet 1991;38:476–80.
59. Schenck A, Bardoni B, Moro A, Bagni C, Mandel JL. A highly conserved protein family interacting with the fragile X mental retardation protein (FMRP) and displaying selective interactions with FMRP-related proteins FXR1P and FXR2P. Proc Natl Acad Sci USA 2001;3:3.
60. Hall A. Rho GTPases and the actin cytoskeleton. Science 1998;279:509–14.
61. Fischer M, Kaech S, Knutti D, Matus A. Rapid actin-based plasticity in dendritic spines. Neuron 1998;20:847–54.
62. Reiss AL, Lee J, Freund L. Neuroanatomy of fragile X syndrome: the temporal lobe. Neurology 1994;44:1317–24.
63. Kates WR, Abrams MT, Kaufmann WE, Breiter SN, Reiss AL. Reliability and validity of MRI measurement of the amygdala and hippocampus in children with fragile X syndrome. Psychiatry Res 1997;75:31–48.
64. Reiss AL, Aylward E, Freund LS, Joshi PK, Bryan RN. Neuroanatomy of fragile X syndrome: the posterior fossa. Ann Neurol 1991;29:26–32.
65. Reiss AL, Freund L, Tseng JE, Joshi PK. Neuroanatomy in fragile X females: the posterior fossa. Am J Hum Genet 1991;49:279–388.
66. Mostofsky SH, Mazzocco MM, Aakalu G, Warsofsky IS, Denckla MB, Reiss AL. Decreased cerebellar posterior vermis size in fragile X syndrome: correlation with neurocognitive performance. Neurology 1998;50:121–30.
67. Reiss AL, Abrams MT, Greenlaw R, Freund L, Denckla MB. Neurodevelopmental effects of the FMR-1 full mutation in humans. Nat Med 1995;1:159–67.
68. Kwon H, Menon V, Eliez S, et al. Functional neuroanatomy of visuospatial working memory in fragile x syndrome: relation to behavioral and molecular measures. Am J Psychiatry 2001;158:1040–51.

69. Menon V, Kwon H, Eliez S, Taylor AK, Reiss AL. Functional brain activation during cognition is related to FMR1 gene expression. Brain Res 2000;877:367–70.
70. Mazzocco MM. Advances in research on the fragile X syndrome. Ment Retard Dev Disab Res Rev 2000;6:96–106.
71. Ashley CT, Sutcliffe JS, Kunst CB, et al. Human and murine FMR-1: alternative splicing and translational initiation downstream of the CGG-repeat. Nat Genet 1993;4:244–51.
72. Consortium D-BFX. Fmr1 knockout mice: a model to study fragile X mental retardation. The Dutch-Belgian Fragile X Consortium. Cell 1994;78:23–33.
73. Kooy RF, D'Hooge R, Reyniers E, et al. Transgenic mouse model for the fragile X syndrome. Am J Med Genet 1996;64:241–5.
74. D'Hooge R, Nagels G, Franck F, et al. Mildly impaired water maze performance in male Fmr1 knockout mice. Neuroscience 1997;76:367–76.
75. Chen L, Toth M. Fragile X mice develop sensory hyperreactivity to auditory stimuli. Neuroscience 2001;103:1043–50.
76. Musumeci SA, Bosco P, Calabrese G, et al. Audiogenic seizures susceptibility in transgenic mice with fragile X syndrome. Epilepsia 2000;41:19–23.
77. Miller LJ, McIntosh DN, McGrath J, et al. Electrodermal responses to sensory stimuli in individuals with fragile X syndrome: a preliminary report. Am J Med Genet 1999;83:268–79.
78. Comery TA, Harris JB, Willems PJ, et al. Abnormal dendritic spines in fragile X knockout mice: maturation and pruning deficits. Proc Natl Acad Sci USA 1997;94:5401–4.
79. Irwin SA, Idupulapati M, Mehta AB, et al. Abnormal dendritic and dendritic spine characteristics in fragile-X patients and the mouse model of fragile-X syndrome. Soc Neurosci Abstr 1999;25:2548.
80. Godfraind JM, Reyniers E, De Boulle K, et al. Long-term potentiation in the hippocampus of fragile X knockout mice. Am J Med Genet 1996;64:246–51.
81. Paradee W, Melikian HE, Rasmussen DL, Kenneson A, Conn PJ, Warren ST. Fragile X mouse: strain effects of knockout phenotype and evidence suggesting deficient amygdala function. Neuroscience 1999;94:185–92.
82. Wu ZL, Thomas SA, Villacres EC, et al. Altered behavior and long-term potentiation in type I adenylyl cyclase mutant mice. Proc Natl Acad Sci USA 1995;92:220–4.
83. Sakimura K, Kutsuwada T, Ito I, et al. Reduced hippocampal LTP and spatial learning in mice lacking NMDA receptor epsilon 1 subunit. Nature 1995;373:151–5.
84. Bakker CE, de Diego Otero Y, Bontekoe C, et al. Immunocytochemical and biochemical characterization of FMRP, FXR1P, and FXR2P in the mouse. Exp Cell Res 2000;258:162–70.
85. Peier AM, McIlwain KL, Kenneson A, Warren ST, Paylor R, Nelson DL. (Over)correction of FMR1 deficiency with YAC transgenics: behavioral and physical features. Hum Mol Genet 2000;9:1145–59.
86. Kooy RF, Reyniers E, Verhoye M, et al. Neuroanatomy of the fragile X knockout mouse brain studied using in vivo high resolution magnetic resonance imaging. Eur J Hum Genet 1999;7:526–32.

3

Modeling Cognitive Disorders

From Genes to Therapies

Rui M. Costa, Ype Elgersma, and Alcino J. Silva

1. INTRODUCTION

The goal of the Human Genome Project was to map and sequence the entire human genome. It was with great anticipation that the scientific community awaited the completion of the human genome project, as this information will revolutionize modern medicine in ways that we are only starting to realize. Of immediate consequence is the enormous impact that the completed sequence will have on the lengthy and extremely laborious process of mapping and cloning disease loci. There is no doubt that the availability of the sequence will shorten and simplify this process, and that in the next 10 years many of the genes underlying the approx 12,000 genetic diseases known will be mapped and perhaps cloned.

The identification of the genes responsible for inherited disorders is a key first step toward understanding the biological processes affected. With these genes at hand it is then possible to generate animal models, which are powerful tools to unravel the etiology of each disorder and therefore to devise treatments. Even though there are numerous encouraging prospects, and a few successes, many of the studies of animal models of brain genetic disorders are in their infancy, and they have yet to yield useful therapies. Here, we review how molecular, physiological, and behavioral studies in animals are starting to elucidate the molecular and cellular basis for cognition. We also discuss how these multilevel integrative studies in animal models can shed light on the etiology of the cognitive deficits associated with genetic disorders in humans. We focus on the role of mouse genetics and use as an example the work that has been done with mouse models of neurofibromatosis type 1 (NF1), one of the most common single-gene disorders to cause

From: *Contemporary Clinical Neuroscience:*
Genetics and Genomics of Neurobehavioral Disorders
Edited by: G. S. Fisch © Humana Press Inc., Totowa, NJ

learning deficits. We also discuss how these studies can lead to insights into possible therapies.

2. APPROACHES TO STUDY COGNITION IN ANIMAL MODELS OF DISEASE

To understand cognition it is important to develop models that are not restricted to one level of analysis, but integrate knowledge from molecular, cellular, systems, and behavioral neuroscience. For example, hypotheses about the role of neurofibromin (the protein encoded by the *NF1* locus) function in learning and memory should incorporate information about signaling processes regulated by this protein, the cellular processes that it mediates, and how these processes shape the circuits that control behavior. This multilayer approach is very powerful because hypotheses can be constrained easily. Until recently, however, it has been difficult to test the impact of most molecular processes in learning and memory because of the lack of specific agents capable of disrupting candidate molecular and cellular processes. The introduction of gene targeting to the study of cognitive processes has circumvented this limitation *(1–3)*, and it is now possible to disrupt almost any molecular process of interest in the brain. There are powerful new strategies to identify genes involved in specific cellular processes (e.g., genes required for long-term changes in synaptic function), and once cloned, these genes can be manipulated in different ways in mice.

2.1. Using Mouse Genetics to Integrate Molecular and Cellular Mechanisms of Cognition

Traditionally, cognitive studies in animals have attempted to make causal links between the animal's behavior, the brain regions recruited, the circuits involved, the physiological mechanisms activated, and the molecular processes that support these mechanisms. This is clearly a complex and lengthy process, but fortunately the history of neuroscience has demonstrated that it is possible to make significant progress even before all of the desirable links between behavior, neuroanatomy, circuitry, and neuronal and molecular processes have been identified. The work summarized in this chapter elucidates how multilevel, integrative studies in animals, mainly in genetically modified mice, helped to establish a connection between molecules, activity-dependent neuronal changes, and different phases of memory. The majority of the work published attempting to integrate knowledge about the molecular and cellular/circuit changes mediating learning has focused predominantly on the role of synaptic plasticity, especially long-term potentiation (LTP) and long-term depression (LTD), on learning and memory. However, studies relating other cellular modifications, such as changes in excitability, inhibition, and structure (e.g., the formation/remodeling of new synapses), with learning and memory have started to enlarge the initial scope of the field. Further work, using more specific molecular tools, should help to establish a more complete and comprehensive model of the molecular and cellular changes underlying learning and memory. For our discussion here, we will use as an example the work that has been done trying to integrate genetics, synaptic plasticity, and behavior.

One of the most studied properties of learning is associativity. During learning, previously unrelated information becomes bound by a series of associative links that reflect an individual's experience. Interestingly, the induction of LTP, one of the best understood forms of synaptic plasticity, depends on the activation of a glutamate-gated receptor with associative properties. The *N*-methyl-D-aspartate receptor (NMDAR) requires two distinct events for activation: postsynaptic depolarization that removes a magnesium block, and presynaptically released glutamate. These properties suggested that the NMDAR may be a coincidence detector for associative learning *(4)*. This hypothesis has been tested using manipulations that affect NMDAR function. Only two methods are available to manipulate molecules experimentally: pharmacology and genetics. A critical role for the NMDAR in learning and memory (L&M) has been suggested by both pharmacological blockade *(5–8)* (but *see 9,10*), and more recently by genetic lesions. For example, mice with a null mutation of the NMDA receptor subunit NR2A require more synaptic stimulation than controls for induction of similar levels of hippocampal LTP. These mutants also need more training than controls for induction of similar levels of contextual conditioning, a form of learning sensitive to hippocampal lesions *(11)*, establishing interesting parallels between NMDA function, the threshold for LTP induction, and learning. Accordingly, mice with a CA1-specific deletion of the NMDAR1 also have impaired LTP induction in the hippocampal CA1 subregion and deficits in spatial learning *(12)*, another form of learning highly dependent on hippocampal function. Conversely, a manipulation that results in an increased time window for coincidence detection in the NMDAR results in increased LTP and spatial learning *(13)*. Note that not all manipulations that result in increased LTP result in increased learning. For example, manipulations that cause increased LTP but disrupted LTD result in learning deficits *(14,15)*. Also, it is important to state that LTP, as commonly studied in hippocampal slices, is only a model system for the far more complex and highly regulated long-term synaptic changes that may accompany learning in vivo in structures such as the hippocampus. LTP measured in vitro does not always reflect faithfully its in vivo counterpart, nor does it capture fully its properties. Even LTP measured in vivo is only an experimental approximation of synaptic changes that may accompany learning, as the induction conditions used almost certainly do not simulate those present during learning. Nevertheless, measurements of LTP in hippocampal slices are a highly useful model. It is also worthwhile mentioning that stable decreases (i.e., LTD) in synaptic strength could also be involved in learning, and that many of the arguments supporting a role for LTP in learning could also be made for LTD.

At the circuit level, models of hippocampal function have suggested that associative synaptic changes could underlie the formation of a spatial map *(16)*. Single-unit studies in the hippocampus have demonstrated that hippocampal neurons can increase their firing rates when animals are in specific places in the environment (place fields) *(16)*, as if the hippocampus had a map of the animal's surroundings. Recent pharmacological studies with CPP(+/–) [3-(2-carboxypiperazin-4-yl-propyl-1-phosphonic acid)], an NMDAR antagonist, suggested that the function of this receptor is required for the stability (but not the induction) of place-specific neuronal firing in the hippocampus *(17)*. In addition, a CA1-specific deletion of the NMDAR1, which results in deficits in both CA1 LTP and in spatial learning *(18)*, was shown to alter the properties of spatial-coding neuronal ensembles in CA1. Indeed, place fields of these mutants are enlarged, and have decreased spatial specificity. More importantly, the firing covariance between cell pairs with overlapping place fields is reduced in these mutants, indicating that ensemble coding of space is severely disrupted *(19)*.

The influx of Ca^{2+} through the NMDAR channel activates the calcium/calmodulin (Ca^{2+}/CaM)-dependent kinase II (α-CaMKII), a kinase enriched in postsynaptic densities that can has two particular properties interesting for synaptic plasticity and learning. First, it can act as a stimulus frequency detector; second, it can have autonomous activity that outlasts the duration of the stimulus. A number of pharmacological and genetic studies have demonstrated that this kinase modulates synaptic plasticity in a variety of different organisms. Ca^{2+}/CaM is required for the activation of α-CaMKII and for its translocation to the membrane *(20)*. Following activation, this oligomeric kinase can become autophosphorylated at threonine (T) 286, which allows it to continue to be active even at basal levels of calcium *(21,22)*. Therefore, the autophosphorylation of this kinase has been proposed to serve as a molecular memory for recent synaptic activity *(23)*. Indeed, a number of pharmacological and genetic studies have demonstrated that this kinase modulates synaptic plasticity in a variety of different organisms. To test the role of the autonomous activity of this kinased, a mutant mouse was derived in which T286 of α-CaMKII was replaced with alanine (A), an amino acid that cannot be phosphorylated *(24)*. Interestingly, the T286A mutant mice showed impaired NMDAR-dependent LTP synaptic plasticity in the CA1 region of hippocampus and in the neocortex *(24,25)*. Consistent with the NMDAR-blocking studies mentioned before, the α-CaMKII T286A mutation disrupted the permanence, but not the generation of place fields in the hippocampal pyramidal region *(26)*, and lead to impaired spatial learning *(24)*. Together, the studies reviewed in the preceding suggest that both NMDAR and α-CaMKII function are required for LTP, the formation of space-specific neuronal ensembles, and spatial learning. However, this does not preclude that different molecular and cellular changes are also involved in these processes.

Memories, as well as synaptic changes, can last for weeks or months or they can decay and dissipate within minutes or hours. The events described in the preceding (NMDAR activation followed by autophosphorylation of CaMKII) are probably involved only in the earliest stages of memory formation. What are the molecular changes required for the stability of synaptic changes and memory? There is considerable evidence that long-term memory requires the synthesis of new proteins *(27)*. In particular, cyclic AMP and calcium-dependent activation of transcription factors (of the cAMP response element-binding protein [CREB] family) have been implicated in the stability of synaptic changes and memory *(27–29)*. Mice lacking the isoforms α and δ of CREB have impaired long-term memory and synaptic plasticity *(30)*. More recently, it has been shown that reducing CREB-dependent transcription specifically during training results in long-term memory deficits *(31)*. Consistently, transgenic mice expressing an inhibitory form of the regulatory subunit of cAMP protein kinase A (PKA), which is involved in CREB activation, show unstable long-term synaptic changes and long-term memory *(32,33)*. Conversely, overexpression of CREB in the amygdala, a region thought to be necessary for associative learning during fear conditioning, results in enhanced long-term but not short-term memory *(34)*. However, CREB does not seem to be the only transcription factor involved in memory. For example, disruptions of the transcription factors Zif268 (with gene targeting) or CEB/P (with antisense methods) also disrupt memory *(35,36)*.

At the systems level, it has been proposed that certain memories (i.e., spatial memories) are initially processed and stored in the hippocampus, but that eventually they are stored in the cortex *(37,38)*. It is possible that they are transferred from the hippocampus to the cortex for storage, or that they are processed in both places and stored permanently only in the cortex. Studies in mice using noninvasive functional brain imaging indicated that indeed hippocampal metabolic activity was higher during spatial tests of recent memory than in tests of remote memory, whereas cortical metabolic activity was stronger for remote memories *(39)*. Recent studies have shed some light on the molecular and cellular processes that underlie this reorganization of memory over time. Mice carrying a heterozygous mutation in the α-CaMKII gene have intact recent memories but disrupted remote memories *(40)*. Remarkably, synaptic plasticity is spared in the hippocampus but impaired in the cortex, which is consistent with the fact that cortical plasticity is required for this restructuring of memory over time.

To demonstrate that long-term changes in plasticity have a role in learning, it is crucial to document that these synaptic changes do take place during learning in relevant circuits. This is difficult to accomplish, perhaps because the number of synaptic sites necessary for a particular memory representation may be small, and because in most cases it is unclear where exactly these synaptic changes could be recorded. Direct observations of synaptic changes during learning have been made in simpler invertebrate systems in which the key sensory and motor pathways are known. In invertebrate systems such as *Aplysia*, it was possible to isolate the central nervous system, mimic the conditioned and unconditioned stimulus by direct neuronal stimulation, record the conditioned response, and monitor the strength of key synapses. Thus, these reduced preparations have identified a number of presynaptic and postsynaptic mechanisms that support short-, and long-term changes in synaptic function underlying nonassociative and associative learning in *Aplysia (41,42)*. Not surprisingly, similar studies have been far more difficult in mammalian systems. However, recent results have brought us a step closer to direct observations of synaptic plasticity during mammalian learning. The amygdala has a critical role in emotional memory, but until recently there was no direct evidence of synaptic changes in the amygdala during the formation of emotional memories *(43–45)*. In Pavlovian fear conditioning, an animal learns to fear a conditioned stimulus, for example, a tone, after its association with an unconditioned stimulus, such as a foot shock. Two groups have shown that tone fear conditioning leads to increases in the strength of synapses between neurons of the auditory thalamus and the lateral amygdala *(46,47)*, one of the sites where information about the conditioned and unconditioned stimuli converge *(48)*. Electrophysiological studies in vivo showed that pairing the tone with shock increases the field potentials triggered by the tone in the lateral amygdala *(47)*. Importantly, this increase is proportional to the magnitude of the conditioned response (freezing). It is not present when the shock and the tone are unpaired during training, and it is stable. Experiments with brain slices also uncovered evidence for training-dependent increases in the strength of auditory thalamus–lateral amygdala synapses in conditioned rats *(46)*.

How do we know that changes in synaptic plasticity observed during learning are indeed critical for learning? If information is encoded by increases in synaptic strength, then an artificially induced increase in synaptic strength prior to training should prevent further synaptic strength increases brought about by training, and thus block learning. Consistent with this hypothesis, previous studies showed that saturation of hippocampal synapses with tetanic stimuli prevents hippocampal-dependent learning *(49)*. However, these studies were not easily reproducible, perhaps because complete saturation of hippocampal synapses is difficult, and remaining unsaturated synapses could have sufficed to support learning in some of the tasks used in these experiments *(50)*. A recent study circumvented this problem by lesioning one hippocampus and using a more comprehensive protocol for saturating the synapses of the spared hippocampus *(51)*. Thus, these results show that saturating the strength of hippocampal synapses prevents hippocampal-dependent learning, suggesting that changes in synaptic strength underlie learning. Conversely, learning-induced synaptic strengthening in the cortex has been shown to preclude further LTP induction and to facilitate LTD *(52)*.

The aforementioned examples illustrate an important dilemma in making connections between phenomena as complex as molecular modifications, synaptic plasticity, neuronal ensemble coding, and learning. Because the modulation of synaptic function is likely to affect a number of functions in the brain other than learning and memory, it is not surprising that the relationship between synaptic plasticity and learning is complex. Therefore, it is not surprising that not all manipulations that affect synaptic plasticity affect learning and memory. There are several examples of genetic manipulations that disrupt LTP but not learning *(53–55)*. Several factors can account for this discrepancy. For example, manipulations that affect synaptic plasticity in a particular brain area may not affect it somewhere else and therefore behavior remains unaltered *(54)*. Also, the same molecular manipulation can completely abolish synaptic plasticity in vitro without having the same effects in vivo *(55,56)*. In addition, forms of synaptic plasticity that are not dependent on the molecule manipulated *(53)* or other cellular changes such as cell excitability, inhibition, and structural changes can support learning. As mentioned earlier, further research unraveling the molecular changes underlying such processes, and the behavioral effects of disrupting them, should create a more complete model of the cellular and molecular basis for cognition. Therefore, it is important to note that it is impossible to assess the merit of the connection between a particular mechanism, such as synaptic plasticity, and learning with single experiments. Only the collective weight of different types of experiments (such as observation, mimicry, and disruption) can establish a connection between synaptic changes and learning.

2.2. Spatial and Temporal Control over Genetic Manipulations

To understand better when and where a particular molecular process is involved in memory, it is useful to create mouse models that allow spatial and temporal control over the genetic manipulation. Several systems have been successfully used in mouse cognitive genetics. For instance, to delete a specific gene or sequence in a particular brain area, one can take advantage of the fact that the enzyme Cre-recombinase will recognize specific 34-basepair sequences called *loxP* sites, and thus will delete areas of DNA that are between *loxP* sites *(57)*. Hence, a sequence of interest can be flanked by *loxP* sites (floxed) using homologous recombination in embryonic stem cells, and specific spatial and temporal control of the deletion can be achieved by controlling Cre expression *(18)*. The control of Cre expression can be accomplished in several ways; for instance, by generating transgenic mice that express (inducibly or not) Cre under a specific promoter *(18)*, or by the neuroanatomically guided injection of Cre-expressing virus *(58)*. For example, crossing targeted mice with the NMDAR1 floxed and transgenic mice expressing Cre specifically in CA1 postnatally *(18)* results in a CA1-specific deletion of the NMDAR1 *(12)* (NMDAR1 null homozygous mutants have neonatal lethality *[59]*). With these mice it was posssible to study the specific role of CA1 NMDAR in synaptic plasticity, spatial representations, and learning. The same method was used to show that forebrain neuronal deletion of presenilin 1 (PS1), in a mouse model of familial Alzheimer's disease, produces spatial learning deficits *(60)*. Similarly to the Cre/*loxP* system, the recombinase Flp can also be used to excise sequences between Flp recognition target (FRT) sites *(61,62)*.

Several inducible approaches have been used to control transgene expression in mice. Doxycycline, a tetracycline analogue that binds the tetracycline transactivator (tTA), can be used to control transcription from the tTA-responsive tet promoter, in cells that express both tTA and the tet promoter *(63,64)*. This system was used, for example, to control transcription of a constitutively active form of α-CaMKII in the mouse forebrain, and to demonstrate further the role of α-CaMKII in synaptic plasticity *(65)*, hippocampal spatial-encoding circuits *(66)*, and spatial learning *(65)*. This method produces reliable activation/repression of transgene expression but the time course of the effect is quite long (days) *(65)*, making it difficult to use in certain learning and memory studies. Other systems, such as the control of protein activity/expression through hormone ligand-binding domains (LBD), can act much faster (hours) *(31)*. Fusion of proteins with the LBD of the estrogen receptor efficiently regulates the activity of protein kinases and transcription in mammalian cells *(67)*. The activity of such fusion proteins is not regulated at the transcriptional level, but via its intracellular state. In the absence of the hormone, the LBD and its fusion partner may be bound by heat shock proteins, and thus remain inactive *(67)*. It has been shown that fusions of the *loxP*/Cre or FLP site-specific recombinase with the LBD of a steroid receptor confer hormone-dependent regulation to the activity of those recombinases *(57,68,69)*. Estrogen receptor mutants have been isolated that are unable to bind their natural ligands, but instead are activated by other ligands, such as 4-hydroxytamoxifen *(70)*. Thus, LBD of this mutant receptor, when fused with Cre, stimulates recombinase activity in human and mouse cell lines in response to 4-hydroxytamoxifen, but not in response to estradiol *(68)*. In a recent study addressing the role of CREB in learning and memory, inducible repression of CREB-dependent transcription was achieved by fusing the 4-hydroxytamoxifen LBD with a dominant-negative form of CREB *(31)*. The aforementioned studies elucidate the usefulness of spatial and temporal control of genetic manipulations in molecular and cellular studies of learning and memory. These methods will also be very powerful in defining where and when a disease process affects cognitive function in mice.

2.3. Using Epistatic and Pharmacogenetic Interactions to Unravel the Signaling Pathways Disrupted in Disease

One of the most challenging processes in the study of a genetic disorder is to determine which signaling pathways are affected by a specific mutation, and most importantly, which of the affected signaling pathways is/are responsible for a particular symptom. A powerful way of addressing these challenges is to take advantage of genetic epistatic interactions, that is, the influence of the genotype at one locus on the effect of a mutation at another locus. Epistatic interactions have been used successfully to dissect molecular pathways in different research areas such as development and oncobiology, and in species as diverse as mice and flies. Epistatic interactions can also be used to study the molecular pathways responsible for cognitive dysfunction. For example, in the case of NF1 (*see* Subheading 3.1.), the spatial learning phenotype of *Nf1* mutant mice is exacerbated by heterozygous NMDA null mutations, which *per se* do not cause any detectable phenotype (Fig. 1) *(71)*. Conversely, these learning deficits can be rescued by heterozygous null mutations in *Ras* genes *(72)*, indicating that increased *Ras* activity is probably at the core of the learning disabilities associated with the disease (Fig. 1).

Pharmacogenetic approaches can also take advantage of epistatic molecular interactions to determine if molecules responsible for a particular phenomenon are in the same pathway. These approaches have been applied recently to the study of learning and memory. For example, dosages of a mitogen-activated/extracellular-signal-regulated kinase (MEK) inhibitor (SL327) that do not affect contextual learning in WT mice induce a learning deficit in K-*ras* heterozygous mice *(73)*, indicating that *Ras* signaling through the MEK/mitogen-activated protein kinase (MAPK) pathway is essential for this kind of learning. Together with biochemical analysis that confirm the specificity of the manipulations, epistatic interactions can be used advantageously in the study of animal models to understand better the etiology of the disease and to identify possible therapeutic methods.

3. FROM GENES TO THERAPIES

3.1. Modeling Cognitive Disorders in Mice

The advent of mouse gene targeting opened the promising possibility of generating and studying mouse models of genetic disorders, with the hope that this would render understanding of the basic dysfunctional phenomena and generate possible therapeutic strategies. But what has been accomplished using this approach? The majority of the mouse models of cognitive disorders generated are models for Alzheimer's disease. Alzheimer's disease is a neurodegenerative disorder that leads to progressive cognitive decline. Mouse models have helped to develop a better understanding of the pathophysiology of the disease (for review *see 74*) and have recently led to the hope of therapeutic interventions. Immunization with amyloid-β (the peptide responsible for plaque formation), or peripheral administration of

---

Fig. 1. Taking advantage of epistatic interactions in the study of mouse models of cognitive disorders. Probe trial data in the hidden version of the water maze. Previous studies showed that *Nf1*[+/−] mice have abnormal spatial learning when tested in the hidden version of the water maze, a task known to be sensitive to hippocampal lesions In the hidden version of the water maze animals learn to locate a submerged platform in a pool filled with opaque water. Learning is assessed in a probe trial, where the platform is removed and the mice were allowed to search for it. Animals learn the task when they spend significantly more time in the quadrant

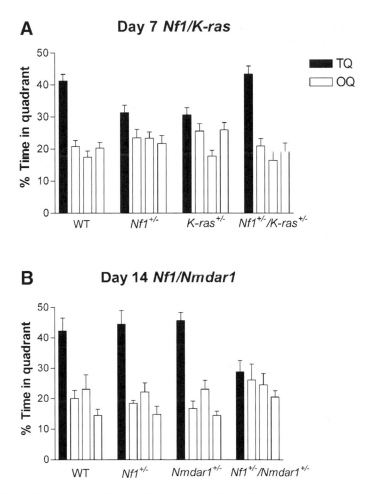

Fig. 1. (*Continued*) where the platform was during training (training quadrant [TQ], *black bars*) than in the other quadrants (OQ, *white bars*). Searching 25% in each quadrant represents chance performance. (**A**) Results from a probe trial given after 7 d of training. The $Nf1^{+/-}$ mice are impaired in the hidden version of the water maze, as they spend significantly less time searching in the TQ than WT mice. K-$ras^{+/-}$ mice are also impaired. The K-$ras^{+/-}$ mutation rescues the spatial learning deficits of the $Nf1^{+/-}$ mice, as $Nf1^{+/-}$/ K-$ras^{+/-}$ mice search more time in the TQ than $Nf1^{+/-}$ mice and are indistinguishable from WT. (**B**) Additional training can alleviate the deficits of $Nf1^{+/-}$ mice. With 14 d of training, $Nf1^{+/-}$ mice search as selectively in the TQ as WT mice. However, a heterozygous mutation in the *Nmdar1*, that *per se* does not cause a deficit, accentuates the deficits of the $Nf1^{+/-}$ mice. Even after 14 d of training, $Nf1^{+/-}$/$Nmdar1^{+/-}$ mice search significantly less time in the TQ than WT, $Nf1^{+/-}$, and $Nmdar1^{+/-}$ mice. Mice in both experiments are from the 129T2/SvEmsJ-C57B/6N genetic background. In each experiment, mice from all four genotypes are isogenic littermates.

antibodies against amyloid-β, can attenuate the formation of plaques (a hallmark of Alzheimer's pathology) in mouse models of Alzheimer *(75,76)*. Mouse models have also been particularly important for the understanding of inherited disorders affecting cognitive function.

Mental retardation is a common cognitive problem that could affect up to 2–3% of the human population *(77)*. The fragile X syndrome is the most common inherited disorder causing mental retardation (approx 1–4000 males, for review see *78–80*). The fragile X syndrome is commonly caused by CGG-repeat expansion in the 5' untranslated region of the fragile X mental retardation gene *(FMR1)*. This results in abnormal methylation which in turn silences gene expression *(80)*.

FMR1 is highly conserved among vertebrates *(81)*, so studies of *FMR1* function in species other than humans could render useful insights into the pathophysiology of the disease. Mouse models of fragile X have been generated either by insertion of a null mutation in the *Fmr1* gene *(82)* or by transgenic insertion of the CGC repeats *(83)*. Mice with a targeted deletion of the *Fmr1* gene exhibit mild cognitive deficits *(82,84–87)*. Other observed phenotyes, such as hyperactivity, attention deficits, and hyperarousal *(88)*, have also been observed in the mouse models (Frankland and Silva, *unpublished data*). Trinucleotide-repeat instability has been more difficult to model in mice. Recently, however, a mouse model with moderate repeat instability was created *(83)*, bringing hope that it will help shed light onto this process. Therefore, mouse models of fragile X are a useful tool to study the molecular and cellular causes of the mental retardation associated with the disease. The FMR1 protein seems to be associated with RNA metabolism *(79,80)*. RNA localization and dendritic translation have been proposed to be crucial for neuronal plasticity *(89)*. Therefore, studies of FMR1 function may not only provide insights into dysfunction *(90)*, but also help to clarify normal processes of neuronal function.

Learning disabilities are another form of cognitive impairment in humans. Neurofibromatosis type 1 (NF1) is the most common single-gene disorder causing learning disabilities in humans (approx 1/4000 individuals worldwide) *(91,92)*. Mutations in the *NF1* gene result in abnormal cell growth and differentiation which cause a variety of symptoms typically including benign neurofibromas, hyperpigmentation of melanocytes, and hamartomas of the iris *(91–94)*. They also result in learning disabilities that occur in 30–60% of patients with NF1 *(95,96)*. Visual–spatial function appears to be the most compromised in NF1 patients, although problems with language skills, executive function, attention, and motor coordination are also common *(95–105)*. The *NF1* gene encodes a 250-kDa protein (neurofibromin) with several known biochemical functions. This protein has a GAP (GTPase-activating) domain that accelerates the inactivation of Ras by stimulating its GTPase activity *(106–108)*. In addition, studies in *Drosophila melanogaster* suggest that neurofibromin modulates the rutabaga-encoded adenylyl cyclase *(109,110)*. Neurofibromin has also been shown to associate with microtubules *(111)*, suggesting that it may be involved in the regulation of multiple signaling pathways in the brain. It is therefore unclear which are the molecular and cellular consequences of *NF1* mutations in the brain. Because the mouse and human neurofibromin are highly conserved, studies of mouse models could help to unravel the mechanisms underlying the different phenotypes associated with NF1. Indeed, the effects of *NF1* mutations in both humans and mice show interesting parallels and have been useful for the understanding of the disorder (*see* next subheading). We will use the study of mouse models of NF1 to illustrate the strategies and the problems that can arise when using animal models to study the molecular and cellular mechanisms of cognitive dysfunction.

3.2. Parallels Between the Effects of Mutations in Mice and Humans

One of the first steps in building an animal model of a genetic disease is to determine the similarities between the effects of the particular mutation in mice and humans. It is important to verify if the proteins have the same functional domains and expression across species. Also, it is crucial to identify those aspects of the disorder that are recapitulated and those that are not. In the case of NF1, the mouse and human neurofibromin are highly homologous (98% sequence similarity) *(112)*, and so are the promoter sequences of the gene, suggesting that both the biochemistry of the protein and the transcriptional regulation of the gene are conserved across species *(112,113)*. In mice, and very likely in humans, the complete loss of neurofibromin is lethal *(114,115)*. Aged mice heterozygous for a targeted disruption of the *Nf1* gene (*Nf1*[+/–]) have an increased incidence of phaeo-chromocytomas, and myeloid leukemias, two phenotypes also observed in NF1 patients. It is important to note, however, that these mice do not show all of the tumor types that are characteristic of neurofibromatosis type I *(114,115)*. Better mouse models of tumor development in NF1 have been developed more recently *(116,117)*. Also, as described for NF1 patients *(118)*, *Nf1*[+/–] mice can develop low levels of region-specific astrogliosis *(119)* indicating changes in brain physiology.

There are also a number of similarities between the behavioral effects of the *NF1* mutations in mice and in humans. First, in both species, the *NF1* mutation seems to affect some brain functions more than others. For instance, it does not seem to disrupt simple associative learning, for example, fear conditioning, but it does impair specifically some more complex forms of learning, such as spatial learning. Second, both in humans and mice, *NF1* mutations do not affect cognition in all carriers, and the effect of these mutations can be compensated for with remedial training *(71,97–102)*. Third, the severity of the NF1 phenotype seemingly is affected by genetic variation, which exacerbates the condition of NF1 patients without having a noticeable impact on normal siblings *(120)*. Consistent with this, we previously showed that a heterozygous mutation of the *Nmdar* increases the severity of the learning deficits of *Nf1*$^{+/-}$ mice without affecting learning in littermate controls *(71)*. Finally, in agreement with the observation of motor coordination problems in a significant percentage of NF1 patients, *Nf1*$^{+/-}$ mutants also show impaired motor skills.

3.3. What Constitutes a Good Animal Model?

The most common misconception concerning animal models of genetic disorders is that they must reproduce all of the principal distinctive features of the disorder. For example, *Nf1*$^{+/-}$ mice do not develop all of the same types of tumors commonly seen in NF1 patients *(114,115)*. Nevertheless, as we describe here, these mutant mice have played a key role in our growing understanding of the biology underlying this disorder. It is important to stress that the paramount feature of all models in science is that they simplify the complexity of the phenomena studied. Inevitably, this simplification process eliminates some of the interesting and important complexity of the original phenomena. Clearly, the discarded complexity should not be ignored. Instead, it is important to always remember that the model at hand it is a required step to deal with the otherwise unyielding complexity of the original phenomena. For example, NF1 patients have a complex cluster of cognitive and neurological symptomology that is hard to interpret in any compelling neuroscience framework *(97–102)*. NF1 patients may show (1) neurological lesions, such as optic pathway gliomas *(91,92)*; (2) learning disabilities, which occur in 30% to 45% of the patients even in the absence of any apparent neural pathology *(105)*; (3) motor impairments *(91,92)*; and (4) attention deficits. The learning disabilities may include lower mean IQ scores, visual–perceptual problems, impairments in spatial cognitive abilities *(97–102)*, and a variety of other deficits of seemingly prefrontal and parietal origin. Also, brain magnetic resonance imaging (MRI) studies revealed areas of increased signal intensity in T2-weighted images in NF1 patients. These phenomena are referred to as unidentified bright objects

(UBOs). They occur throughout the brain, and some studies have reported a correlation between the presence of UBOs and learning impairments in NF1 patients *(105,121,122)* (but *see 123–125*). These UBOs are present in children, but tend to disappear in adulthood. Unfortunately, the neuroanatomic basis for UBOs is still unclear. They may reflect areas of abnormal brain parenchyma, either hamartomas, heterotopias, or local areas of brain dysplasia. Interestingly, postmortem studies revealed areas of astroglioisis in selected brain regions *(118)*. Astrogliosis is a common marker of brain pathology and it is often seen in the brains of patients with neurodegenerative disorders, such as Alzheimer's and Parkinson's disease *(126,127)*.

It is clear, even from this incomplete description of brain pathology associated with NF1, that it would be unrealistic to expect that a mouse model of this disease could recapitulate this complex human symptomology. The successful study of the learning deficits of the $Nf1^{+/-}$ mice are in part due to the greater simplicity of this animal model, which eased the interpretation of the results. For example, the absence of optic and other brain tumors in the $Nf1^{+/-}$ mice permitted us to study the effects of the $Nf1$ mutation on brain function independently of its confounding effects on tumor formation. Therefore, to dismiss this particular mouse model because it did not reproduce faithfully the full neuronal complexity of the human disorder would have been unfortunate. For example, much has been made about the lack of tangles and neurodegeneration in the brains of mice with various human amyloid precursor protein (APP) mutations correlated with Alzheimer's disease *(128)*. These mice develop plaques (another neuroanatomical landmark of Alzheimer's disease) and they show exacerbated age-related cognitive decline *(128)*, but do not show tangle formation. These and other results have been instrumental in showing that the debilitating cognitive deficits associated with Alzheimer's disease may not be due solely to neuronal death. It is possible that physiological changes precipitated by the abnormal APP products lead to cognitive deficits and to other physiological changes that trigger the aggressive neurodegeneration associated with this disease. Importantly, the Alzheimer's disease mouse models at hand will be useful for the study of the pathophysiological states that precede neurodegeneration. This presumptive predegenerative stage of the disease may be the best time for preventive intervention.

3.4. Validity of Modeling Human Cognitive Deficits in Mice

The cognitive deficits associated with NF1 may include deficits in receptive and perceptive language *(129)* (but *see 130*), clearly a phenotype that is impossible to study directly in mice. Therefore, it is possible that studies in mice may never elucidate the mechanisms of these putative language deficits. Also, other problems such as executive dysfunction have been poorly studied in mice. Consequently, the results of studies in mouse models, which have been focused mainly on hippocampal and amygdalar function, should be taken with some caution when generalized to human cognitive problems. However, it could be that the cellular and molecular mechanisms underlying the spatial learning deficits in NF1 may be similar to the ones underlying the language deficits in NF1 patients. Molecular and cellular studies of learning and memory have revealed a surprising conservation of molecular mechanisms of learning across species, and therefore it would not be surprising that different brain regions also use similar learning mechanisms. For example, many studies have demonstrated the involvement of calmodulin-induced kinases, PKA, phosphodiesterases, CREB, and many other molecular components, including neurofibromin, in the modulation of synaptic plasticity and learning in several species and brain regions tested *(131,132)*. Consequently, although it is inappropriate to model language deficits in mice, learning and memory mechanisms studied in mice may have commonalities with language processing in humans. Therefore, animal model studies targeting these basic learning mechanisms may also apply to higher level cognitive phenomena, such as language.

3.5. *From Genotype to Phenotype:* Multiple Effects of Multi-Functional Proteins

It is well known that individual mutations may have targeted effects in the complex functional repertoire of a protein. For example, studies of homozygous null α-CaMKII mutants revealed profound impairments in presynaptic short-term plasticity, and in postsynaptically induced long-term plasticity, including LTP and LTD *(131)*. Interestingly, a mutation that substituted threonine for alanine at position 286 of this kinase resulted in profound impairments in LTP, but in seemingly normal presynaptic plasticity *(133)*. As discussed previously, autophosphorylation at threonine 286 allows this kinase to be active even in the absence of calcium *(134)*. Thus, these results indicate that although the autophosphorylation and continued activity of α-CaMKII is critical for the induction of LTP, it does not seem to be essential for the modulation of neurotransmitter release *(133)*. Consequently, treatments directed at reversing the postsynaptic deficits caused by this kinase may not necessarily be effective against the presynaptic abnormalities of the mutants. Therefore, in treating diseases caused by mutations in multifunctional proteins, it will be important to characterize the mutation of each patient. Newly developed methods, such as automated sequencing and microarrays, are facilitating the lengthy and difficult process of tracking mutations in disease loci.

NF1 is another example of an inherited disorder in which insight about the genotype of the patient could be useful for devising the correct treatment. For example, the neurofibromin type II isoform is the consequence of alternative splicing events in the *NF1* gene that result in the inclusion of exon 23a. This inclusion results in a protein with higher affinity for Ras, but lower GTPase activity *(135)*. Thus, the expression of the neurofibromin type II isoform may actually decrease the overall GTPase activity encoded by the *NF1* gene because of competition with other isoforms with higher GTPase function. Therefore, deletions of exon 23a should lead to lower Ras signaling, while deletions of the GAP domain should result in higher Ras signaling. Interestingly, both manipulations result in learning deficits *(136)* suggesting that either decreases or increases in Ras signaling disrupt learning. This implies that treatments that decrease Ras signaling could actually worsen the condition of patients with exon 23a-like deletions.

The functional complexity outlined in the preceding may also underlie the apparent discrepancy between the biochemical function of neurofibromin in *Drosophila* and mice. Work with homozygous mutations in *Drosophila* has shown that neurofibromin mediates the modulation of potassium currents by the neuropeptide PACAP3 (pituitary adenylyl cyclase-activating polypeptide) at the neuromuscular junction *(109)*, and that it is required for Pavlovian conditioning *(110)*. Both of these functions seem to depend on the ability of neurofibromin to regulate adenylate cyclase, and not on its role as a Ras GAP *(109,110)*. In contrast, the role of neurofibromin in mouse spatial learning (Fig. 1) *(72)* and in *Drosophila's* circadian rhythms *(137)* seems to depend on its ability to regulate Ras signaling.

In mice, neurofibromin seems to be critical for adenylate cyclase in homozygous mutants but not in heterozygous *(138)*. Interestingly, there is also evidence of increased activation of the Ras/MAPK pathway in brains of homozygous *(139)* and heterozygous *Nf1* mutants (Cui, Costa, and Silva, *unpublished data*). In *Nf1* heterozygous null mutants, genetic and pharmacological studies have shown that its ability to regulate Ras signaling is critical for its role on synaptic plasticity and learning (Fig. 1). Either a drug that decreases Ras signaling or mutations that reduce the levels of two different isoforms of Ras can reverse the learning deficits caused by the *Nf1* heterozygous null mutation *(72)*. In addition, a mutation that specifically disrupts the Ras-GAP activity of neurofibromin resulted in learning impairments in patients *(140)*. This suggests that the up-regulation of Ras activity alone could underlie the learning impairments in both mice and humans. It is possible that the levels of neurofibromin in heterozygous null mutants (with approximately half of normal levels) are sufficient to regulate adenylate cyclase, but not sufficient to control Ras signaling. Consequently, only *Nf1* homozygous mutations may reveal the functional importance of the role of neurofibromin in regulating adenylate cyclase. Nevertheless, it is critical to determine which of these functions should be the target of clinical trials and treatments for neurofibromatosis type 1. It is possible that this type of complexity of phenotypes and treatments will be the norm rather than the exception in human genetic studies. On careful analysis, most inherited disorders, even the seemingly "simple" Mendelian traits, turn out to be far more complex than suspected *(141)*.

3.6. The Importance of Genetic Background

Almost every mutation studied is sensitive to changes in genetic background. Not surprisingly, the overall consequences of altering a single protein in cells are dependent on the functional state of other proteins. Proteins do not work alone but in large biochemical complexes and cascades, in which the importance of each step is directly dependent on many other simultaneous molecular events. For example, the effects of deleting a given kinase are likely to be more severe in cells in which the relevant opposing phosphatases are more active. Thus, just as any other experimental variable, genetic background has to be carefully controlled for and could affect results both in the laboratory and clinic. In the laboratory, the simplest way to control for genetic background is to derive and maintain mutations in a specific genetic background *(142–144)*, a common practice in studies with yeast, *Drosophila*, and *C. elegans*. By maintaining mutations in a homogeneous background it is easier to study and cross-reference studies in different laboratories. Heterogeneous uncontrolled genetic backgrounds (resulting from uncontrolled crosses between inbred lines) introduce unknown genetic variables that segregate randomly in pedigrees and confound the interpretation of experiments. Alternatively, mutations can be studied in outbred genetic backgrounds that resemble more the reality of genetic background in humans. This would allow researchers to study the robustness, penetrance, and pleiotropy of phenotypes, but at the cost of increasing variability.

Importantly, there is also extensive evidence for the important effects of genetic background in humans. For example, an *NF1* mutation that disrupts learning in one patient may not have any noticeable effect on another. Studies have shown that only approximately half of the patients affected with NF1 show learning impairments *(97–102)*. Similar results are observed for other aspects of the NF1 phenotype, such as tumor formation. Some patients are afflicted with a large tumor burden, while others remain unaffected. Although there are several possible causes for partial penetrance in this and other disorders, it is likely that genetic background plays a critical role *(141)*.

Recently, our studies showed that the C57Bl6/N genetic background occludes the spatial learning deficits (but not their working memory deficits) previously described for the *Nf1* mutants (Fig. 2) *(71)*. Importantly, isogenic first-generation (F1) mutants obtained from a cross between C57Bl6/N and 129T2/SvEmsJ recapitulate the learning phenotype described earlier (Fig. 2) *(71)*. This demonstrates that the cognitive deficits previously described for the *Nf1* mice were not due to other uncontrolled factors, such as independently assorting loci unrelated to the *Nf1* locus. Other studies have also reported effects of genetic background on tumor development in mice with *Nf1* mutations *(Nf1$^{+/-}$/Trp53$^{+/-}$) (145)*. In our laboratory alone, we have several other cases that clearly demonstrate how genetic background can alter the cognitive phenotype of mutations. For example, both the electrophysiological and behavioral phenotypes of the α-CaMKII mutants studied in our laboratory are sensitive to genetic background *(146)*. The phenotype of mouse models of fragile X mental retardation is also dependent on genetic background *(86,87)*. However, the influence of genetic background on a particular phenotype can also be useful. Humans have an uncontrollable, but determinable genetic background. Therefore genetic background effects may identify protective genes that could be used to develop prognostic and therapeutic tools.

3.7. *Establishing Protein Function:* Implications for Therapeutic Intervention

Because the phenotypes of mutations can change in different genetic backgrounds, how can we ever determine the "function" of a protein? If it is difficult to assign functions to proteins, how can we ever depend on rational drug development efforts? As stated in the preceding, the function of proteins cannot be determined in isolation, and must be defined in a specific genetic/functional context. In addition, to determine the function of a protein it is important to include, in addition to genetic data, a variety of other data from other experimental approaches. Genetic data alone are not sufficient. Most genetic experiments delete or lesion specific molecular components, and there is a long history in biology that clearly demonstrates that function cannot be derived from lesion studies alone. Surprisingly, there are no commonly agreed on criteria to assign functions to proteins. We have previously proposed a set of simple criteria *(147)* to accomplish this. We will illustrate these criteria with a specific example: CaMKII's role in LTP,

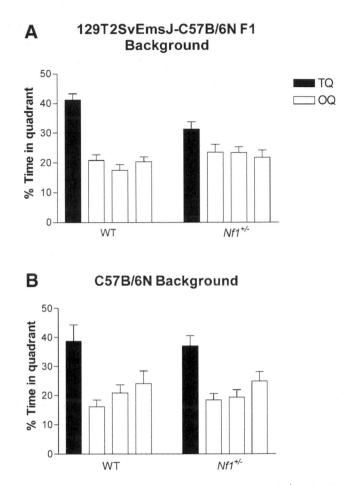

A   **129T2SvEmsJ-C57B/6N F1**
          Background

B   **C57B/6N Background**

Fig. 2. The importance of genetic background. (**A**) *Nf1+/−* mice in the hybrid 129T2/SvEmsJ-C57B/6N F1 genetic background have impaired spatial learning in the hidden version of the water maze (*see* Fig. 1). During a probe trial *Nf1+/−* mice search significantly less time in the TQ than WT mice. (**B**) *Nf1+/−* mice in the C57B/6N genetic background do not show an impairment the hidden version of the water maze (although they are still impaired in a working memory version of the water maze; data not shown). Even under demanding training conditions, *Nf1+/−* mice in the C57B/6N background learn as well as WT animals. In each experiment, mice from both genotypes are isogenic littermates. Training quadrant (TQ), *black bars*; other quadrants (OQ), *white bars*.

a cellular model of learning and memory. First, disruption of or changes in CaMKII should affect LTP (disruption). Second, CaMKII activation should be observed during LTP (observation). Third, induction or enhancement of

CaMKII activation should, under certain circumstances, either promote or facilitate LTP (mimicry). In addition to these three criteria, there should be a credible model of how CaMKII modulates LTP. Interestingly, all four criteria have been met for the role of CaMKII in LTP, which is reflected in the general consensus in the field about the key role played by this kinase in synaptic plasticity *(148)*. These criteria may be not only useful guidelines on how to assign function to proteins, but also in deciding when to choose a protein's function for rational drug studies.

3.8. What Is the Ideal Level of Analysis in Animal Models of Cognitive Dysfunction?

Because the ultimate goal of animal studies of human disorders is to devise drug (most likely) treatments, one could argue that molecular approaches are key to studies of animal models. However, our experience has suggested that studies at other levels of biological complexity (i.e., neurophysiology and behavior) complement and confirm molecular findings. For example, our studies suggested that hippocampal function is affected by *Nf1* mutations. Interestingly, recent hippocampal physiological studies revealed LTP impairments, probably caused by enhanced γ-aminobutyric acid-A (GABA-A) inhibition, due to deregulation of Ras signaling. This convergence of information is a powerful tool in determining the validity of a hypothesis. Furthermore, a sound multilevel understanding of the biological effects of *Nf1* mutations may be extremely helpful in developing a rational approach to treating the disorder. This multilevel information may be also instructive when complications develop, or when designing treatments for patients with other conditions.

4. SUMMARY

Recent excitement with the human genome project stems partly from the belief that the identification of the genes underlying the nearly 12,000 known genetic disorders will bring us closer to the development of therapies. However, it is still unclear how genetic information can be translated into treatments for inherited disorders. Here, we review how molecular, physiological, and behavioral studies in mouse models can improve our understanding of genetic disorders that affect cognitive function. We also discuss the nature and usefulness of animal models of brain disorders. We use as an example research in an animal model of neurofibromatosis type 1 (NF1), one of the most common single-gene disorders to cause learning deficits, because similar issues are likely to impact the study of other neurological and psychiatric disorders.

REFERENCES

1. Silva AJ, Stevens CF, Tonegawa S, Wang Y. Deficient hippocampal long-term potentiation in alpha-calcium-calmodulin kinase II mutant mice. Science 1992;257:201–6.
2. Silva AJ, Paylor R, Wehner JM, Tonegawa S. Impaired spatial learning in alpha-calcium-calmodulin kinase II mutant mice. Science 1992;257:206–11.
3. Grant SG, O'Dell TJ, Karl KA, Stein PL, Soriano P, Kandel ER. Impaired long-term potentiation, spatial learning, and hippocampal development in *fyn* mutant mice. Science 1992;258:1903–10.
4. Bliss TV, Collingridge GL. A synaptic model of memory: long-term potentiation in the hippocampus. Nature 1993;361:31–9.
5. Morris RGM, Anderson E, Lynch GS, Baudry M. Selective impairment of learning and blockade of long-term potentiation by an *N*-methyl-D-aspartate receptor antagonist, AP5. Nature 1986;319:774–6.
6. Miserendino MJ, Sananes CB, Melia KR, Davis M. Blocking of acquisition but not expression of conditioned fear-potentiated startle by NMDA antagonists in the amygdala. Nature 1990;345:716–8.
7. Maren S, Aharonov G, Stote DL, Fanselow MS. *N*-methyl-D-aspartate receptors in the basolateral amygdala are required for both acquisition and expression of conditional fear in rats. Behav Neurosci 1996;110:1365–74.
8. Gewirtz JC, Davis M. Second-order fear conditioning prevented by blocking NMDA receptors in amygdala. Nature 1997;388:471–4.
9. Bannerman DM, Good MA, Butcher SP, Ramsay M, Morrix RGM. Distinct components of spatial learning revealed by prior training and NMDA receptor blockade. Nature 1995;378:182–6.
10. Saucier D, Cain DP. Spatial learning without NMDA receptor-dependent long-term potentiation. Nature 1995;378:186–9.
11. Kiyama Y, Manabe T, Sakimura K, Kawakami F, Mori H, Mishina M. Increased thresholds for long-term potentiation and contextual learning in mice lacking the NMDA-type glutamate receptor epsilon1 subunit. J Neurosci 1998;18:6704–12.
12. Tsien JZ, Huerta PT, Tonegawa S. The essential role of hippocampal CA1 NMDA receptor-dependent synaptic plasticity in spatial memory. Cell 1996;87:1327–38.
13. Tang YP, Shimizu E, Dube GR, et al. Genetic enhancement of learning and memory in mice. Nature 1999;401:63–9.
14. Migaud M, Charlesworth P, Dempster M, et al. Enhanced long-term potentiation and impaired learning in mice with mutant postsynaptic density-95 protein. Nature 1998;396:433–9.
15. Zeng H, Chattarji S, Barbarosie M, et al. Forebrain-specific calcineurin knockout selectively impairs bidirectional synaptic plasticity and working/episodic-like memory. Cell 2001;107:617–29.
16. O'Keefe J, Dostrovsky J. The hippocampus as a spatial map. Preliminary evidence from unit activity in the freely-moving rat. Brain Res 1971;34:171–5.

17. Kentros C, Hargreaves E, Hawkins RD, Kandel ER, Shapiro M, Muller RV. Abolition of long-term stability of new hippocampal place cell maps by NMDA receptor blockade. Science 1998; 280:2121-6.
18. Tsien JZ, Chen DF, Gerber D, et al. Subregion- and cell type-restricted gene knockout in mouse brain. Cell 1996;87:1317–26.
19. McHugh TJ, Blum KI, Tsien JZ, Tonegawa S, Wilson MA. Impaired hippocampal representation of space in CA1-specific NMDAR1 knockout mice. Cell 1996;87:1339–49.
20. Shen K, Meyer T. Dynamic control of CaMKII translocation and localization in hippocampal neurons by NMDA receptor stimulation. Science 1999;284:162–6.
21. Meyer T, Hanson PI, Stryer L, Schulman H. Calmodulin trapping by calcium-calmodulin-dependent protein kinase. Science 1992;256:1199–202.
22. De Koninck P, Schulman H. Sensitivity of CaM kinase II to the frequency of Ca^{2+} oscillations. Science 1998;279:227–30.
23. Lisman JE, Goldring MA. Feasibility of long-term storage of graded information by the Ca^{2+}/calmodulin-dependent protein kinase molecules of the postsynaptic density. Proc Natl Acad Sci USA 1988;85:5320–4.
24. Giese KP, Fedorov NB, Filipkowski RK, Silva AJ. Autophosphorylation at Thr286 of the alpha calcium-calmodulin kinase II in LTP and learning. Science 1998;279:870–3.
25. Glazewski S, Giese K, Silva A, Fox K. The role of alpha-CaMKII autophosphorylation in neocortical experience-dependent plasticity. Nat Neurosci 2000;3:911–8.
26. Cho YH, Giese KP, Tanila H, Silva AJ, Eichenbaum H. Abnormal hippocampal spatial representations in alpha CaMKIIT286A and CREB alphadelta mice. Science 1998;279:867–9.
27. Matthies H. In search of cellular mechanisms of memory. Prog Neurobiol 1989;32:277–349.
28. Bailey CH, Bartsch D, Kandel ER. Toward a molecular definition of long-term memory storage. Proc Natl Acad Sci USA 1996;93:13445–52.
29. Silva AJ, Kogan JH, Frankland PW, Kida S. CREB and memory. Annu Rev Neurosci 1998;21:127–48.
30. Bourtchuladze R, Frenguelli B, Blendy J, Cioffi D, Schutz G, Silva AJ. Deficient long-term memory in mice with a targeted mutation of the cAMP-responsive element-binding protein. Cell 1994;79:59–68.
31. Kida S, Josselyn SA, Ortiz SP, et al. CREB required for the stability of new and reactivated memories. Nat Neurosci 2002;5:348–55.
32. Abel T, Nguyen PV, Barad M, Deuel TA, Kandel ER, Bourtchouladze R. Genetic demonstration of a role for PKA in the late phase of LTP and in hippocampus-based long-term memory. Cell 1997;88:615–26.
33. Bourtchouladze R, Abel T, Berman N, Gordon R, Lapidus K, Kandel ER. Different training procedures recruit either one or two critical periods for contextual memory consolidation, each of which requires protein synthesis and PKA. Learn Mem 1998;5:365–74.

34. Josselyn SA, Shi C, Carlezon WA, Jr, Neve RL, Nestler EJ, Davis M. Long-term memory is facilitated by cAMP response element-binding protein overexpression in the amygdala. J Neurosci 2001;21:2404–12.

35. Jones MW, Errington ML, French PJ, et al. A requirement for the immediate early gene Zif268 in the expression of late LTP and long-term memories. Nat Neurosci 2001;4:289–96.

36. Taubenfeld SM, Milekic MH, Monti B, Alberini CM. The consolidation of new but not reactivated memory requires hippocampal C/EBP beta. Nat Neurosci 2001;4:813–8.

37. Squire LR, Alvarez P. Retrograde amnesia and memory consolidation: a neurobiological perspective. Curr Opin Neurobiol 1995;5:169–77.

38. McClelland JL, McNaughton BL, O'Reilly RC. Why there are complementary learning systems in the hippocampus and neocortex: insights from the successes and failures of connectionist models of learning and memory. Psychol Rev 1995;102:419–57.

39. Bontempi B, Laurent-Demir C, Destrade C, Jaffard R. Time-dependent reorganization of brain circuitry underlying long-term memory storage. Nature 1999;400:671–5.

40. Frankland PW, O'Brien C, Ohno M, Kirkwood A, Silva AJ. Alpha-CaMKII-dependent plasticity in the cortex is required for permanent memory. Nature 2001;411:309–13.

41. Byrne JH, Kandel ER. Presynaptic facilitation revisited: state and time dependence. J Neurosci 1996;16:425–35.

42. Murphy GG, Glanzman DL. Mediation of classical conditioning in *Aplysia californica* by long-term potentiation of sensorimotor synapses. Science 1997;278:467–71.

43. LeDoux JE. Emotion: clues from the brain. Annu Rev Psychol 1995;46:209–35.

44. Davis M, Falls WA, Campeau S, Kim M. Fear-potentiated startle: a neural and pharmacological analysis. Behav Brain Res 1993;58:175–98.

45. Rogan MT, LeDoux JE. LTP is accompanied by commensurate enhancement of auditory-evoked responses in a fear conditioning circuit. Neuron 1995;15:127–36.

46. McKernan MG, Shinnick-Gallagher P. Fear conditioning induces a lasting potentiation of synaptic currents in vitro. Nature 1997;390:607–11.

47. Rogan MT, Staubli UV, LeDoux JE. Fear conditioning induces associative long-term potentiation in the amygdala. Nature 1997;390:604–7.

48. Romanski LM, Clugnet MC, Bordi F, LeDoux JE. Somatosensory and auditory convergence in the lateral nucleus of the amygdala. Behav Neurosci 1993;107:444–50.

49. McNaughton BL. Long-term synaptic enhancement and short-term potentiation in rat fascia dentata act through different mechanisms. J. Physiol 1982;324:249–62.

50. Barnes CA, Jung MW, McNaughton BL, Korol DL, Andreasson K, Worley PF. LTP saturation and spatial learning disruption: effects of task variables and saturation levels. J Neurosci 1994;14:5793–806.

51. Moser EI, Krobert KA, Moser MB, Morris RGM. Impaired spatial learning after saturation of long-term potentiation. Science 1998;281:2038–42.

52. Rioult-Pedotti MS, Friedman D, Donoghue JP. Learning-induced LTP in neocortex. Science 2000;290:533–6.
53. Zamanillo D, Sprengel R, Hvalby O, et al. Importance of AMPA receptors for hippocampal synaptic plasticity but not for spatial learning. Science 1999;284:1805–11.
54. Huang YY, Kandel ER, Varshavsky L, et al. A genetic test of the effects of mutations in PKA on mossy fiber LTP and its relation to spatial and contextual learning. Cell 1995;83:1211–22.
55. Nosten-Bertrand M, Errington ML, Murphy KPSJ, et al. Normal spatial learning despite regional inhibition of LTP in mice lacking Thy-1. Nature 1996;379:826–9.
56. Errington ML, Bliss TVP, Morris RJ, Laroche S, Davis S. Long term potentiation in awake mutant mice. Nature 1997;387:666–7.
57. Metzger D, Clifford J, Chiba H, Chambon P. Conditional site-specific recombination in mammalian cells using a ligand-dependent chimeric Cre recombinase. Proc Natl Acad Sci USA 1995;92:6991–5.
58. Brooks AI, Muhkerjee B, Panahian N, Cory-Slechta D, Federoff HJ. Nerve growth factor somatic mosaicism produced by herpes virus-directed expression of cre recombinase. Nat Biotechnol 1997;15:57–62.
59. Forrest D, Yuzaki M, Soares H, et al. Targeted disruption of NMDA receptor 1 gene abolishes NMDA response and results in neonatal death. Neuron 1994;13:325–38.
60. Yu H, Saura CA, Choi SY, et al. APP processing and synaptic plasticity in presenilin-1 conditional knockout mice. Neuron 2001;31:713–26.
61. Dymecki SM. Flp recombinase promotes site-specific DNA recombination in embryonic stem cells and transgenic mice. Proc Natl Acad Sci USA 1996;93:6191–6.
62. Dymecki SM. A modular set of Flp, FRT and lacZ fusion vectors for manipulating genes by site-specific recombination. Gene 1996;171:197–201.
63. Gossen M, Bujard H. Tight control of gene expression in mammalian cells by tetracycline-respective promoters. Proc Natl Acad Sci USA 1992;89:5547–51.
64. Furth PA, St Onge L, Boger H, et al. Temporal control of gene expression in transgenic mice by a tetracycline-responsive promoter. Proc Natl Acad Sci USA 1994;91:9302–6.
65. Mayford M, Bach ME, Huang YY, Wang L, Hawkins RD, Kandel ER. Control of memory formation through regulated expression of a CaMKII transgene. Science 1996;274:1678–83.
66. Rotenberg A, Mayford M, Hawkins RD, Kandel ER, Muller RU. Mice expressing activated CaMKII lack low frequency LTP and do not form stable place cells in the CA1 region of the hippocampus. Cell 1996;87:1351–61.
67. Picard D. Steroid-binding domains for regulating functions of heterologous proteins in cis. Trends Cell Biol 1993;3:278–80.
68. Feil R, Brocard J, Mascrez B, LeMeur M, Metzger D, Chambon P. Ligand-activated site specific recombination in mice. Proc Natl Acad Sci USA 1996;93:10887–90.
69. Logie C, Stewart AF. Ligand-regulated site-specific recombination. Proc Natl Acad Sci USA 1995;92:5940–4.

70. Danielian PS, White R, Hoare SA, Fawell SE, Parker MG. Identification of residues in the estrogen receptor that confer differential sensitivity to estrogen and hydroxytamoxifen. Mol Endocrinol 1993;7:232–40.
71. Silva AJ, Frankland PW, Marowitz Z, et al. A mouse model for the learning and memory deficits associated with neurofibromatosis type I. Nat Genet 1997;15:281–4.
72. Costa RM, Federov NB, Kogan JH, et al. Mechanism for the learning deficits in a mouse model of neurofibromatosis type 1. Nature 2002;16:16.
73. Ohno M, Frankland PW, Chen AP, Costa RM, Silva AJ. Inducible, pharmaco-genetic approaches to the study of learning and memory. Nat Neurosci 2001;4:1238–43.
74. Janus C, Westaway D. Transgenic mouse models of Alzheimer's disease. Physiol Behav 2001;73:873–86.
75. Schenk D, Barbour R, Dunn W, et al. Immunization with amyloid-beta attenuates Alzheimer-disease-like pathology in the PDAPP mouse. Nature 1999;400:173–7.
76. Bard F, Cannon C, Barbour R, et al. Peripherally administered antibodies against amyloid beta-peptide enter the central nervous system and reduce pathology in a mouse model of Alzheimer disease. Nat Med 2000;6:916–9.
77. Daily DK, Ardinger HH, Holmes GE. Identification and evaluation of mental retardation. Am Fam Physician 2000;61:1059–67, 1070.
78. Fisch GS. What is associated with the fragile X syndrome? Am J Med Genet 1993;48:112–21.
79. Bardoni B, Mandel JL, Fisch GS. FMR1 gene and fragile X syndrome. Am J Med Genet 2000;97:153–63.
80. Jin P, Warren ST. Understanding the molecular basis of fragile X syndrome. Hum Mol Genet 2000;9:901–8.
81. Ashley CT, Sutcliffe JS, Kunst CB, et al. Human and murine FMR-1: alternative splicing and translational initiation downstream of the CGG-repeat. Nat Genet 1993;4:244–51.
82. Oostra BA, Bakker CE, Reyniers E, et al. FMR1 knockout mice: a model to study fragile X mental retardation. Am J Hum Genet 1994;55:A46.
83. Bontekoe CJ, Bakker CE, Nieuwenhuizen IM, et al. Instability of a (CGG)98 repeat in the Fmr1 promoter. Hum Mol Genet 2001;10:1693–9.
84. Kooy RF, D'Hooge R, Reyniers E, et al. Transgenic mouse model for the fragile X syndrome. Am J Med Genet 1996;64:241–5.
85. D'Hooge R, Nagels G, Franck F, et al. Mildly impaired water maze performance in male Fmr1 knockout mice. Neuroscience 1997;76:367–76.
86. Paradee W, Melikian HE, Rasmussen DL, Kenneson A, Conn PJ, Warren ST. Fragile X mouse: strain effects of knockout phenotype and evidence suggesting deficient amygdala function. Neuroscience 1999;94:185–92.
87. Dobkin C, Rabe A, Dumas R, El Idrissi A, Haubenstock H, Brown WT. Fmr1 knockout mouse has a distinctive strain-specific learning impairment. Neuroscience 2000;100:423–9.
88. Munir F, Cornish KM, Wilding J. A neuropsychological profile of attention deficits in young males with fragile X syndrome. Neuropsychologia 2000;38:1261–70.

89. Steward O, Schuman EM. Protein synthesis at synaptic sites on dendrites. Annu Rev Neurosci 2001;24:299–325.

90. Comery TA, Harris JB, Willems PJ, et al. Abnormal dendritic spines in fragile X knockout mice: maturation and pruning deficits. Proc Natl Acad Sci USA 1997;94:5401–4.

91. Gutmann DH, Collins FS. von Recklinghausen neurofibromatosis. In: The metabolic and molecular basis of inherited disease, 7th ed. New York: McGraw Hill, 1994;14:1–19.

92. Huson SM, Hughes RAC. The neurofibromatoses: a pathogenic and clinical overview. London: Chapman & Hall, 1994:204–52.

93. Viskochil D. Neurofibromatosis 1. Am J Med Genet 1999;89:V–VIII.

94. Cichowski K, Jacks T. NF1 tumor suppressor gene function: narrowing the GAP. Cell 2001;104:593–604.

95. North K. Neurofibromatosis type 1. Am J Med Genet 2000;97:119-27.

96. Ozonoff S. Cognitive impairment in neurofibromatosis type 1. Am J Med Genet 1999;89:45–52.

97. Eliason MJ. Neurofibromatosis: implications for learning and behavior. Dev Behav Pediatr 1986;7:175–9.

98. Eliason MJ. Neuropsychological patterns: neurofibromatosis compared to developmental learning disorders. Neurofibromatosis 1988;1:17–25.

99. Varnhagen C, Lewin S, Das JP, Bowen P, Ma K, Klimek M. Neurofibromatosis and psychological processes. Dev Behav Pediatr 1988;9:257–65.

100. Eldridge R, Denckla MB, Bien E, et al. Neurofibromatosis type 1 (Recklinghausen's Disease): neurologic and cognitive assessment with sibling controls. Am J Dis Child 1989;143:833–7.

101. North K. Neurofibromatosis type 1: review of the first 200 patients in an Australian clinic. J Child Neurol 1993;8:395–402.

102. North K, Joy P, Yuille D, Cocks N, Hutchins P. Cognitive function and academic performance in children with neurofibromatosis type 1. Dev Med Child Neurol 1995;37:427–36.

103. Chapman CA, Waber DP, Bassett N, Urion DK, Korf BR. Neurobehavioral profiles of children with neurofibromatosis 1 referred for learning disabilities are sex-specific. Am J Med Genet 1996;67:127–32.

104. Zoller ME, Rembeck B, Backman L. Neuropsychological deficits in adults with neurofibromatosis type 1. Acta Neurol Scand 1997;95:225–32.

105. North K, Joy P, Yuille D, et al. Specific learning disability in children with neurofibromatosis type I: significance of MRI abnormalities. Neurology 1994;44:878–83.

106. Martin GA, Viskochil D, Bollag G, et al. The GAP-related domain of the neurofibromatosis type 1 gene product interacts with *ras* p21. Cell 1990;63:843–9.

107. Xu GF, Lin B, Tanaka K, et al. The catalytic domain of the neurofibromatosis type 1 gene product stimulates ras GTPase and complements ira mutants of *S. cerevisiae*. Cell 1990;63:835–41.

108. Ballester R, Marchuk D, Bouguski M, et al. The NF1 locus encodes a protein functionally related to mammalian GAP and yeast IRA proteins. Cell 1990;63:851–9.

109. Guo HF, The I, Hannan F, Bernards A, Zhong Y. Requirement of *Drosophila* NF1 for activation of adenylyl cyclase by PACAP38-like neuropeptides. Science 1997;276:795–8.
110. Guo HF, Tong J, Hannan F, Luo L, Zhong Y. A neurofibromatosis-1-regulated pathway is required for learning in Drosophila. Nature 2000;403:895–8.
111. Xu H, Gutmann DH. Mutations in the GAP-related domain impair the ability of neurofibromin to associate with microtubules. Brain Res 1997;759:149–52.
112. Bernards A, Snijders AJ, Hannigan GE, Murthy AE, Gusella JF. Mouse neurofibromatosis type 1 cDNA sequence reveals high degree of conservation of both coding and non-coding mRNA segments. Hum Mol Genet 1993;2:645–50.
113. Hajra A, Martin-Gallardo A, Tarle SA, et al. DNA sequences in the promoter region of the NF1 gene are highly conserved between human and mouse. Genomics 1994;21:649–52.
114. Jacks T, Shih TS, Schmitt EM, Bronson RT, Bernards A, Weinberg RA. Tumour predisposition in mice heterozygous for a targeted mutation in Nf1. Nat Genet 1994;7:353–61.
115. Brannan CI, Perkins AS, Vogel KS, et al. Targeted disruption of the neurofibromatosis type-1 gene leads to developmental abnormalities in heart and various neural crest-derived tissues. Genes Dev 1994;8:1019–29.
116. Cichowski K, Shih TS, Schmitt E, et al. Mouse models of tumor development in neurofibromatosis type 1. Science 1999;286:2172–6.
117. Vogel KS, Klesse LJ, Velasco-Miguel S, Meyers K, Rushing EJ, Parada LF. Mouse tumor model for neurofibromatosis type 1. Science 1999;286:2176–9.
118. Nordlund ML, Rizvi TA, Brannan CI, Ratner N. Neurofibromin expression and astrogliosis in neurofibromatosis (type 1) brains. J Neuropathol Exp Neurol 1995;54:588–600.
119. Rizvi TA, Akunuru S, de Courten-Myers G, Switzer RC, 3rd, Nordlund ML, Ratner N. Region-specific astrogliosis in brains of mice heterozygous for mutations in the neurofibromatosis type 1 (Nf1) tumor suppressor. Brain Res 1999;816:111–23.
120. Easton D, Ponder M, Huson S, Ponder B. An analysis of variation in expression of neurofibromatosis (NF) type 1 (NF1): evidence for modifying genes. Am J Hum Genet 1993;53:305–13.
121. Denckla MB, Hofman K, Mazzocco MM, et al. Relationship between T2-weighted hyperintensities (unidentified bright objects) and lower IQs in children with neurofibromatosis-1. Am J Med Genet 1996;67:98–102.
122. Hofman KJ, Harris EL, Bryan RN, Denckla MB. Neurofibromatosis type 1: the cognitive phenotype. J Pediatr 1994;124:S1–8.
123. Duffner PK, Cohen ME, Seidel FG, Shucard DW. The significance of MRI abnormalities in children with neurofibromatosis. Neurology 1989;39:373–8.
124. Ferner RE, Chaudhuri R, Bingham J, Cox T, Hughes RA. MRI in neurofibromatosis 1. The nature and evolution of increased intensity T2 weighted lesions and their relationship to intellectual impairment. J Neurol Neurosurg Psychiatry 1993;56:492–5.

125. Legius E, Descheemaeker MJ, Steyaert J, et al. Neurofibromatosis type 1 in childhood: correlation of MRI findings with intelligence. J Neurol Neurosurg Psychiatry 1995;59:638–40.
126. Overmyer M, Helisalmi S, Soininen H, Laakso M, Riekkinen P, Sr, Alafuzoff I. Astrogliosis and the ApoE genotype. An immunohistochemical study of postmortem human brain tissue. Dement Geriatr Cogn Disord 1999; 10:252–7.
127. Renkawek K, Stege GJ, Bosman GJ. Dementia, gliosis and expression of the small heat shock proteins hsp27 and alpha B-crystallin in Parkinson's disease. NeuroReport 1999;10:2273–6.
128. Hsiao K. Transgenic mice expressing Alzheimer amyloid precursor proteins. Exp Gerontol 1998;33:883–9.
129. Dilts CV, Carey JC, Kircher JC, et al. Children and adolescents with neurofibromatosis 1: a behavioral phenotype. J Dev Behav Pediatr 1996;17:229–39.
130. Cutting LE, Koth CW, Denckla MB. How children with neurofibromatosis type 1 differ from "typical" learning disabled clinic attenders: nonverbal learning disabilities revisited. Dev Neuropsychol 2000;17:29–47.
131. Silva AJ, Giese KP, Fedorov NB, Frankland PW, Kogan JH. Molecular, cellular, and neuroanatomical substrates of place learning. Neurobiol Learn Mem 1998;70:44–61.
132. Kandel ER, Pittenger C. The past, the future and the biology of memory storage. Philos Trans Roy Soc Lond [B] Biol Sci 1999;354:2027–52.
133. Giese KP, Fedorov NB, Filipkowski RK, Silva AJ. Autophosphorylation at Thr286 of the α calcium-calmodulin kinase II in LTP and learning. Science 1998;279:870–3.
134. Braun PA, Schulman H. The multifunctional calcium/calmodulin-dependent protein kinase: from form to function. Annu Rev Physiol 1995;57:417–45.
135. Anderson LB, Ballester R, Marchuk DA, et al. A conserved alternative splice in the van Recklinghausen neurofibromatosis (NF1) gene produces two neurofibromin isoforms, both of which have GTPase-activating protein activity. Mol Cell Biol 1993;13:487–95.
136. Costa RM, Yang T, Huynh DP, et al. Learning deficits, but normal development and tumor predisposition, in mice lacking exon 23a of Nf1. Nat Genet 2001;27:399–405.
137. Williams JA, Su HS, Bernards A, Field J, Sehgal A. A circadian output in *Drosophila* mediated by neurofibromatosis-1 and Ras/MAPK. Science 2001;293:2251–6.
138. Tong J, Hannan F, Zhu Y, Bernards A, Zhong Y. Neurofibromin regulates G protein-stimulated adenylyl cyclase activity. Nat Neurosci 2002;14:14.
139. Zhu Y, Romero MI, Ghosh P, et al. Ablation of NF1 function in neurons induces abnormal development of cerebral cortex and reactive gliosis in the brain. Genes Dev 2001;15:859–76.
140. Klose A, Ahmadian MR, Schuelke M, et al. Selective disactivation of neurofibromin GAP activity in neurofibromatosis type 1. Hum Mol Genet 1998;7:1261–8.

141. Dipple K, McCabe E. Phenotypes of patients with simple Mendelian disorders are complex traits: thresholds, modifiers, and systems dynamics. Am J Hum Gent 2000;66:1729–35.
142. Silva A, et al. Mutant mice and neuroscience: recommendations concerning genetic background. Banbury conference on genetic background in mice. Neuron 1997; 19:755–9.
143. Wehner JM, Silva A. Importance of strain differences in evaluations of learning and memory processes in null mutants. Ment Retard Dev Disab Res Rev 1996;2:243–8.
144. Wehner JM, Bowers BJ, Paylor R. The use of null mutant mice to study complex learning and memory processes. Behav Genet 1996;26:301–12.
145. Reilly KM, Loisel DA, Bronson RT, McLaughlin ME, Jacks T. Nf1;Trp53 mutant mice develop glioblastoma with evidence of strain-specific effects. Nat Genet 2000;26:109–13.
146. Silva AJ, Giese KP. Gene targeting: a novel window into the biology of learning and memory. In: Martinez J, Kesner R, eds. Neurobiology of learning and memory. San Diego, CA: Academic Press, 1998:89–142.
147. Elgersma Y, Silva AJ. Molecular mechanisms of synaptic plasticity and memory. Curr Opin Neurobiol 1999;9:209–13.
148. Malenka RC, Nicoll RA. Long-term potentiation—a decade of progress? Science 1999;285:1870–4.

4

What Can the Study of Behavioral Phenotypes Teach Us About the Pathway from Genes to Behavior?

Jonathan Flint

1. INTRODUCTION

During the last decade, the study of behavioral phenotypes has generated a great deal of interest that has focused on genetically determined syndromes associated with mental retardation. As Hodapp and Dykens *(1)* report, there has been a 10-fold or greater increase in the number of articles published on the etiologies of genetic syndromes associated with mental retardation in the 1990s compared to the 1980s. The increase does not merely reflect advances in molecular genetics, but also includes a growing awareness that behavioral disorders are not a nonspecific outcome of mental retardation. It is well known that mental retardation is associated with an increased risk of behavioral disorder: epidemiological work carried out a quarter of a century ago indicated that 30% of mentally retarded children had some form of psychopathology, compared to 6% of controls *(2)*. Part of the increased risk is due to the presence of behavioral phenotypes that are relatively specific and characteristic of individual genetic syndromes.

Identifying and describing the characteristics of behavioral patterns specific to a syndrome are undoubtedly helpful for those actively engaged in the care of syndromal patients. Behavioral problems can be detected more easily and earlier, with the opportunity to anticipate and possibly prevent future problems, for example, self-injury in Lesch–Nyhan syndrome. It can also be a comfort to relatives and caregivers to learn that the severe behavioral disorder they have to deal with is an expression of the genotype and not to be blamed on their handling of the patient. However, it should be borne in mind that the psychopathology may, at least in part, be a consequence of mental retardation *(2)*.

From: *Contemporary Clinical Neuroscience:*
Genetics and Genomics of Neurobehavioral Disorders
Edited by: G. S. Fisch © Humana Press Inc., Totowa, NJ

Delineating behavioral phenotypes has another aim, that of understanding the relationship between behavior and genetic variant. The hope is that molecular techniques, in conjunction with careful phenotypic characterization, would lead to new clues about the biological basis of behavior. These findings would, in turn, lead to the discovery of the biochemical pathways and cellular mechanisms that mediate the behavioral phenotype. The field has now progressed to point where we should be able to decide if that hope can be realized, and for this reason I have chosen a question to head this chapter. How we can best answer it?

The data we have that address this question come from three areas of research. The first is the psychological characterization of patients of known genotype. The ability to classify patients by molecular type has enabled ever more detailed investigation of the relationship between genetic variant and phenotype. The second is the molecular investigation of the gene product. As I will show, in many cases this work is directing us to those proteins and biochemical pathways that are most likely to mediate a behavioral phenotype. Finally, there is the behavioral characterization of mouse knockouts. Over the last 10 years many animal models of human mental retardation syndromes have been made, by reproducing in mice the genetic defect discovered in humans. These animals allow not only functional exploration at a cellular and biochemical level but also behavioral characterization of a mutant.

2. PSYCHOLOGICAL CHARACTERIZATION OF BEHAVIORAL PHENOTYPES

Defining and characterizing behavioral phenotypes is not easy. As Einfeld and Hall have pointed out, inadequate attention to establishing and abiding by criteria for recognizing a behavioral phenotype can result in the misidentification of syndrome-specific behaviors *(3)*. A classical example is the belief that Down syndrome confers gifts of mimicry and musicality *(4)*, a view discredited by more recent studies (for a review of the older literature *see* 5). The psychological characterization of Down syndrome also provides a good example of the value of defining a behavioral phenotype: recognizing the presence of a dementia in Down syndrome provided insights into the biology of Alzheimer's disease *(6)*.

Einfeld and Hall suggest that evidence for establishing a behavioral phenotype should meet the following criteria: The study should be case controlled; chance must be ruled out as an explanation for the association; ascertainment bias must be considered; validated measures should be used; and, if in no association is found, the probability of a false-negative result should be estimated *(3)*. Undoubtedly this is a counsel of perfection, which may not be achievable in practice; many syndromes are rare, making it difficult to collect enough cases to attain sufficient power to establish an association with confidence. Nevertheless, detailed investigation of syndromes continues to provide insights into the unusual phenotypes that are sometimes associated with genetic syndromes. More important for our understanding of the relationship between genotype and phenotype has been the ability to explain variation within a syndrome by the type of molecular lesion and the investigation of longitudinal changes in behavioral phenotypes.

Molecular and behavioral variation has been correlated in the Prader–Willi (PWS) and Angelman syndromes (AS). PWS has attracted much attention because of the unusual genetic mechanism that gives rise to it *(7)*. The two syndromes have characteristic and distinct neurobehavioral profiles. In AS, retardation is severe (very few affected individuals develop expressive language) and there is ataxia, seizures, hyperactivity, and paroxysmal laughter. By contrast, in PWS mental retardation may be only mild and there is a specific behavioral abnormality: hyperphagia resulting in severe obesity. In addition, there are high rates of obsessive–compulsive behaviors. Almost three quarters of individuals with PWS have non-food-related compulsive behaviors and more than 90% exhibit repetitive skin picking *(8,9)*. Most cases of PWS are due to a deletion of DNA in 15q11–q13, but about a quarter of cases arise because of the patient has inherited two maternal copies of chromosome 15 (rather than the usual situation of one maternal and one paternal). Conversely, acquiring two paternal copies of chromosome 15 results in AS. This phenomenon is called uniparental disomy (UPD). The chromosomal region is said to bear a parent of origin imprint, of which the molecular signature is a difference in DNA methylation.

It now appears that the different molecular causes of PWS and AS have consequences for the behavioral phenotype. Cases with UPD have on average higher IQ, fewer speech problems, and less severe compulsions than those with deletions *(10)*. Intriguingly, in AS, in which imprinting operates in the opposite direction, paternal UPD is associated with a less severe phenotype: fewer seizures and better language skills *(11)*.

Unfortunately, there has been much less success in associating genetic and phenotypic variation in other syndromes. It might be expected that research on fragile X syndrome would be instructive, but convincing evidence has been difficult to come by. There is certainly scope for the appropriate studies, given the variability in the molecular basis of fragile X, the variable clinical picture, and the fact that the syndrome is relatively common, so that suitable sample sizes can be obtained. Fragile X syndrome is due primarily to an expansion of a trinucleotide repeat in the 5' untranslated region of gene coding for an RNA binding protein that exists in six isoforms. Two types of expansion are recognized. The full mutation consists of >200 trinucleotide repeats. Premutations consist of between 60 and 200 repeats. The full mutation is abnormally methylated on the X chromosome of males and the active X chromosome of females.

The full mutation causes mental retardation in all males and in about 60% of females, but there is extensive phenotypic variation in both sexes. In most cases there is a poor relationship between the degree of cognitive impairment and the presence of a full or premutation, almost certainly due to the presence of mosaicism. Levels of protein provide a much better index *(12)*. Mildly impaired fragile X males have been described in whom unmethylated expansions are found in a large proportion of cells *(13)*. Furthermore, levels of mosaicism vary between tissues *(14)*, so that it is not possible to draw conclusions easily from findings in leucocytes. This probably explains the weak correlation between proportion of active X chromosomes carrying the mutation in females and the degree of cognitive impairment *(15)*.

There is a second way in which the psychological characterization of behavioral phenotypes has advanced our knowledge of the relationship between behavior and genes. Evidence of a genetically determined behavioral phenotype appears to support the hypothesis that the brain is a modular system, paralleling the view from lesion and functional imaging work that different brain regions perform specific functions. Were this to be true, it might be possible to define genetic correlates of specific brain systems. For example, a grammar module might be encoded in part genetically and involve specialized innately determined brain areas.

The investigation of infants with Williams syndrome has been used to address this question *(16)*. Williams syndrome is due to a microdeletion on chromosome 7q and has a characteristic cognitive profile. Most composite IQ scores range between 45 and 60, with seemingly good verbal and relatively deficient visual–spatial abilities *(17,18)*. The importance of the Williams syndrome cognitive profile is that it provides evidence of an innate neural system, mediating some aspects of language.

An innate module is expected to be present from birth, so in genetic disorders it is assumed that the pattern of abilities and impairments will be maintained throughout development. Longitudinal analysis can be used to see if this assumption is true. Paterson and colleagues *(16)* administered tests of vocabulary recognition and number skills to toddlers, age-matched controls, and children with Down syndrome who had similar IQ scores. The prediction from the findings in adults is that children with Williams syndrome should perform better on the vocabulary test than on the number skills test. However, the researchers found the opposite: toddlers with Williams syndrome did better than children with Down syndrome on the number task, and performed equally well on the vocabulary test.

The importance of this result is that it challenges the simple assumption that behavioral phenotypes reflect the action of discrete neural systems or brain modules. The data do not argue against the existence of such modules, but rather that the relationship between modules, genes, and phenotype is likely to be very complex. Careful investigation of a phenotype, however, may reveal modules that are more tractable to dissection than others. One of the problems in the psychological characterization of genetic syndromes has been continuing difficulty in finding appropriate measures. For example, Jarrold and colleagues examined short-term memory difficulties in Down and Williams syndromes. Their evidence for working memory deficits provides an explanation for the cognitive profile that does not involve a defect in a specific language system. Neither does it support the view that working memory can be dissociated into separate subsystems *(19,20)*.

3. MOLECULAR CATEGORIZATION OF BEHAVIORAL PHENOTYPES

Molecular characterization of the mental retardation syndromes continues to provide novel insights into the relationship between gene and behavior. There are four disorders in which we are beginning to see a molecular explanation for cognitive and behavioral deficits emerge and that is in the study of fragile X, Prader–Willi syndrome, nonsyndromic X-linked mental retardation, and neurofibromatosis type 1. I discuss these first and then briefly turn to data that show the converse, that in some syndromes a molecular explanation will probably not be particularly useful. I argue that in those cases in which a transcriptional regulator is found to be the cause of mental retardation, the site of genetic action is too far removed from the cognitive and behavioral abnormalities for the genetic and biochemical information to be useful for understanding the biology of behavior.

3.1. Fragile X and Synaptic Regulation of Protein Synthesis

Most gray matter in human cortex consists of dendrites, the processes that emerge from bodies of neurons and provide the site for synapses, yet their size and complexity has impeded experimental investigation. Recently, however, it has been possible to demonstrate that dendrites perform computational tasks *(21)*, transforming presynaptic inputs into a signal delivered to the cell's axon. The relative computational autonomy of dendrites in conjunction with another discovery, that dendrites control local protein production, is critical for the development of long-lasting synaptic change and a putative molecular substrate of learning and memory *(22–25)*. New protein synthesis requires mRNA and it is now clear that newly synthesized mRNAs target dendrites *(26,27)*. The importance of this observation is that the fragile X protein (FMRP) is synthesized in dendrites.

Although the genetic basis of fragile X was uncovered 10 years ago *(28–31)*, the function of the gene product has remained unclear. FMRP is known to export mRNA from the nucleus, but how this might relate to the cognitive phenotype has not yet been articulated. In normal brain, FMRP is found in nearly all neurons. It can bind RNA, including its own transcript, and it has been postulated that the FMRP has a role in the machinery of translation. Because it shuttles between nucleus and cytoplasm, it may be involved in mRNA export *(32,33)*. Functional studies yield few clues. FMR1 knockout mice manifest macroorchidism and mildly impaired spatial learning abilities *(34)*. Biochemical and immunofluorescence studies reveal a tight colocalization of FMR protein with cytoplasmic ribosomes, as observed for translation factors *(35–37)*.

Greenough and colleagues, investigating the mechanisms whereby synapses are formed in response to experience, discovered that FMRP is involved in the synaptic regulation of protein synthesis *(38)*. They found that stimulation of a preparation of presynaptic terminals resulted in a rapid rise in the association of ribsosomes with mRNAs and a concomitant increase in protein synthesis. Arguing that only a subset of mRNAs would be involved in this response, the researchers searched for a message that was enriched in the presynaptic terminals. They found a striking increase in polyribosomal association for one clone, which turned out to be the transcriptional product of the fragile X gene *(39)*. Subsequently, they showed that FMRP levels are elevated in animals learning new motor skills *(40)*, and that humans with fragile X syndrome show immature dendritic spine morphology *(41,42)*. There is also evidence that neurotransmitter evoked protein synthesis is reduced in vivo *(38)*, strengthening the suggestion that one role of FMRP in normal brains is to regulate the localized translational response to synaptic stimulation. This in turn would explain the mental retardation observed in the phenotype.

3.2. snoRNAs in Prader–Willi Syndrome

Molecular dissection of the Prader–Willi syndrome has been frustrated by attempts to determine whether the phenotype can be accounted for by abnormal expression of a single gene, or whether it is a function of several genes in the critical region on chromosome 15q. However, there is now some evidence to suggest that the defect in PWS is mediated by abnormal RNA editing due to misregulation of guide RNAs.

The nucleolus contains a large number of small RNAs, termed small nucleolar RNAs (snoRNAs); the majority of these snoRNAs function in the posttranscriptional modification of rRNA nucleotides. It is now clear however, that snoRNAs are involved in more than ribosome biogenesis. Recently, three brain-specific snoRNAs, which are subject to genomic imprinting in mice and humans, have been discovered within the 15q11 critical region for PWS *(43)*. The function of these snoRNAs is not clear, but one has a sequence similarity to the mRNA encoded by the gene for the serotonin receptor 2C. The sequence matches a conserved region subject to both alternative splicing and adenosine-to-inosine editing. Because of the known involvement of serotonin in appetite control and cognition, this finding raises the intriguing possibility that the defect in PWS involves a defect in serotonin neurotransmission.

3.3. Regulators of Rho- and Rab-GTPase Proteins

One of the most remarkable discoveries to have emerged from the molecular study of mental retardation syndromes is that mutations in the Ras signaling pathway occur in different X-linked conditions. Of course, given that there are so many mental retardation syndromes whose genetic basis is not known, it is possible that, by chance, we have a biased set of results, that, in fact, once all the genes are found the causes will be heterogeneous. Nevertheless it is a striking observation, already suggesting mechanisms involved in the pathogenesis of intellectual disability.

The Ras proteins form a superfamily of small GTP-binding proteins (or G-proteins) that participate in signal pathways crucial for a wide variety of biological functions *(44)*. There are two main classes of G-proteins, the heterotrimeric G-proteins that associate with receptors of the seven transmembrane domain superfamily and are involved in signal transduction, and the small cytoplasmic G-proteins. The Gα-subunit of the heterotrimeric G-proteins dissociates from the βγ-subunits when GTP is bound, and in this state will interact with various second messenger systems, either inhibiting (Gi) or stimulating (Gs). The Gα-subunit has slow GTPase activity and once the GTP is hydrolyzed it reassociates with the βγ-subunits. The small G-proteins are a diverse group of monomeric GTPases that include Ras, Rab, Rac, and Rho, and that play an important part in regulating many intracellular processes including cytoskeletal organization and secretion. Their GTPase activity is regulated by activators (GAPs) and inhibitors (GIPs) that determine the duration of the active state.

Central to the activity of G-proteins is the ratio of their GTP/GDP-bound forms, the former being the activated one. This ratio is subject to complex regulation. The main known regulators of this ratio are guanine-nucleotide exchange factors (GEF), GTPase-activating proteins (GAPs), and guanine nucleotide dissociation inhibitors (GDIs). The ras superfamily of kinases includes rho- and rab-subfamilies, which are implicated in regulation of the actin cytoskeleton and vesicle exocytosis respectively. Members of the former family, small G-proteins RhoA, Rac, and Cdc42, are key actors in signal transduction regulating actin cytoskeleton *(45,46)* and dendritic spine formation *(47)*. The most abundant of the latter is Rab3, which is expressed only in neurons and neuroendocrine cells.

Mutations in genes affecting different components of the Rho signaling pathway have been found in patients with nonsyndromic mental retardation. Two proteins, oligophrenin-1 (OPHN1) *(48)* and ARHGEF6 *(49)*, directly affect the Rho activation cycle. OPHN1 encodes a Rho-GAP protein that stimulates the intrinsic GTPase activity of Rho, Rac, and Cdc42. The *ARHGEF6* gene encodes a small cytoplasmic protein homologous to GEF for Rho-GTPases that activate them by exchanging Rho-bound GDP for GTP. The third gene found mutated in X-linked mental retardation (MRX) families is *PAK3* (in MRX30) *(50)*. *PAK3* may well be a downstream effector of the Rho-GTPases Rac and Cdc42 putting the message forward to the actin cytoskeleton *(51)* and to transcriptional activation.

The second subfamily of Rab-GTPases has a similar activation cycle and is also implicated in MR. D'Adamo et al. *(52)* found GDI1 to be mutated in two MRX families. GDI1 inhibits GDP dissociation from Rab3a by binding to GDP-bound Rab proteins and appears to be crucial in maintaining the balance between the GTP- and GDP-bound forms of Rab3. Rab3a is a small GTP-binding protein that functions in the recruitment of synaptic vesicles for exocytosis *(53,54)* and it is essential for long-term potentiation (LTP) in hippocampal neurons *(55)*. All Rab proteins are hydrophobic by nature and need GDI to mediate membrane attachment and retrieval *(56)*. Rab exists exclusively as a soluble complex with GDI in the cytoplasm, where it forms a reservoir to deliver Rab to the membrane during assembly of a transport vesicle.

How might the biology of the small GTP-binding proteins explain human cognitive function? Perhaps mutations in these genes disrupt normal development of axonal connections. This would fit with the known cell biology of the Rho GTPases *(44)*. Growth cones of developing axons find their way through the brain by sampling molecular signals, helped by GTPases *(47)*, whereas Cdc 42 and Rac1 are involved in the formation of lamellipodia and filopodia *(57)*; inhibition of Rho, Rac and Cdc42 also reduces dendrite formation *(58)*. Perhaps cognitive dysfunction in these MR families is due to a failure of neural networks involved in cortical development.

The second possibility (not exclusive of the first) is that synaptic function is compromised. This view is supported by the function of Rab3a. It is expressed only in neurons and neuroendocrine cells and localizes to secretory vesicles *(53,59)*. Synaptic vesicles contain Rab3a, which is the most abundant Rab protein in the brain. In one model, exocytosis of synaptic vesicles leads to the dissociation of Rab3a from the vesicle. Because Rab3a-deficient mice have no fundamental deficits in synaptic vesicle exocytosis the protein is not essential to the process but is required to maintain a normal reserve of synaptic vesicles. By disrupting RAB3a traffic, the GDI1 mutation is expected to alter neurotransmitter release, which might, in turn, account for the intellectual impairment.

Why is the effect of the mutation specific? Both the developmental and synaptic transmission account of Rho GTPase involvement must explain why only neurons involved in cognitive systems are disrupted. One likely explanation is that the mutations only partly disrupt the brain system on which they operate, but it could also be that compensatory mechanisms, effective in other cell types, fail when it comes to neuronal processes involved in cognitive processing.

There is also evidence that cognitive defects associated with neurofibromatosis type 1 (NF1) derive from an effect on the Ras pathway. NF1 is a common familial tumor syndrome with an incidence of 1/3500. It is a Mendelian autosomal dominant trait affecting primarily brain and skin. Some 30% to 65% of the affected children have learning difficulties but only 4–8% have mental retardation *(60,61)*. Individuals with NF1 seem to have impaired visual–spatial perceptual skills but language skills are also affected, and these impairments tend to co-occur. Owing to a lack of IQ matching in studies, it is not clear whether the language impairment is a specific consequence of NF1. Children with NF1 are at increased risk of having learning problems but the cognitive profile of NF1 includes both verbal and nonverbal impairments.

The *NF1* gene is large, consisting of 60 exons; most mutations are truncating, either significantly reducing or completely abolishing the protein or mRNA. Alternative splicing gives rise to several different transcripts whose differential functions are not well understood. However, neurofibromin has a GAP-related domain, NF1GRD, linking it to signal transduction pathways *(62)*. Klose and colleagues *(63)* identified a loss of function point mutation in neurofibromin molecule that results in a proline-for-arginine substitution at amino acid 1276 of neurofibromin. The effect is to disable the Ras-GTPase activating function (RasGAP function). In the family they described, affected children with this mutation had an IQ range of 80–89 and impairment in both language and motor development. This tells us that RasGAP activity is needed for the development of these functions. Possibly intact neurofibromin acts as a control element for Ras-GTP so that dosage-dependent loss of the neurofibromin's RasGAP activity leads to higher levels of activated Ras-GTP. Neurofibromin is also associated with microtubules, which links it to cytoskeleton and signal transduction pathways *(62)*.

3.4. Transcriptional Regulators as an Indirect Cause of Cognitive Impairment

Genes whose products influence the expression of other genes are known as transcriptional regulators. They can determine the point in development or the tissue in which the gene is expressed, often by binding to regulatory sequences or interacting with the transcriptional machinery of their target genes. It should come as no surprise that transcriptional regulators would be found in the molecular analysis of mental retardation. So many mental retardation syndromes have a complex phenotype, involving multisystem abnormalities, that mutations in genes that have broad effects were good candidates. The genetic basis of two syndromes is now known to be mutations in genes that alter gene expression by altering the structure of chromatin.

Gene transcription is in part controlled by the extent to which the DNA is made accessible to the transcriptional machinery. DNA does not exist in a free state in the cell; it is closely associated with a complex of proteins called chromatin, which we now know is intricately involved in DNA metabolism *(64)*. DNA has to be free of nucleosomes for it to be accessible to transcription factors and the large complex of proteins that constitute RNA polymerase. Understanding that which controls chromatin packaging will therefore reveal one way of controlling gene expression. For this reason there has been much interest in characterizing proteins that remodel chromatin and consequently influence many biochemical pathways, including the control of genes involved in the development and activity of the central nervous system. Rett syndrome and the α-thalassemia mental retardation syndrome (ATRX) are both due to mutations in transcriptional activators that affect chromatin structure.

Rett syndrome is an X-linked pervasive neurodevelopmental disorder, that affects 1/10,000–15,000 females *(65)*. The phenotype in affected females is distinctive, with developmental arrest at the age of 6–18 mo. From then on, girls progressively lose purposeful hand use as well as all communication skills. Autistic features emerge and classically they show hand wringing and other repetitive hand movements. After rapid deterioration, a stable period is reached and most girls survive into adulthood.

The genetic basis of Rett syndrome is a mutation in MECP2 *(66)*, a protein that binds to one of the constituents of chromatin *(67)*. The biochemistry of MECP2 has been studied and it is known that the protein binds methylated CpG-nucleotides throughout the chromosome. Methylation of CpG dinucleotides is important in tissue-specific gene expression *(68)*. The action of MECP2 appears to be to recruit Sin3a and histone deacetylase to form a repressor complex bound to DNA that deacetylates the tails of histones H3 and H4, leading to chromatin compaction *(69–71)*. This inhibits the transcriptional machinery and represses target gene expression. Note that there is nothing to explain specificity of gene regulation here.

MECP2 has a multitude of downstream targets, which currently remain unknown. Therefore it is not obvious how its loss leads to neuronal dysfunction. The symptoms are primarily those of a neurological syndrome, but MECP2 is expressed in most of the tissues. So why is the brain so vulnerable to these mutations? The presence of alternative transcripts might provide a solution, as they show a differential expression pattern *(72)*. The gene is highly expressed in fetal brain, where the largest 10-kb transcript is the predominant isoform.

Pleiotropic effects are also seen in ATRX syndrome *(73)*. This disorder is X-linked and patients have severe mental retardation, α-thalassemia, characteristic facial appearance, profound developmental delay, neonatal hypotonia, and genital abnormalities. The mutated gene belongs to the SNF2 family of proteins and contains a PHD finger (a putative zinc binding domain), and a motif that relates ATRX to a group of proteins called helicases *(74)*. Other members of this group are known to bind to chromatin and ATRX may be involved in chromatin remodeling, considered to be a crucial step in the control of gene expression. Recent findings suggest that ATRX may be part of the complexes that histone deacetylase forms with proteins that have a methyl-binding domain, such as MECP2 *(75)*. Again, as with Rett syndrome, understanding the biochemistry of the ATRX protein casts no light on the origins of the cognitive impairment. We will need to know far more about the downstream effects of both mutations to relate behavioral phenotype to genetic lesion.

4. ANIMAL MODELS OF BEHAVIORAL PHENOTYPES

A key tool for attributing function to genes is the creation of animal models by transgenesis. Therefore, the fact that several syndromes with behavioral phenotypes have been modeled in animals should allow a test of whether transgenesis is propitious, and these are listed in Table 1. The list

Table 1
Phenotypes of Mouse Models of Genetic Syndromes
That Have a Behavioral Phenotype

Syndrome	Mutational basis	Phenotype	Water maze
Fragile X	Fragile X gene knockout	Abnormal	Decreased spatial abilities marginal motor deficits *(108)*
	Fragile X gene knockout	Abnormal	Different navigational pattern in cross maze only in FVB-129 background *(110)*
	Fragile X gene knockout	Abnormal	Slight differences in early stages of training *(111)*
	YAC transgene	Abnormal	No differences *(86)*
Prader–Will	*SNRPN* gene Knockout Deletion	Appears normal *(112)* Poor feeding *(113)*	
Angelman	*UBE3A* gene knockout	Abnormal	
Lesch–Nyhan	*HPRT* and *APRT* gene knockout	No Abnormality *(83)*	
Rett	*MECP2* gene knockout	Inertia and hind limb clasping, breathing irregularities *(115,116)*	
22q11 deletion	Proline dehyrodgenase gene knockout	Impaired prepulse inhibition *(117)*	
Rubinstein–Taybi	CREB BP gene truncation	Deficient long-term memory *(92)*	No difference *(92)*
Neurfibromatosis	Neurofibromin gene exon 23a deletion	Abnormal	Impaired spatial learning *(118)*
Down Syndrome	Ts65dn	Abnormal	Impaired nonspatial and spatial learning *(119)*
Down Syndrome	Ts1Cje	Abnormal	Impaired spatial learning *(120)*

Table 1 (continued)

Fear conditioning	Discrimination task box	Light–dark	Open field	Conditioned emotional response
Non significant decrease in freezing *(109)*	Knockouts perform better-than controls *(85)*			No significant differences *(109)*
No differences *(110)*				
Less freezing in knock-out mice *(111)*		Increased trans- itions *(86)*	Increased activity *(86)*	
No differences *(86)*		Decreased trans- itions *(86)*	Decreased activity *(86)*	
Impaired contextual learning *(114)*				
			Reduced activity *(116)*	
Normal contextual con- ditioning; decreased cued conditioning *(92)*				
	Impaired *(118)*			

includes single gene mutations (fragile X, Lesch–Nyhan, Rett, Rubinstein–Taybi, and neurofibromatosis), segmental aneusomies (Prader–Willi syndrome, velo–cardio–facial syndrome), and trisomies (Down syndrome).

Overall, one must admit that animal models have provided very few new insights into the pathogenesis of behavioral phenotypes. In fact, most of the lessons have been negative, telling us either we are looking in the wrong direction or that we do not know how best to interrogate the animal model. In this respect, the example of Lesch–Nyhan syndrome is instructive. Lesch–Nyhan syndrome is an X-linked recessive disorder that can lay claim to having a classical behavioral phenotype, as Nyhan used the term behavioral phenotype in describing the compulsive self-injurious behavior *(76,77)*. The self-inflicted injuries associated with the disorder are frequently of such severity as to result in extensive loss of tissue, and to require arm splints or teeth extraction to prevent self-mutilation *(78)*.

Lesch–Nyhan syndrome arises from a lack or very low levels of hypoxanthine phosphoribosyltransferase (HPRT), an enzyme that resynthesizes the components of nucleic acids from their breakdown products. There are three purine bases involved (adenine, guanine, and hypoxanthine) and the enzymes that salvage them are different: adenine phosphoribosyltransferase (APRT) works on adenine, while HPRT works on guanine and hypoxanthine. Following the discovery of the metabolic basis of the disorder there were numerous investigations into the purine pathway of the nervous system. It emerged that basal ganglia cells produce HPRT with high specific activity and that *de novo* synthesis of purines is low, so that the cells are peculiarly dependent on the salvage pathway. Dopamine levels in the basal ganglia were <30%of normal in Lesch–Nyhan patients *(79)*, suggesting that there could be a connection between purine concentrations and the establishment of dopaminergic transmission in the basal ganglia. This might in turn account for the behavioral phenotype.

The mouse model of Lesch–Nyhan syndrome was expected to investigate the relationship between disordered purine metabolism and self-injury. However there appeared to be nothing wrong with the knockouts *(80,81)*. One explanation was that activities of the enzymes were different in mice, so that APRT could take on some of the function of HPRT, even in the basal ganglia. Subsequently, Wu and Melton *(82)* developed a pharmacological method for inactivating APRT in mice and reported that APRT inhibitors produced self-mutilation in HPRT-deficient mice. This seemed to resolve the question: purine metabolism was directly related to self-injury and possibly also to the other stereotypic behaviors seen in Lesch–Nyhan patients. However, Engle and colleagues have shown that the effect must be more complex than this *(83)*. They crossed APRT- and HRPT-deficient mice and examined the double mutant. Without either enzyme, the animal was expected to show the same phenotype as the HPRT knockouts treated with inhibitors. However, although the doubly deficient mice excrete adenine, as the mutant should, no additional abnormalities or any self-injurious behavior was detected. Subsequent investigation has also not replicated finding of self-injurious behavior with an inhibitor of APRT *(84)*.

Table 1 also shows the difficulty of using behavioral results from the mouse work to interpret the human behavioral phenotype. The most detailed investigation has been carried out for the fragile X mutant mouse, which initially was reported to have impaired visual–spatial discrimination *(34)*. Subsequently, Fisch et al. *(85)* have shown that the deficit does not extend to other cognitive phenotypes, as would be expected for a model of mental retardation. They showed that knockouts actually performed better than controls on a discrimination task.

In an interesting advance, Peier and colleagues *(86)* created a transgenic mouse that contains the human fragile X locus on a yeast artificial chromosome (YAC). They then crossed this transgenic animal with the knockout to see whether the phenotype could be rescued. To evaluate the functional impact of the YAC transgene, they performed a wide battery of tests, including those used by other groups (such as the Morris water maze), but in addition used tests of emotional behavior. They report that the fragile X gene influences anxiety-related responses. They drew this conclusion from unconditioned tests of exploration, the light–dark box and open field, where knockout animals were seen to explore novel environments more than controls while a YAC transgene, overexpressing FMRP, explored less than controls. However, they found no significant differences in tests of conditioned fear. Interpreting this mixed set of results is difficult, but highlights the need for complex and focused investigations. As the researchers point out, it is inconsistent with the observation that fragile X patients are more prone to anxiety than controls.

In one instance, the availability of a mouse model has made it possible to test for a cognitive phenotype that has not been looked for in humans. Rubinstein–Taybi syndrome is an autosomal dominant condition characterized by growth retardation, characteristic dysmorphic features, broad thumbs and toes, and mental retardation *(87)*. It is due to mutations in a coactivator molecule known as CREB binding protein (CBP) that interacts with the protein that binds to the cAMP binding response element (CREB). It also interacts with other transcription factors and nuclear receptors *(88–90)*. Although this description suggests that is unlikely that the gene would have a direct effect on a cognitive or behavioral phenotype, there is evidence from other mouse transgenes for the involvement of the CREB pathway in memory. CREB has been implicated in the activation of protein synthesis required for long-term facilitation, a cellular model of memory in *Aplysia*. Intriguingly, Silva and colleagues found that mice with a targeted disruption of the α and δ isoforms of CREB have profoundly deficient long-term memory, while short-term memory is normal *(91)*. These results implicate CREB- dependent transcription in mammalian long-term memory.

To date, no one has reported the necessary psychometric studies of patients with Rubinstein–Taybi syndrome to see if the same observation holds in humans. However, it can be performed in the mouse model. Oike and colleagues *(92)* constructed a mouse that has a truncated CBP protein. (Mice homozygous for the CBP null mutation have only a mild phenotype, suggesting that the phenotype is not due to hemizygosity of the gene *[93]*). They carried out behavioral tests similar to that of Silva's team *(91)* and confirmed that their mutant does indeed have abnormal long-term but normal short-term memory. These results should encourage study of memory in Rubinstein–Taybi patients.

A similarly imaginative use of an animal model has implicated proline dehydrogenase as a mediator of psychotic symptoms in the 22q11 deletion syndrome. A behavioral phenotype that includes schizophrenia has been described for patients with 22q11 deletions (sometimes referred to also as the velo–cardio–facial syndrome) *(94)*. Working from the observation that abnormally high levels of proline had been reported in a patient with a 22q11 deletion *(95)*, and that proline dehyrogenase, the first enzyme in the catabolism of proline, lies in the deleted region, Karayirogou and colleagues created a proline dehyrogenase knockout. They chose to investigate sensorimotor gating in the mutant mouse, as information filtering is suspected to be defective in schizophrenia *(96–98)*. In the test, a loud noise is used to startle the animal. Once the baseline response is known, startle is measured when the animal has received an auditory prepulse, a softer noise that is presented some 100 ms before the startling stimulus. Normally, mice show a reduction in startle, so the phenomenon is called prepulse inhibition; it is one of the few neuropsychological tests in which mice and humans are evaluated in a similar fashion. Investigators found that prepulse inhibition was defective in knockout mice and point to similar findings in humans as an indication that the gene is involved in the behavioral phenotype.

5. CONCLUSION

The study of behavioral phenotypes is now no longer a recondite interest. The characterization of phenotypes continues to attract interest and there is an expectation that, together with advances in the molecular and biochemical study of genetic syndromes that give rise to behavioral and cognitive abnormalities, it may be possible to understand how genes influence behavior and cognition. The evidence I have reviewed in this chapter is reason for optimism in this respect.

It is important to make explicit two assumptions in the literature on genetic effects on behavioral phenotypes. The first is that there will be cases in which the genetic effect on behavior will be close enough to the genetic lesion for it to make sense to study gene products with no, or negligible, reference to environmental and other mediators of genetic expression. For example, mental retardation in some conditions can be considered a nonspecific consequence of brain malformation, as in syndromes such as MASA (mental retardation, asphasia, spastic paraplegia, and adducted thumbs) and X-linked lissencephaly *(99–101)*. Or, it may be progressive destruction of neuronal tissue, as in Alexander disease *(102,103)* and in neuronal ceroid lipofuscinosis syndrome *(104,105)*. By contrast, in conditions where there are no noticeable alterations in brain structures or when postmortem histopathological analysis appears normal, the cause of cognitive impairment is difficult to find and may relate more directly to the genetic lesion. The assumption here is that these cases represent examples of relatively immediate genetic action and may therefore be more productive subjects for investigating how genes influence behavior.

Finding immediate genetic action on behavior is fraught with problems. Genetic mutations operate throughout development: the mutation could disrupt the expression of a series of developmental genes that in turn determine tissue-specific regulation in the adult of proteins directly controlling the phenotype of interest. Second, mutations are influenced by interactions with other genes. This can happen in a number of ways. The phenotype of a mutation will be affected by unlinked genetic variants (as is well known in other organisms) *(106,107)*. Alternatively, the phenotype may arise as a consequence of changes far downstream from the mutation. There may be a large number of different pathways affected, each with its own specific outcome. If these interact, attributing the final cause to the mutation, although true, does not tell us much about the immediate processes that give rise to the phenotype.

Despite these caveats, however, we have seen that there is evidence for relatively immediate genetic effects and that, to some extent, the phenotype can be a guide. Investigation of nonsyndromic mental retardation has pointed to the importance of Rho- and Rab-GTPase proteins, while mutations in transcriptional regulators are the cause of the complex phenotypes seen in Rett and ARTX syndromes. Regulators of Rho- and Rab-GTPase may be what we are looking for, causally much closer to the cognitive impairment than the transacting factors MECP2 and ATRX.

We have also seen that recent advances in our understanding of two syndromal causes of mental retardation, fragile X and Prader–Willi, reveal mechanisms for genetic effects that appear to be relatively immediate causes of cognitive impairment. The striking finding that FMRP is involved in the synaptic regulation of protein synthesis, together with the realization that protein synthesis in dendrites may be a critical step in learning and memory, provides the first glimpse of how mental retardation arises in the fragile X syndrome. Thus we can give qualified support to the first of the assumptions and expect that further progress in the molecular characterization of these syndromes will be helpful in explaining the genesis of behavioral and cognitive phenotypes.

The second assumption is that behavioral phenotypes are examples of innately determined brain systems that represent, in a fractionated pattern, the modularity often assumed to underlie brain function. There is sufficient evidence from neuroimaging and brain lesion studies to support the modular hypothesis in the adult brain, but the extent to which it pertains throughout development is still unknown. One view is that early in life the brain is not specialized and acquires modularity only during development. In this respect, investigating the genetic determination of specific cognitive and behavioral phenotypes can be immensely instructive, as has been shown with work on Williams syndrome. In this case, the results question the view that there is an innate language model. The data do not imply that it will be impossible to find direct genetic correlates for brain systems. In fact, it may simply be that we do not yet know which behavioral systems we should be correlating with genetic variation. But they do show that the correlation will be complex and will continue to be a fruitful line of investigation for many years to come.

REFERENCES

1. Hodapp RM, Dykens EM. Strengthening behavioral research on genetic mental retardation syndromes. Am J Ment Retard 2001;106:4–15.
2. Rutter M, Tizard J, Yule W, Graham P, Whitmore K. Research report: Isle of Wight studies 1964–1974. Psychol Med 1976;6:313–32.
3. Einfeld SL, Hall W. When is a behavioral phenotype not a phenotype? Dev Med Child Neurol 1994;36:467–70.
4. Belmont JM. Medical behavioral research: retardation. In: Fellis NR, ed. International review of research in mental retardation, Vol 5. New York: Academic Press, 1971;1–81.
5. Flint J, Yule W. Behavioral phenotypes. In: Rutter MR, Taylor E, Hersov L, eds. Child and adolescent psychiatry. Oxford: Blackwell Scientific, 1994;666–87.

6. Whalley LJ. The dementia of Down's syndrome and its relevance to aetiological studies of Alzheimer's disease. Ann NY Acad Sci 1982;396:39–53.
7. Nicholls RD, Saitoh S, Horsthemke B. Imprinting in Prader–Willi and Angelman syndromes. Trends Genet 1998;14:194–200.
8. Dykens EM, Leckman JF, Casidy SB. Obsessions and compusions in Prader–Willi syndrome. J Child Psychol Psychiatry 1996;37:995–1002.
9. Dykens EM, Cassidy SB. Prader–Willi syndrome, In: Goldstein SR, Reynolds CR, eds. Handbook of neurodevelopmental and genetic disorders in childhood. New York: Guildford Press, 1999:525–54.
10. Dykens EM, Cassidy SB, King BH. Maladaptive behavior differences in Prader–Willi syndrome due to paternal deletion versus maternal uniparental disomy. Am J Ment Retard 1999;104:67–77.
11. Smith A, Marks R, Haan E, Dixon J, Trent RJ. Clinical features in four patients with Angelman syndrome resulting from paternal uniparental disomy. J Med Genet 1997;34:426–9.
12. Tassone F, Hagerman RJ, Ikle DN, et al. FMRP expression as a potential prognostic indicator in fragile X syndrome. Am J Med Genet 1999;84:250–61.
13. de Vries BB, Jansen CC, Duits AA, et al. Variable FMR1 gene methylation of large expansions leads to variable phenotype in three males from one fragile X family. J Med Genet 1996;33:1007–10.
14. Taylor AK, Tassone F, Dyer PN, et al. Tissue heterogeneity of the FMR1 mutation in a high-functioning male with fragile X syndrome. Am J Med Genet 1999;84:233–9.
15. de Vries BB, Wiegers AM, Smits AP, et al. Mental status of females with an FMR1 gene full mutation. Am J Hum Genet 1996;58:1025–32.
16. Paterson SJ, Brown JH, Gsodl MK, Johnson MH, Karmiloff-Smith A. Cognitive modularity and genetic disorders. Science 1999;286:2355–8.
17. Francke U. Williams–Beuren syndrome: genes and mechanisms. Hum Mol Genet 1999;8:1947–54.
18. Bellugi U, Lichtenberger L, Mills D, Galaburda A, Korenberg JR. Bridging cognition, the brain and molecular genetics: evidence from Williams syndrome. Trends Neurosci 1999;22:197–207.
19. Jarrold C, Baddeley AD, Hewes AK. Genetically dissociated components of working memory: evidence from Down's and Williams syndrome. Neuropsychologia 1999;37:637–51.
20. Jarrold C, Baddeley AD, Phillips C. Down syndrome and the phonological loop: the evidence for, and importance of, a specific verbal short-term memory deficit. Downs Syndr Res Pract 1999;6:61–75.
21. Single S, Borst A. Dendritic integration and its role in computing image velocity. Science 1998;281:1848–50.
22. Kang H, Schuman EM. A requirement for local protein synthesis in neurotrophin-induced hippocampal synaptic plasticity. Science 1996;273:1402–6.
23. Schuman EM. mRNA trafficking and local protein synthesis at the synapse. Neuron 1999;23:645–8.
24. Ouyang Y, Rosenstein A, Kreiman G, Schuman EM, Kennedy MB. Tetanic stimulation leads to increased accumulation of $Ca^{(2+)}$/calmodulin-dependent

protein kinase II via dendritic protein synthesis in hippocampal neurons. J Neurosci 1999;19:7823–33.

25. Aakalu G, Smith WB, Nguyen N, Jiang C, Schuman EM. Dynamic visualization of local protein synthesis in hippocampal neurons. Neuron 2001; 30:489–502.
26. Steward O, Worley PF. A cellular mechanism for targeting newly synthesized mRNAs to synaptic sites on dendrites. Proc Natl Acad Sci USA 2001;98:7062–8.
27. Steward O, Worley PF. Selective targeting of newly synthesized Arc mRNA to active synapses requires NMDA receptor activation. Neuron 2001; 30:227–40.
28. Yu S, Pritchard M, Kremer E, et al. Fragile X genotype characterized by an unstable region of DNA. Science 1991;252:1179–81.
29. Pieretti M, Zhang F, Fu Y-H, et al. Absence of expression of the *FMR-1* gene in fragile X syndrome. Cell 1991;66:817–22.
30. Verkerk AJMH, Pieretti M, Sutcliffe JS, et al. Identification of a gene (*FMR-1*) containing a CGG repeat coincident with a breakpoint cluster region exhibiting length variation in fragile X syndrome. Cell 1991;65:905–14.
31. Oberle I, Rousseau F, Heitz D, et al. Instability of a 550 base pair DNA segment and abnormal methylation in fragile X-syndrome. Science 1991;252: 1097–102.
32. Eberhart DE, Malter HE, Feng Y, Warren ST. The fragile X mental retardation protein is a ribonucleoprotein containing both nuclear localization and nuclear export signals. Hum Mol Genet 1996;5:1083–91.
33. Tamanini F, Meijer N, Verheij C, et al. FMRP is associated to the ribosomes via RNA. Hum Mol Genet 1996;5:809–13.
34. Consortium TD-BFX. Fmr1 knockout mice: a model to study fragile X mental retardation. Cell 1994;78:23–33.
35. Feng Y, Absher D, Eberhart DE, Brown V, Malter HE, Warren ST. FMRP associates with polyribosomes as an mRNP, and the I304N mutation of severe fragile X syndrome abolishes this association. Mol Cell 1997;1:109–18.
36. Feng Y, Gutekunst CA, Eberhart DE, Yi H, Warren ST, Hersch SM. Fragile X mental retardation protein: nucleocytoplasmic shuttling and association with somatodendritic ribosomes. J Neurosci 1997;17:1539–47.
37. Khandjian EW, Corbin F, Woerly S, Rousseau F. The fragile X mental retardation protein is associated with ribosomes. Nat Genet 1996;12:91–3.
38. Greenough WT, Klintsova AY, Irwin SA, Galvez R, Bates KE, Weiler IJ. Synaptic regulation of protein synthesis and the fragile X protein. Proc Natl Acad Sci USA 2001;98:7101–6.
39. Weiler IJ, Irwin SA, Klintsova AY, et al. Fragile X mental retardation protein is translated near synapses in response to neurotransmitter activation. Proc Natl Acad Sci USA 1997;94:5395–400.
40. Irwin SA, Swain RA, Christmon CA, Chakravarti A, Weiler IJ, Greenough WT. Evidence for altered fragile-X mental retardation protein expression in response to behavioral stimulation. Neurobiol Learn Mem 2000;74:87–93.
41. Irwin SA, Galvez R, Greenough WT. Dendritic spine structural anomalies in fragile-X mental retardation syndrome. Cereb Cortex 2000;10:1038–44.

42. Hinton VJ, Brown WT, Wisniewski K, Rudelli RD. Analysis of neocortex in three males with the fragile X syndrome. Am J Med Genet 1991;41:289–94.
43. Cavaille J, Buiting K, Kiefmann M, et al. Identification of brain-specific and imprinted small nucleolar RNA genes exhibiting an unusual genomic organization. Proc Natl Acad Sci USA 2000;97:14311–6.
44. Van Aelst L, D'Souza-Schorey C. Rho GTPases and signalling networks. Genes Dev 1997;11:2295–322.
45. Mackay DJ, Hall A. Rho GTPases. J Biol Chem 1998;273:20,685–8.
46. Hall A. Rho GTPases and the actin cytoskeleton. Science 1998;279:509–14.
47. Luo L, Hensch TK, Ackerman L, Barbel S, Jan LY, Jan YN. Differential effects of the Rac GTPase on Purkinje cell axons and dendritic trunks and spines. Nature 1996;379:837–40.
48. Billuart P, Bienvenu T, Ronce N, et al. Oligophrenin-1 encodes a rhoGAP protein involved in X-linked mental retardation. Nature 1998;392:923–6.
49. Kutsche K, Yntema H, Brandt A, et al. Mutations in ARHGEF6, encoding a guanine nucleotide exchange factor for Rho GTPases, in patients with X-linked mental retardation. Nat Genet 2000;26:247–50.
50. Allen KM, Gleeson JG, Bagrodia S, et al. PAK3 mutation in nonsyndromic X-linked mental retardation. Nat Genet 1998;20:25–30.
51. Sells MA, Knaus UG, Bagrodia S, Ambrose DM, Bokoch GM, Chernoff J. Human p21-activated kinase (Pak1) regulates actin organization in mammalian cells. Curr Biol 1997;7:202–10.
52. D'Adamo P, Menegon A, Lo Nigro C, et al. Mutations in GDI1 are responsible for X-linked non-specific mental retardation. Nat Genet 1998;19:134–9.
53. Geppert M, Bolshakov VY, Siegelbaum SA, et al. The role of Rab3A in neurotransmitter release. Nature 1994;369:493–7.
54. Fischer von Mollard G, Stahl B, Li C, Sudhof TC, Jahn R. Rab proteins in regulated exocytosis. Trends Biochem Sci 1994;19:164–8.
55. Castillo PE, Janz R, Sudhof TC, Tzounopoulos T, Malenka RC, Nicoll RA. Rab3A is essential for mossy fibre long-term potentiation in the hippocampus. Nature 1997;388:590–3.
56. Wu SK, Zeng K, Wilson IA, Balch WE. Structural insights into the function of the Rab GDI superfamily. Trends Biochem Sci 1996;21:472–6.
57. Nobles C, Hall A. Rho, Rac and Cdc42 GTPases regulate the assembly of multimolecular focal complexes associated with actin stress fibres, lamellipoia and filopodia. Cell 1995;81:53–62.
58. Threadgill R, Bobb K, Ghosh A. Regulation of dendriic growth and remodelling by Rho, Rac and Cdc42. Neuron 1997;19:625–34.
59. Sudhof TC. The synaptic vesicle cycle: a cascade of protein–protein interactions. Nature 1995;375:645–53.
60. North K. Neurofibromatosis type 1. Am J Med Genet 2000;97:119–27.
61. Ozonoff S. Cognitive impairment in neurofibromatosis type 1. Am J Med Genet 1999;89:45–52.
62. Scheffzek K, Ahmadian MR, Wiesmuller L, et al. Structural analysis of the GAP-related domain from neurofibromin and its implications. EMBO J 1998;17:4313–27.

63. Klose A, Ahmadian MR, Schuelke M, et al. Selective disactivation of neurofibromin GAP activity in neurofibromatosis type 1. Hum Mol Genet 1998;7:1261–8.

64. Wolffe AP, Guschin D. Review: chromatin structural features and targets that regulate transcription. J Struct Biol 2000;129:102–22.

65. Hagberg B, Goutieres F, Hanefeld F, Rett A, Wilson J. Rett syndrome: criteria for inclusion and exclusion. Brain Dev 1985;3:372–3.

66. Amir RE, Van den Veyver IB, Wan M, Tran CQ, Francke U, Zoghbi HY. Rett syndrome is caused by mutations in X-linked MECP2, encoding methyl-CpG-binding protein 2 [see comments]. Nat Genet 1999;23:185–8.

67. Lewis JD, Meehan RR, Henzel WJ, et al. Purification, sequence, and cellular localization of a novel chromosomal protein that binds to methylated DNA. Cell 1992;69:905–14.

68. Bird AP, Wolffe AP. Methylation-induced repression—belts, braces, and chromatin. Cell 1999;99:451–4.

69. Nan X, Ng HH, Johnson CA, et al. Transcriptional repression by the methyl-CpG-binding protein MeCP2 involves a histone deacetylase complex. Nature 1998;393:386–9.

70. Jones PL, Veenstra GJ, Wade PA, et al. Methylated DNA and MeCP2 recruit histone deacetylase to repress transcription. Nat Genet 1998;19:187–91.

71. Wade PA, Jones PL, Vermaak D, et al. Histone deacetylase directs the dominant silencing of transcription in chromatin: association with MeCP2 and the Mi-2 chromodomain SWI/SNF ATPase. Cold Spring Harb Symp Quant Biol 1998;63:435–45.

72. Wan M, Lee SS, Zhang X, et al. Rett syndrome and beyond: recurrent spontaneous and familial MECP2 mutations at CpG hotspots. Am J Hum Genet 1999;65:1520–9.

73. Gibbons RJ, Higgs DR. Molecular-clinical spectrum of the ATR-X syndrome. Am J Med Genet 2000;97:204–12.

74. Picketts DJ, Higgs DR, Bachoo S, Blake DJ, Quarrell OW, Gibbons RJ. ATRX encodes a novel member of the SNF2 family of proteins: mutations point to a common mechanism underlying the ATR-X syndrome. Hum Mol Genet 1996;5:1899–907.

75. Gibbons RJ, McDowell TL, Raman S, et al. Mutations in ATRX, encoding a SWI/SNF-like protein, cause diverse changes in the pattern of DNA methylation. Nat Genet 2000;24:368–71.

76. Nyhan WL. Behavior in the Lesch–Nyhan syndrome. J Autism Child Schizophr 1976;6:235–52.

77. Nyhan WL. Behavioral phenotypes in organic genetic disease. Pediatr Res 1972;6:1–9.

78. Christie R, Bay C, Kaufman IA, Bakay B, Borden M, Nyhan WL. Lesch–Nyhan disease: clinical experience with nineteen patients. Dev Med Child Neurol 1982;24:293–306.

79. Lloyd KG, Hornykiewicz O, Davison L. Biochemical evidence of dysfunction of brain neurotransmitter in the Lesch–Nyhan syndrome. N Engl J Med 1981;305:1106–11.

80. Kuehn MR, Bradley A, Robertson EJ, Evans MJ. A potential animal model for Lesch–Nyhan syndrome through introduction of HPRT mutations into mice. Nature 1987;326:295–8.

81. Hooper ML, Hardy K, Handyside A, Hunter S, Monk M. HPRT-deficient (Lesch–Nyhan) mouse embryos derived from germline colonization by cultured cells. Nature 1987;326:292–5.

82. Wu CL, Melton DW. Production of a model for Lesch–Nyhan syndrome in hypoxanthine phosphoribosyltransferase-deficient mice. Nat Genet 1993; 3:235–40.

83. Engle SJ, Womer DE, Davies PM, et al. HPRT-APRT-deficient mice are not a model for Lesch–Nyhan syndrome. Hum Mol Genet 1996;5:1607–10.

84. Edamura K, Sasai H. No self-injurious behavior was found in HPRT-deficient mice treated with 9-ethyladenine. Pharmacol Biochem Behav 1998;61:175–9.

85. Fisch GS, Hao HK, Bakker C, Oostra BA. Learning and memory in the FMR1 knockout mouse. Am J Med Genet 1999;84:277–82.

86. Peier AM, McIlwain KL, Kenneson A, Warren ST, Paylor R, Nelson DL. (Over)correction of FMR1 deficiency with YAC transgenics: behavioral and physical features. Hum Mol Genet 2000;9:1145–59.

87. Rubinstein JH. Broad thumb-hallux (Rubinstein–Taybi) syndrome 1957–1988. Am J Med Genet (Suppl) 1990;6:3–16.

88. Petrij F, Giles HR, Dauwerse HG, et al. Rubinstein-Taybi syndrome caused by mutations in the transcriptional co-activator CNP. Nature 1995;376:348–51.

89. Kamei Y, Xu L, Heinzel T, et al. A CBP integrator complex mediates transcriptional activation and AP-1 inhibition by nuclear receptors. Cell 1996;85:403–14.

90. Kwok RP, Lundblad JR, Chrivia JC, et al. Nuclear protein CBP is a coactivator for the transcription factor CREB. Nature 1994;370:223–6.

91. Bourtchuladze R, Frenguelli B, Blendy J, Cioffi D, Schutz G, Silva AJ. Deficient long-term memory in mice with a targeted mutation of the cAMP-responsive element-binding protein. Cell 1994;79:59–68.

92. Oike Y, Hata A, Mamiya T, et al. Truncated CBP protein leads to classical Rubinstein–Taybi syndrome phenotypes in mice: implications for a dominant-negative mechanism. Hum Mol Genet 1999;8:387–96.

93. Tanaka Y, Naruse I, Maekawa T, Masuya H, Shiroishi T, Ishii S. Abnormal skeletal patterning in embryos lacking a single Cbp allele: a partial similarity with Rubinstein–Taybi syndrome. Proc Natl Acad Sci USA 1997;94:10,215–20.

94. Karayiorgou P, Morris MA, Morrow B, et al. Schizophrenia susceptibility associated with interstitial deletions of chromosome 22q11. Proc Natl Acad Sci USA 1995;17:7612–6.

95. Jaeken J, Goemans N, Fryns JP, Francois I, de Zegher F. Association of hyperprolinaemia type I and heparin cofactor II deficiency with CATCH 22 syndrome: evidence for a contiguous gene syndrome locating the proline oxidase gene. J Inherit Metab Dis 1996;19:275–7.

96. Swerdlow NR, Braff DL, Taaid N, Geyer MA. Assessing the validity of an animal-model of deficient sensorimotor gating in schizophrenic-patients. Arch Gen Psychiatry 1994;51:139–54.

97. Geyer MA, Swerdlow NR, Mansbach RS, Braff DL. Startle response models of sensorimotor gating and habituation deficits in schizophrenia. Brain Res Bull 1990;25:485–98.

98. Swerdlow NR, Braff DL, Masten VL, Geyer MA. Schizophrenic-like sensorimotor gating abnormalities in rats following dopamine infusion into the nucleus-accumbens. Psychopharmacology 1990;101:414–20.

99. Leventer RJ, Pilz DT, Matsumoto N, Ledbetter DH, Dobyns WB. Lissencephaly and subcortical band heterotopia: molecular basis and diagnosis. Mol Med Today 2000;6:277–84.

100. Vits L, Van Camp G, Coucke P, et al. MASA syndrome is due to mutations in the neural cell adhesion gene L1CAM. Nat Genet 1994;7:408–13.

101. Jouet M, Rosenthal A, Armstrong G, et al. X-linked spastic paraplegia (SPG1), MASA syndrome and X-linked hydrocephalus result from mutations in the *L1* gene. Nat Genet 1994;7:402–7.

102. Messing A, Goldman JE, Johnson AB, Brenner M. Alexander disease: new insights from genetics. J Neuropathol Exp Neurol 2001;60:563–73.

103. Brenner M, Johnson AB, Boespflug-Tanguy O, Rodriguez D, Goldman JE, Messing A. Mutations in GFAP, encoding glial fibrillary acidic protein, are associated with Alexander disease. Nat Genet 2001;27:117–20.

104. Holmberg V, Lauronen L, Autti T, et al. Phenotype-genotype correlation in eight patients with Finnish variant late infantile NCL (CLN5). Neurology 2000;55:579–81.

105. Peltonen L, Savukoski M, Vesa J. Genetics of the neuronal ceroid lipofuscinoses. Curr Opin Genet Dev 2000;10:299–305.

106. Crawley JN, Belknap JK, Collins A, et al. Behavioral phenotypes of inbred mouse strains: implications and recommendations for molecular studies. Psychopharmacology (Berl) 1997;132:107–24.

107. de Belle JS, Heisenberg M. Expression of *Drosophila* mushroom body mutations in alternative genetic backgrounds: a case study of the mushroom body miniature gene (mbm). Proc Natl Acad Sci USA 1996;93:9875–80.

108. D'Hooge R, Nagels G, Franck F, et al. Mildly impaired water maze performance in male Fmr1 knockout mice. Neuroscience 1997;76:367–76.

109. Van Dam D, D'Hooge R, Hauben E, et al. Spatial learning, contextual fear conditioning and conditioned emotional response in Fmr1 knockout mice. Behav Brain Res 2000;117:127–36.

110. Dobkin C, Rabe A, Dumas R, El Idrissi A, Haubenstock H, Brown WT. Fmr1 knockout mouse has a distinctive strain-specific learning impairment. Neuroscience 2000;100:423–9.

111. Paradee W, Melikian HE, Rasmussen DL, Kenneson A, Conn PJ, Warren ST. Fragile X mouse: strain effects of knockout phenotype and evidence suggesting deficient amygdala function. Neuroscience 1999;94:185–92.

112. Yang T, Adamson TE, Resnick JL, et al. A mouse model for Prader–Willi syndrome imprinting-centre mutations. Nat Genet 1998;19:25–31.

113. Tsai TF, Jiang YH, Bressler J, Armstrong D, Beaudet AL. Paternal deletion from Snrpn to Ube3a in the mouse causes hypotonia, growth retardation and

partial lethality and provides evidence for a gene contributing to Prader–Willi syndrome. Hum Mol Genet 1999;8:1357–64.

114. Jiang YH, Armstrong D, Albrecht U, et al. Mutation of the Angelman ubiquitin ligase in mice causes increased cytoplasmic p53 and deficits of contextual learning and long-term potentiation. Neuron 1998;21:799–811.

115. Chen RZ, Akbarian S, Tudor M, Jaenisch R. Deficiency of methyl-CpG binding protein-2 in CNS neurons results in a Rett-like phenotype in mice. Nat Genet 2001;27:327–31.

116. Guy J, Hendrich B, Holmes M, Martin JE, Bird A. A mouse Mecp2-null mutation causes neurological symptoms that mimic Rett syndrome. Nat Genet 2001;27:322–6.

117. Gogos JA, Santha M, Takacs Z, et al. The gene encoding proline dehydrogenase modulates sensorimotor gating in mice. Nature Genet 1999;21:434–9.

118. Costa RM, Yang T, Huynh DP, et al. Learning deficits, but normal development and tumor predisposition, in mice lacking exon 23a of Nf1. Nat Genet 2001;27:399–405.

119. Reeves RH, Irving NG, Moran TH, et al. A mouse model for down-syndrome exhibits learning and behavior deficits. Nat Genet 1995;11:177–84.

120. Sago H, Carlson EJ, Smith DJ, et al. Ts1Cje, a partial trisomy 16 mouse model for Down syndrome, exhibits learning and behavioral abnormalities. Proc Natl Acad Sci USA 1998;95:6256–61.

121. Smith DJ, Stevens ME, Sudanagunta SP, et al. Functional screening of 2 Mb of human chromosome 21q22.2 in transgenic mice implicates minibrain in learning defects associated with Down's syndrome. Nat Genet 1997;16:28–36.

122. Shinohara T, Tomizuka K, Miyabara S, et al. Mice containing a human chromosome 21 model behavioral impairment and cardiac anomalies of Down's syndrome. Hum Mol Genet 2001;10:1163–75.

II

Autosomal Disorders and Neurobehavioral Dysfunction

5

The Central Nervous System
in Neurofibromatosis Type 1

Nancy Ratner and Kathryn North

1. INTRODUCTION

Neurofibromatosis 1 (NF1) is the most common single-gene disorder that affects the human nervous system. The estimated prevalence is two to three cases per 10,000 individuals (*1–2*, reviewed in *3*).

NF1 is associated with a wide variety of physical manifestations, but the most common consequence of the disorder in childhood, and often the major concern of the parent of a child with NF1, is cognitive impairment. A wide range of learning disabilities occurs in 40–60% of children with NF1 that can lead to academic underachievement, behavioral problems, failure to complete higher education, and the limitation of career choice. In addition, a combination of factors including altered physical appearance, school failure, difficulties with social interaction, and the stigma of having a chronic disorder contribute to low self-esteem and poor self-image in individuals with NF1.

The *NF1* gene on human chromosome 17 is usually classified as a tumor suppressor gene. Although this explains the high frequency of benign and malignant tumors, the effects of the disorder on higher cortical function and the relationship between *NF1* gene mutations, cognitive deficits, and intracranial pathology are less well understood. Understanding how loss of the NF1 gene product, neurofibromin, affects the function of the brain will provide insight into the pathogenesis of cognitive impairment and learning disabilities in the general population.

This chapter summarizes our current understanding of the frequency and nature of cognitive deficits and learning disability in children with NF1. We also review, in light of their relevance to the cognitive and behavioral manifestations of NF1, anatomical and biochemical abnormalities of the central

From: *Contemporary Clinical Neuroscience:*
Genetics and Genomics of Neurobehavioral Disorders
Edited by: G. S. Fisch © Humana Press Inc., Totowa, NJ

nervous system associated with NF1, and the cellular and molecular basis of the disease.

1.1. NF1 Disease Manifestations

NF1 is inherited in an autosomal dominant manner with equal sex incidence. By adulthood nearly all NF1 patients show diagnostic neurocutaneous signs of NF1 including café au lait spots, axillary freckling, neurofibromas (benign peripheral nerve tumors), and iris hamartomas (Lisch nodules) (*3–5*; Table 1). NF1 is also a multisystem disorder with disease manifestations affecting the eyes, the bony skeleton, the endocrine system, blood vessels, and the central and peripheral nervous system. Common complications of NF1 include short stature, plexiform neurofibromas, scoliosis, and headache. Less frequent complications of NF1 include epilepsy, intracranial tumors, hydrocephalus, tibial dysplasia, sphenoid wing dysplasia, renal artery stenosis, pheochromocytoma, and malignant peripheral nerve sheath tumor (MPNST) (*3,6–9*). In addition to learning disabilities, the central nervous system (CNS) manifestations of NF1, which are discussed in detail in the following subheadings, include optic nerve pathway tumors (mainly pilocytic astrocytoma), T2-hyperintensities on MRI , increased size of white matter tracts, and macrocephaly.

Although NF1 patients are at risk for significant morbidity, most patients are mildly or moderately affected and live healthy and productive lives. Several population-based studies and a recent analysis of death certificates (*10–13*) demonstrate a reduction in life span of about 15 years, primarily due to pediatric myeloid leukemia, and adult malignant soft tissue sarcoma (MPNST). Malignant brain tumors, which are very rare in the general population, are more prevalent in NF1, however, the actual incidence is unknown (*13*). Females with NF1 may be at a slightly higher risk of cancer than males (*14*).

1.2. The NF1 Gene

The *NF1* gene was identified in 1990 (*15–17*, reviewed in *18*). It spans a 365-kb length of genomic DNA on human chromosome 17q11.2. The large size of the *NF1* locus is thought to underlie its high mutation frequency (1×10^{-4}–6.5×10^{-5}) (*19,20*). Its 60 exons are known and intron/exon boundaries mapped, although significant stretches of intron remain unsequenced (*21*). Mutations in NF1 patients occur throughout the gene with no evidence of hotspots (*20,22–25*). Loss of NF1 protein in cells causes NF1 disease, as

Table 1
Frequency of Clinical Features of NF1

Disease features	Percent affected
Major disease features >six cafe au lait spots[a]	>95
Axillary freckling[a]	65–84
Cutaneous neurofibromas[a]	
0–9 years	14
10–19 years	44
20–29 years	85
>30 years	95
Plexiform neurofibromas[a]	
All lesions	25
Large lesions of the nead and neck	1–4
Lisch nodules[a]	
0–4 years	22
5–9 years	41
10–19 years	82
>20 years	96
Other disease features	
MRI T2-hyperintensities	60–70
Short stature (height <3rd centile)	≅30
Macrocephaly (head circumference >97th centile)	≅45
Scoliosis	12–20%
Optic pathway gliomas[a]	
All lesions	15–20
Symptomatic	5–7
Neurological manifestations	
Headache	10–20
Epilepsy	3–5
Aqueduct stenosis	2.5
Bone lesions[a]	
Dysplasia of the long bones	3
Sphenoid wing dysplasia	<1
Malignant peripheral nerve sheath tumors	1–4
Renal artery stenosis	1–2
Noonan syndrome-like facies	7

Frequency of each disease manifestation derived from four major studies *(2,7–9)*—apart from figures for optic pathway gliomas *(114)* and MRI T2-hyperintensities *(89)*.

[a]Used as diagnostic criteria (two or more or one with a first-degree affected relative) as defined in Mulvihill et al. *(4)*.

NF1 mutations are deletions, rearrangements, mRNA splicing defects, and missense mutations that predict absent or dysfunctional protein *(20,22,23,26)*. NF1 is classified as a tumor suppressor gene because mutations in both *NF1* alleles are detectable in benign and malignant tumors associated with NF1 *(27–30)*. Several alternatively spliced *NF1* exons exist and at least one of these may have special relevance to cognition (*31* [*see* Subheading 6.2.3.]).

Phenotypic variability is as great within a family whose members all have the same *NF1* mutation, as it is between families. This makes it highly unlikely that particular *NF1* mutations cause specific disease phenotypes. Nonetheless it is still debated whether the association of specific phenotypes, such as learning problems, might be linked with increased frequency to particular mutations but be obscured by the plethora of mutations that exist throughout the gene. Specific modifiers of major NF1 phenotypes are believed to account for some of variability among patients with the same mutation *(32)*. Although no modifiers of cognitive phenotypes have been identified, two genes have been implicated in enhancing severity of the overall NF1 phenotype *(33)* or predisposing to mutation of the *NF1* gene *(34,35)*. One instance in which some correlation between genotype and phenotype has been observed is in patients with deletions of the whole *NF1* gene (including three genes embedded in intron 27b and 13 surrounding genes) *(36,37)*. Of NF1 patients with large deletions, 10–30% exhibit severe learning disabilities or mental retardation in association with facial dysmorphism and early onset or increased frequency of neurofibromas *(38,39)*. Conversely, of NF1 patients with this severe phenotype, about 11% have deletions *(40,41)*. In principle, severe phenotypes could be due to the absence of one *NF1* allele, a contiguous gene syndrome involving deletion of one or more genes adjacent to the *NF1* locus, or the loss of a substantial portion of a chromosome. The high percentage of these patients with large deletions argues for a role of one or more of the surrounding genes. The severe phenotype observed in patients lacking large deletions could be due to separate mutations or polymorphisms in the relevant surrounding genes.

2. THE NF1 COGNITIVE PHENOTYPE

Until the late 1980s, there were few systematic studies of cognitive deficits in NF1. No formal diagnostic criteria were available for NF1 and there was no clear distinction between NF1, NF2, and other forms of neurofibromatosis (e.g., segmental NF), all of which have different implications for cognitive development. Early reports of intellectual function gave marked overestimates of the incidence of mental retardation because studies included only patients with severe disease manifestations, introducing a significant ascertainment bias. The inclusion of patients with intracranial tumors and infrequent use of standardized psychometric assessment also limited interpretation of data concerning intellectual function in NF1 prior to the early 1980s. Furthermore, in the absence of standardized psychometric assessment, academic achievement was wrongly interpreted as a measure of intelligence. These methodological problems were partially addressed during the 1990s, providing a more accurate picture of the NF1 cognitive phenotype (reviewed in *42–44*).

2.1. Mental Retardation

Mental retardation is not a common feature of NF1, but its actual incidence in NF1 is unknown. Ideally, to exclude ascertainment bias, estimates should be based on population studies in which standardized objective measures of IQ are performed. In addition, the consequences of clinical variables, such as intracranial tumors and epilepsy, need to be considered. In a population-based study *(2)* in which formal assessment of IQ was not performed, the incidence of mental retardation (based on retrospective analysis of educational needs) was estimated at 3.2%, only slightly higher than in the general population (2–3%). Despite some ascertainment bias, the results of clinic-based studies with objective psychometric testing are likely to provide a more accurate estimate of the prevalence of mental retardation in patients with NF1. Eleven such studies have been performed resulting in estimates of the prevalence of mental retardation (defined as full-scale IQ more than two standard deviations below the population mean) ranging between 4.8% *(45,46)* and 11% *(47)*. The true incidence likely lies somewhere between these two estimates. Thus, the risk for mental retardation in NF1 is now considered to be approx 2–3 times the risk for the general population.

2.2. IQ in the NF1 Population

Many studies report a lowering of IQ scores in children with NF1 compared to normative data for the population *(45,48–54)*, or to unaffected sibling controls *(55,56)*. The mean IQ score of patients with NF1, as measured on the WISC-R, ranges between 89 and 98, within one standard deviation of the normal population (mean = 100; SD = 15). In a study of 16 children, Varnhagen et al. *(49)* found that cognitive deficit increased as a function of the severity of physical disease manifestations. The effect was most marked on performance IQ and in tests of sequential and simultaneous processing. The small number of patients, however, necessitating the use of nonparametric statistical analysis, limits interpretation of this study. No other study has supported this association and the general consensus is that there is no apparent association between the left shift in IQ and any clinical variable, including socioeconomic status, gender, severity of disease, macrocephaly, or family history of NF1 *(45,53,55,57,58)*. An important exception to this rule is the association between intracranial tumors in NF1 and lowering of IQ *(51)*. Unless stated otherwise, children with intracranial pathology are excluded in all studies cited in the following paragraphs. It is unclear from individual studies whether there is a general lowering of IQ scores in all patients with NF1 or whether only a subset of patients has lowered IQ *(45,59)*. A cluster analysis identified three subgroups of children with NF1 based on intellectual function and academic achievement: those with normal intellectual function and appropriate academic performance for IQ, those with normal intellect and significant specific deficits, and those with mild global deficits and no specificity *(59)*.

2.3. Academic Achievement

Specific learning disability (LD) is typically defined as a significant (2 or more standard deviations) discrepancy between ability (intellect or aptitude) and achievement (performance in reading, spelling, written language, and/ or mathematics). The reported frequency of LD in NF1 ranges between 30% and 65%. As noted by Ozonoff *(43)* and Kayl et al. *(60)*, the variability in these estimates is due to differences in definitions of LD, the lack of appropriate control groups in early studies, and the failure to account for lower intellectual function in the NF1 group.

Among NF1 patients, male gender and lower socioeconomic status (SES IV and V) are associated with poorer performance in tests of academic achievement. In addition, boys with NF1 demonstrate poorer adaptive functioning and social skills and a higher incidence of behavioral problems than girls. This sex difference is consistent with a higher incidence of LD in males in the general population *(61)*. In one study, a family history of NF1 was strongly associated with lower socioeconomic status based on ratings of employment and education. This result is probably a secondary effect of the high incidence of LD in the NF1 population, that is, individuals with NF1 are less likely to complete post secondary school education, and thus fall into lower socioeconomic groups *(46)*.

Early studies of neuropsychological profiles in children with NF1 led researchers to propose that nonverbal learning problems (characterized by difficulty with written work, poor organizational skills, impulsivity, and a decreased ability to perceive social cues) were predominant in the NF1 population. The basis for this proposal was a discrepancy between verbal and performance IQ (VIQ > PIQ) found in two studies *(47,48,62)*, poor performance in tests of spatial memory *(49)*, and consistent deficits in the Judgment of Line Orientation (JLO) *(63)*, a test of visual–spatial function *(48,64)*. More recent studies that include evaluation of language and reading demonstrate that language-based learning problems are at least as common as nonverbal learning deficits in children with NF1 *(45,46,51–53,55,56,58,65)*. Specific verbal deficits include poorer performance on measures of word definition, naming, written vocabulary, phonological awareness, receptive syntactic language, and verbal reasoning and recall *(46,65)*. The discrepancy between VIQ and PIQ is not reproducible across studies and is of questionable significance. The JLO is abnormal in many studies to date, with mean scores for the NF1 study population more than 2 standard deviations below the mean *(48,55,64,66)*. However, when Cutting et al. *(58)* compared NF1 children with IQ matched controls, this test was not significantly different in the two groups.

Poor attentional and organizational skills in children with NF1 affect performance in many areas *(46,53,55)*. Speech (articulation) problems are common (approx 25%) although rarely severe enough to affect intelligibility. Motor coordination is frequently impaired; up to one third of children demonstrate significant impairment in tests of manual dexterity, balance, and ball skills *(46)*.

In summary, there does not appear to be a profile of LD specific to NF1. Academic LD may be associated with depressed performance in verbal tasks such as reading and spelling, and/or nonverbal tasks such as mathematics. Nevertheless, LD is not thought to be secondary to global intellectual impairment in the majority of children with NF1. Performance of memory tasks is not impaired *(56,66)*, and there are no group differences, compared to controls, in neuropsychological measures typically influenced by overall intellectual impairment *(65)*.

2.4. Attention Skills and ADHD

Attentional problems undermine performance in many areas in children with NF1. Research into attention skills has focused mainly on sustained attention. Results from Continuous Performance Tests suggest that children with NF1 have problem concentrating for long periods *(53,65)*. In addition, they have difficulties with selective attention (i.e., the ability to screen out unnecessary information) and divided attention (i.e., the ability to attend to two sources of information at the same time) *(53)*. The capacity to shift attention from one stimulus to another is unclear; two studies have found deficits *(49,67)* whereas a third has not *(68)*.

The predominance of attentional problems in children with NF1 has raised the possibility of ADHD as a diagnostic label for some of these children. In the study by Eliason *(48)*, nearly 50% of the 23 children were diagnosed as "hyperactive" or as having ADHD, 8 of whom were taking stimulant medication. Mothers described these children as highly unpredictable, impulsive, and socially inept. However, this study cohort was referred for learning and/ or behavioral problems and therefore cannot offer information on the prevalence of ADHD or other behavioral problems in the overall population of children with NF1. Estimates of the frequency of attention deficit disorder in NF1 vary between studies from 17.6% *(68)* to 30% *(69)*. In another study, 42% of children with NF1 had ADHD as compared to 13% of siblings without NF1 and 5% of non-NF1 parents *(70)*. In contrast Eldridge et al. *(64)* compared children with NF1 to unaffected siblings and found no differences in ADHD incidence between the two groups. Anecdotal reports suggest a beneficial response to stimulant medication. There are currently no controlled studies demonstrating utility of stimulant medication in NF1, however.

2.5. The Natural History of Cognitive Deficits in NF1

Relatively few researchers have focused on the cognitive abilities of very young children with NF1. Samango-Sprouse et al. *(71)* compared infants and toddlers with NF1 to their age-matched peers. They found that young children with NF1 had lower cognitive abilities with abnormal neuromotor and perceptual–motor development. They also had a flattened affect and a more passive interaction style. Problem-solving skills were monochromatic, with one strategy excessively used. Motor dysfunction included truncal hypotonia, motor-planning deficits, and delayed acquisition of motor skills. They postulated that delays in fine and gross motor development might be early indicators of the visual–perceptual dysfunction seen in school-aged children with NF1. Legius et al. *(52)* also demonstrated that infants from 17 mo to 4 years showed delays in active language development and both gross and fine motor coordination.

Although most research in NF1 has focused on children, several studies have been conducted with adults. Zoller et al. *(67)* found that adults with NF1 had problems in inductive reasoning, visual construction, visual and tactile memory, logical abstraction, cognitive speed, coordination, and mental flexibility. Unlike children with NF1, basic motor speed and vocabulary were not affected in these adults. This suggests that in the NF1 population motor and language deficits resulting from developmental delays resolve with age. Similarly, Lorch et al. *(72)* examined 30 adults with NF1 and found that whereas reading difficulties are not prevalent in adult NF1 individuals (13%), writing difficulties presented problems for a larger percentage of adults (40%). Spelling errors were evident in 50% of patients. Subjectively, patients reported improvements in reading past school age, and that writing production was the most neurologically vulnerable language modality. However, the lack of controls in this study makes these results difficult to interpret.

Although some manifestations of NF1 appear to worsen with age (e.g., number of cutaneous neurofibromas, size of plexiform neurofibromas), the natural history of cognitive deficits in NF1 is unclear. Using cross-sectional data from children and adults with NF1, Riccardi and Eichner *(73)* suggested that IQ scores improve with age. The average IQ for children aged 6–17 years (*n* = 67) was at or near 90, compared to a mean IQ of 99.3 for patients 17 years or older (*n* = 89). Legius et al. *(52)* found that children between 4 and 6 years had a mean IQ of 99, whereas children between 6 and 16 years had a mean IQ of 87.7. Additional research examining developmental changes in children with NF1 supported a negative correlation between age and IQ for children under the age of 16 *(74,75)*. In contrast, Ferner and colleagues *(53)* examined 103 patients and 105 controls between the ages of 6 and 75. They found a sizeable reduction in FSIQ for the NF1 patients, but no discrepancy in IQ in children compared to adults with NF1. Systematic longitudinal studies, with attention to comparability of tests for young children and adults, are necessary to determine whether there are significant differences in cognitive function over the lifetime of individuals with NF1, or whether changes are an artifact produced by shifting from one IQ test to another, for example, from the WISC-R to the WAIS-R.

2.6 Effects of NF1 on Self-Image and Social and Emotional Health

Several studies have demonstrated a detrimental effect of NF1 on the emotional health of NF1 patients. A retrospective study *(76)* found that almost 50% of NF1 patients were distressed by the presence of neurofibromas and had changed their social behavior and manner of dress to hide them. Many individuals experienced anxiety about physical aspects of NF1, had been teased at school about the skin manifestations of the disorder, and felt that NF1 had hindered their ability to form new friendships. Porter Counterman et al. *(77)* found that children with NF1 were often unhappy with their own behavioral conduct and that those with more severe disease manifestations had a diminished sense of self-worth.

The behavioral phenotype of children with NF1 was assessed by administration of the Child Behavior Checklist *(78)* to parents and teachers

(46,56,79). Children with NF1 were reported to have more difficulty with social interactions and getting along with friends and family members than would be expected for their peer group. There was a high frequency of internalizing features, which are often associated with anxiety and depression, and high rates of inattention and impulsivity. Subjects with NF1 were less functionally independent than expected for age and were less involved or less skilled in sports and nonsport activities. On the social problems subscale, common items identified included "frequently teased," "not liked by peers," "acts young," "prefers younger children," and "clumsy." Johnson et al. *(79)* found that decreased psychosocial functioning was not correlated with disfigurement, short stature, or disease severity in children. A quality of life survey on a hospital-based adult population, however, indicated that emotional effects of NF1 correlated with severity of cutaneous disease (other NF1 features were not monitored) *(80)*.

2.7. Implications for Assessment and Management

There have been no systematic studies to date to determine the best way to manage cognitive deficits and LD in children with NF1. Nevertheless, we can draw certain conclusions from studies of the cognitive phenotype to provide guidelines for assessment and intervention. Because children with NF1 are at high risk of LD, this risk should be discussed with parents in the same way that the other manifestations of the disorder are explained during medical assessment and counseling. The diagnostic label of NF1 should alert clinicians, parents, and teachers to the need to monitor for LD. A developmental history and review of school progress should be incorporated in the yearly review of all children with NF1. If any areas of concern are identified a formal educational assessment, including measures of language and motor performance, attention, and academic achievement, should be performed. Children should be followed throughout their school career, as the vulnerabilities identified persist and may manifest only at a later age when demands on performance increase.

Once identified, management of NF1-related LD need not differ from that of LD in other populations, although the underlying diagnosis may assist in obtaining special services. In younger children, hypotonia and motor incoordination may be the predominant problems and referral to an occupational therapist will be beneficial. Remediation in school-age children should focus on providing the child with skills aimed at compensating for areas of weakness. Self-esteem is often poor in children with NF1 owing to both the physical and cognitive manifestations of the disorder. These children will benefit from a modified teaching approach that focuses on their relative strengths and allows them to achieve optimum results on a day-to-day basis.

3. CENTRAL NERVOUS SYSTEM PATHOLOGY IN NF1

The occurrence of cognitive deficits in NF1 has led to an interest in the morphological analysis of NF1 brains. Several studies describe histological abnormalities of the brain in a subset of patients with NF1. Two early studies of the neuropathology of autopsied NF1 brains *(81,82)* found disordered cortical architecture with random orientation of neurons, focal heterotopic neurons, proliferation of glial cells to form well-defined gliofibrillary nodules, and hyperplastic gliosis. In approx 50% of patients the histology of the brain was normal. Nordlund and colleagues *(83)* demonstrated that glial fibrillary acidic protein (GFAP), a marker for astrocytes, was up-regulated in three NF1 brains studied by immunohistochemistry; there was a 4- to 18-fold increase in GFAP levels in the NF1 brains compared to controls. Such an increase reflects reactive astrocytic gliosis—a phenomenon that has been reported in many neurodegenerative diseases including Down syndrome, Alzheimer's disease, and Parkinson disease. Histological examination of these brains demonstrated nonspecific but consistent abnormalities; foci of hypertrophic astrocytes were present in two brains, and an increase in the perivascular spaces was present in all cases. In one brain, focal heterotopias and focal cellular disorganization in the thalamus and neocortex were also evident.

In a recent study, the brains of five NF1 patients with *NF1* whole-gene deletions were evaluated by computed tomography (CT) and magnetic resonance imaging (MRI). Of these, three had structural abnormalities *(84)*. The authors proposed that these result from defects in brain development, perhaps accounting for the profound learning problems and mental retardation in this subset of patients.

3.1. MRI T2-Hyperintensities in NF1 Brains

The use of MRI has permitted the precise definition of intracranial lesions in living subjects. Focal areas of high signal intensity on T2-weighted images (also known as unidentified bright objects [UBOs], unidentified bright signals [UBSs], or neurofibromatosis bright objects [NBOs]) are well described and are considered characteristic of NF1. These lesions are usually isointense on T1-weighted images; they exert no mass effect, there is no surrounding edema, they do not enhance with contrast, and are not visible on CT scan. They most commonly occur in the basal ganglia, cerebellum, brain stem, and subcortical white matter *(85–89)*. They are not associated with focal neurological deficits *(45,90)*. The reported incidence of T2-hyperintensities varies between 43% and 79% (reviewed in *91*) and their frequency decreases with age *(88,89,92–95)*. Thus the variation in the reported frequency of areas of increased T2 signal is probably secondary to the variation in the age range of patients in individual studies.

There has been much speculation as to the nature of areas of increased T2 signal intensity on MRI. They have been considered regions of dysplasia or heterotopia, based on the studies of Rosman and Pearce *(81)* and of Rubinstein *(82)*. However, neither of these studies correlated pathological findings with neuroimaging and the lesions described occurred in different parts of the brain from areas that typically show increased T2 signal on MRI examination. Sevick et al. *(88)* proposed that areas of increased T2 signal intensity represent the formation of chemically abnormal myelin that was subsequently broken down by normal metabolic processes and replaced by myelin with a more stable conformation.

Only one study has correlated histological studies with MRI findings. DiPaolo et al. *(96)* performed autopsies on two pediatric patients with NF1 and histological studies of five areas of brain tissue (two globus pallidus and three midbrain peduncle specimens) that correlated with areas of high T2 signal intensity on MRI examinations performed prior to death. The five areas examined had similar histologic appearances. These consisted of atypical glial infiltrate with "bizarre" hyperchromatic nuclei, foci of microcalcification associated with perivascular gliosis, areas of dysmyelination on specific staining, and spongy change in the white matter (spongiform myelinopathy) at the periphery of the lesions. The latter was thought to be due to intramyelinic edema. It was concluded that the high signal intensity lesions on MRI represented increased fluid within the myelin associated with hyperplastic or dysplastic glial proliferation. These areas were not malignant or premalignant. The MRI changes and associated pathological changes were thought to be unique to NF1, and it was postulated that the abnormal MRI signals might disappear due to resolution of the intramyelinic edema and replacement of abnormal myelin.

4. THE CORRELATION BETWEEN T2-HYPERINTENSITIES AND COGNITIVE DEFICITS

The high frequency of T2-hyperintensities on MRI led to the hypothesis that these lesions are associated with the occurrence of cognitive deficits in children with NF1. Several studies performed to test this hypothesis yielded mixed results. Three initial studies *(86,90,97)* found no association between the presence of MRI T2-hyperintensities and cognitive deficits in patients with NF1. However, these studies included a large number of patients with CNS pathology (such as epilepsy and intracranial tumors), which could have confounding effects on cognitive function *(51)*. Three independent studies using clinic-based study samples and quantitative neuropsychological assessment have found a significant association between lowering of IQ and T2-weighted hyperintensities in children with NF1. North et al. *(45)* studied 40 children with NF1 without other intracranial pathology and found that children with T2-hyperintensities on MRI (T2+) had significantly lower IQ scores than children without these lesions. Scores in tests of language function, visual–motor integration, and coordination were also significantly lower in the T2+ group. The 15 children without areas of abnormal T2 signal on MRI scan did not differ significantly from the general population in any parameter measured. A number of recent studies by Denckla and colleagues also found a significant association between T2-hyperintensities and cognitive dysfunction *(55,98–100)*. The number and volume of T2-hyperintensities were highly correlated with deficits in IQ scores (compared to unaffected siblings), and pilot data suggested an association between impaired visual–spatial function (as demonstrated in the JLO) and the volume of T2-hyperintensities in the most commonly involved site, the basal ganglia. Samango-Sprouse and colleagues *(71)* confirmed an association between intellectual development and T2-hyperintensities in a study of 94 preschool children (age range 18–72 mo). However, the association between T2-hyperintensities and learning disabilities remains controversial. In a study of 28 children with NF1 aged 4–16 years, Legius et al. *(101)* found no significant difference in full-scale IQ score between the T2+ and T2– group. Likewise, Moore and colleagues *(74,102)* found no correlation between cognitive deficits and T2-hyperintensities in a study of 84 patients from a Houston NF clinic. The reason for the contradictory findings in these studies is not known. If, indeed, areas of increased T2 signal on MRI prove to be consistently associated with cognitive deficits in children with NF1 this would have theoretical implications for our understanding of underlying pathogenesis, that is, a radiological marker for risk of cognitive deficits and academic learning disabilities. However, these MRI lesions could not be used as a firm predictor of cognitive deficits in children with NF1. Not all children in the T2+ group had significant school performance problems and several had above average IQs. The possible association between T2-hyperintensities and cognitive deficits in NF1 is of primary interest in helping to understand the pathogenesis of LD in a subset of children with NF1 and hence is likely of theoretical rather than practical import.

Ferner et al. *(53)* and Chapman et al. *(103)* observed that deficits (poor reading skills, impaired short-term memory, verbal and motor disinhibition, compromised social discourse, poorly regulated attention, awkward motor output, and delayed adaptation to complex and unfamiliar tasks) similar to those seen in patients with lesions in frontal and subcortical areas were over-represented in NF1 patients. Consistent with this observation, MRI studies suggest that hyperopacities in the NF1 brain are more common in the anterior and subcortical areas of the brain. These initial observations provided a foundation for further neuropsychological investigations to explore the correlation between anatomical and cognitive deficits in NF1 patients. Some of these are described in the following subheadings.

4.1. Macrocephaly

Macrocephaly has long been recognized as a common feature of children with NF1 *(7,9)*. Macrocephaly *per se* is not directly associated with cognitive deficits in the majority of studies. However, recent studies suggest an association between macrocephalus and specific neuropsychological deficits. Said et al. *(104)* observed that increased brain volume was largely due to an increase in white matter and that children with greater right hemisphere gray matter volume exhibited better visual–spatial skills. In contrast, Moore et al. *(75)* suggested that increased brain volume in children with NF1 was most likely to be due to increased gray matter and that there was a positive correlation between the volume of gray matter and the severity of learning disabilities. There are some differences in experimental design between these two conflicting studies; in addition, Said et al. *(104)* did not include the brain stem and cerebellum in the volumetric analyses. Cutting et al. *(57)* observed that children with NF1 and macrocephaly performed worse on a vocabulary task compared to those without macrocephaly, suggesting a possible underlying mechanism for language deficits. They found no association between macrocephaly and T2-hyperintensities, which suggests that these two brain abnormalities could represent different results of mutation in the *NF1* gene. This study was limited by small sample size, the inclusion of only male subjects, and a definition of macrocephaly that is broader than the usual definition (i.e., >1SD above the mean vs >2 SD). Dubovsky et al. *(105)* compared cognitive function, T2-hyperintensities on MRI, and macrocephaly. In their study, macrocephaly did not correlate with differences in neuropsychometric test scores. All children had T2-hyperintensities; macrocephalic children were more likely to have bilateral T2-hyperintensities or an enlarged corpus callosum, pons, and/or medulla.

The basis of macrocephaly in NF1 is not well understood, although increases in brain volume could in principle be related to a decrease in apoptosis during brain development *(75)*. Steen et al. *(54)* evaluated the brains of 18 children with NF1, 7 with macrocephaly. A quantitative T1 imaging method detected abnormalities in all NF1 subjects, with more extensive abnormalities in subjects with macrocephaly. NF1 children with macrocephaly showed enlarged brain structures and abnormally low brain T1 signals. A reduction of T1 intensity in normocephalic NF1 patients was present only in the corpus callosum while macrocephalic patients had decreased T1 intensity in all white matter tracts. Overall, macrocephalic subjects showed a significant 22% increase in white matter volume. While no significant change in gray matter volume was noted, several macrocephalic NF1 subjects showed a reduction in T1-weighted signal in several gray matter regions. The authors speculate that a pervasive disturbance in brain development and dysplastic myelination underlies macrocephaly. A general decrease in cortical metabolism in NF1 patient brain in positron emission tomography (PET) scans may support this view *(106,107)*.

There is increasing interest in the involvement of the corpus callosum in cognitive dysfunction in NF1. Kayl et al. *(60)* found that children with NF1 had significantly larger corpus callosi compared to controls, and that more severe attention problems in children with both NF1 and ADHD were associated with smaller corpus callosum size. Moore et al. *(75)* also found that corpus callosum size was larger for children with NF1, but found that diminished performance on measures of academic achievement and visual–spatial and motor skills were associated with greater regional corpus callosum size.

4.2. Recent Brain Imaging Studies

Functional brain imaging is beginning to provide additional information concerning MRI T2 lesions and brain dysfunction in NF1. In the mid-1990s, PET scans of T2-hyperintense lesions indicated normal *(107)* or low *(106)* metabolic activity. Proton MR spectroscopy showed normal metabolism *(108,109)*. More recent studies using MRI and MR spectroscopy have revealed a spectrum of abnormalities in NF1 brain, NF1 brain with T2-hyperintense lesions, and areas in the brain from which T2-hyperintensities have disappeared *(110,111)*. These studies conclude that there are two groups of lesions: one with a slight decrease in metabolite ratios, and another with a greater decrease in metabolite ratios, along with a large decrease in *N* acetyl aspartate (NAA) (a neuronal marker). Wang et al. *(112)* showed that in T2-hyperintensities, and in other brain regions, an increase in choline is typical in the thalami of younger NF1 children, with a decrease in NAA prevalent in older individuals. Taken together, it is proposed that early metabolic abnormalities in the NF1 brain lead to focal edema and vacuolization of myelin, which may be visible as T2-hyperintensities, then to destruction of neurons and ultimately to regression of visible lesions. Some support for a widespread myelin disorder model comes from work by Eastwood et al. *(113)*. They compared water diffusibility in MR imaging in NF1 children as compared to normal controls. Strongly significant increases in brain water diffusion were observed in NF1 patient globus pallidus, frontal white matter, and in the brachium pontis; less striking differences were observed in the thalamus and hippocampus. When T2-hyperinsense lesions were specifically sampled even more difference from control values was observed. These data support the idea that the hyperintense lesions are focally severe patches of more widespread myelin disorder.

5. ASTROCYTOMAS IN CHILDREN WITH NF1: *ARE THEY TUMORS?*

Benign optic pathway lesions are observed in at least 15% of NF1 children *(114,115)*. Lesions involving the optic chiasm are more likely to impair vision than prechiasmatic lesions. The lesions have been called tumors and pilocytic astrocytomas, but analyses of progress and clinical outcomes associated with these lesions show that they rarely become malignant *(116,117)*. Indeed, the lesions can regress *(118)*. It is now rare to intervene unless progressive impairment of vision is observed *(114,119)*. Visual acuity in NF1 children can be evaluated using visual-evoked potentials and visual fields tests *(120,121)*.

Benign optic pathway growths observed in NF1 differ from non-NF1 astrocytomas. For example, decreased levels of the tumor suppressor proteins p53, p16, and Rb are common in non-NF1 astrocytomas, but not in NF1 lesions. Epidermal growth factor receptor (EGFR) is highly expressed in some astrocytomas, but not in NF1 lesions *(122)*. Mutations in both *NF1* alleles is common in NF1-associated lesions, but not in sporadic pilocytic astrocytomas *(123,124)*. In addition, unlike astrocytomas in non-NF1 patients, the lesions in NF1 patients generally spare the central part of the optic nerve *(125)*. Taken together these studies support a distinct mechanism of optic pathway tumor formation in NF1 patients.

This leads to the question of whether there are actually differences between T2-hyperintensities and pilocytic astrocytomas in NF1. Both can regress and neither becomes malignant with detectable frequency. Wilkinson et al. *(111)* used magnetic resonance spectroscopy (MRS) to compare T2-hyperintensities and lesions they termed "gliomas" in children with NF1. These were defined as areas of increased T2 signal that developed mass effect, showed enhancement with gadolinium, and/or were surrounded by edema *(126)*. They were not malignant growths. The lesions had very low NA/Cho ratios and increased choline/creatinine (Cho/Cr), in addition to decreased NA per milliliter as compared to "typical" T2-hyperintensities or control brain. This is the same profile previously described for regressing T2-hyperintensities. A case study of a contrast-enhancing lesion followed over time showed that enhancement was temporary *(127)*. A recent study of MR images, including four that enhanced with contrast, suggests that the "tumors" in NF1 children be named "gliomatoses" *(128)*. Such a designation would be consistent with the current limited available pathological evaluations of the optic pathway lesions.

6. NEUROFIBROMIN, THE NF1 GENE PRODUCT

The 2818-amino-acid NF1 gene product, neurofibromin, was identified in 1991 (reviewed in *18,129*). Neurofibromin is an intracellular signaling molecule with two key domains, a central domain called the GAP-related domain (GRD) that shares sequence homology with the GTPase-activating proteins (GAPs)—off signals for Ras proteins—and a more N-terminal domain called the cysteine/serine-rich domain (CSRD, *20,130*).

6.1. The Function of Neurofibromin

6.1.1. Ras-GAP Activity of Neurofibromin

The GRD was identified by homology to other Ras-GAPs (p120^{GAP} in mammalian cells, ira1, ira2, and sar1 in yeast, and GAP1 in *Drosophila* (reviewed in *131*) on sequencing of the NF1 cDNA *(132)*. The GRD is known to interact with p21^{ras} *(133)*. Several patients have missense mutations in the GRD in bases known to affect GAP activity *(20,26,134)*, supporting a key role for Ras-GAP activity in NF1 etiology. Indeed, a mutation in this domain is sufficient to cause disease *(134)*.

Ras-GAPs act as off signals for proteins in the Ras family. Ras proteins are intracellular messengers that become activated by binding GTP subsequent to growth factor stimulation and by the binding of cells to extracellular matrix. Ras activation causes cell proliferation or cell differentiation in a cell-type specific manor, and loss of function at *NF1* correlates with increased cellular GTP-bound Ras in several cell types. Neurofibromin's GAP domain has GAP activity in vitro for N-, H-, and K-Ras and related TC21/R-Ras2 and R-Ras *(135–137)*. An *NF1* splice variant with an altered affinity for Ras-GTP has been identified (reviewed in *22*). Hiatt et al. *(138)* tested the ability of the GAP-related domains of NF1 and p120 to restore normal growth and cytokine signaling in primary cells from *NF1* mutant mice. They found that the neurofibromin, but not the p120, GRD was able to correct the defect. They suggest that the GRDs of neurofibromin and p120 have specific nonoverlapping functions.

6.1.2. Neurofibromin Binds Syndecan and Tubulin

In addition to interacting with Ras proteins, the neurofibromin GRD also binds tubulin (the protein that forms microtubules) and syndecans. Microtubule-associated proteins are involved in stabilizing microtubules and in actively promoting microtubule movement and microtubule-mediated intracytoplasmic transport. Some populations of microtubules have also been implicated in signal transduction pathways involving surface receptors and neurotransmitters. Polymerized microtubules bind neurofibromin via the GRD, and this binding inhibits the Ras-GAP activity of the GRD *(139)*. Mutations in the GRD domain diminish its ability to interact with microtubules *(140)*.

Using a yeast two-hybrid screen, Hsueh et al. *(141)* found that syndecan-2, a transmembrane heparan sulfate proteoglycan, binds to a C-terminal domain of neurofibromin at amino acids 2616–2812. Syndecans 1–4 are a family of transmembrane heparan sulfate proteoglycans that are targeted to numerous intracellular locations on the plasma membrane; all bind neurofibromin. Syndecans might serve as linkers of neurofibromin to intracellular scaffolds and receptor proteins. Taken together, the in vitro interactions with tubulin and sydecan suggest that neurofibromin function in vivo might be modulated based on binding partners and location within the cell.

6.1.3. Function of the CRSD

The neurofibromin CRSD was identified more recently than the GRD through mutational analysis of missense mutations *(20)*. This region of neurofibromin has no proven function but contains an ATP-binding motif and three protein kinase A (PKA) recognition sites (586T, 818S, and 876S) implicating neurofibromin in the response to, or regulation of cAMP-dependent signaling.

Several pieces of evidence support the view that neurofibromin regulates adenylcyclase-mediated signaling and, thus, cAMP levels. Loss of *NF1* in *Drosophila* is correlated with defective cAMP-mediated learning and memory, a defective neuropeptide response, and decreased body size *(142–144)*. Adenylyl cyclase activity is diminished in the fly mutants and in embryonic NF1$^{-/-}$ mouse brain extracts and in cultured NF1$^{-/-}$ embryonic neurons *(145)*. Levels of cAMP are also increased in cultured Schwann cells lacking neurofibromin *(146)*.

Interestingly, Tokuo et al. *(147)* found that the phosphorylation of neurofibromin by pKA is increased by cellular association with N^G, N^G-dimethylarginine dimethylaminohydrolase (DDAH), a regulator of cellular NO/NOS. Neurofibromin binds DDAH via the CSRD and a C-terminal domain containing PKA phosphorylation sites *(147)*. The role of DDAH in cAMP signaling in *NF1* mutant cells and the molecular details of the role of neurofibromin in cAMP cascades warrants further investigation.

6.2. Distribution of Neurofibromin in the CNS

The typical distribution of neurofibromin has been investigated in chicken, mouse, rat, and some human tissues and the pattern of expression is known in detail. In all these species, NF1 accounts for a very low proportion of total cellular protein, even in tissues with the highest neurofibromin expression, such as brain *(148)*. Localization of neurofibromin and *NF1* mRNAs, including alternative splice variants, was expected to identify the cells most likely to be directly affected by *NF1* mutations, and to focus detailed investigations to analyses of particular cell types. However, neurofibromin distribution is complex and there is no absolute correlation of NF1 expression with NF1 disease. That is, neurofibromin is expressed in cells and tissues affected in NF1 disease and in those that appear unaffected. Indeed, some manifestations of NF1 may be due to abnormal interactions between affected cell types.

6.2.1. Distribution During Development

There are no studies describing neurofibromin expression in developing human brains. Neurofibromin is expressed globally in all cells and tissues during rodent development (at least from mid-gestation) and becomes progressively enriched in the developing nervous system *(149–153)*. In avian embryos, *NF1* mRNA is expressed in the neural tube and in the early developing brain *(154)* and neurofibromin is detectable during neural tube closure *(155)*. In the E16 rat, neurofibromin is expressed at high levels in the cortical plate layer of the cerebral cortex, while cells in the ventricular, intermediate, and marginal zones are either negative or only weakly positive *(149,150)*. At this stage of development, cells in the cortical plate are well differentiated compared to other layers where cells are still proliferating. A similar pattern is seen in developing rodent spinal cord, with high levels of expression in the differentiating motor neurons and barely detectable expression in surrounding undifferentiated cells *(149,150)*. These findings suggest that neurofibromin expression correlates positively with differentiation and inversely with cell proliferation in developing neurons.

6.2.2. Subcellular Localization

The subcellular localization of neurofibromin is dependent on cell type. For example, using two anti-neurofibromin antibodies and an identical immunoelectron microscopy protocol, keratinocytes showed plasma membrane neurofibromin localization *(156)*, whereas in cerebellar Purkinje neurons, the majority of neurofibromin was localized to smooth endoplasmic reticulum *(153)*.

In cultured mouse B lymphocytes, neurofibromin can be cocapped with surface immunoglobulin, a convincing demonstration of localization to the plasma membrane *(157)*. In contrast, individual cells from many different cell lines show punctate, cytoplasmic staining that has been attributed to various subcellular structures. Gregory et al. *(158)* demonstrated that neurofibromin is expressed predominantly in the cytoplasm and is associated with microtubules in cultured fibroblasts and in mammalian brain. However, others suggest that punctate staining can be ascribed to mitochondria *(159)*. In subcellular fractionation, neurofibromin can be detected in purified fractions of mitochondria *(159)* as well as cytosol, crude membranes, and nuclei, but is not highly enriched in any of these fractions *(141,159)*. DeClue et al. *(160)* detected NF1 in insoluble fractions, where it complexed with an unidentified 400–500-kDa protein.

These studies show that there are cell-type-specific differences in the subcellular localization of neurofibromin. How neurofibromin localization is regulated and the functional significance of differences among cell types is unknown. Intracellular neurofibromin localization could be determined by specific *NF1* splice variants, or the ratios of the variants, but this remains to be demonstrated. Other mechanisms such as differential expression of neurofibromin binding partners could also influence neurofibromin intracellular localization.

6.2.3. Splice Variants

Most studies analyzing neurofibromin distribution have not discriminated among possible neurofibromin variants generated by alternative splicing, but those that do have found tissue-specific differences in the relative levels of the different forms of *NF1* mRNAs *(150–152,161–163)*. Alternate splicing results in two distinct gene products known as type 1 and type 2 neurofibromin. Type 1 neurofibromin contains sequences encoded by exon 23a that are lacking in the type 2 variant. The specific absence of this alternatively spliced exon has recently been linked to learning problems in mice *(164)*. The GRD of the type 2 variant is less efficient in converting GTP-bound Ras to its GDP-bound form *(132)*.

Another alternately spliced exon of neurofibromin, exon 9a, is expressed almost exclusively in the CNS in humans and rodents *(161)*. Expression of this exon is enriched in the forebrain, is present in neurons, not astrocytes, and its expression increases during CNS neuronal differentiation in vivo and in vitro *(165)*. The identification of a CNS neuron-specific *NF1* isoform supports the hypothesis that neurofibromin has brain-specific functions that may relate to the high incidence of cognitive deficits in NF1 individuals.

6.2.4. Functions of Neurofibromin in Neurons and Glia

In the uninjured adult CNS, neurofibromin is enriched in some neurons and in oligodendrocytes *(148,153)*. Neurons expressing neurofibromin are mainly those that project their axons long distances, such as Purkinje neurons and pyramidal cells *(153)*. Oligodendrocytes, the myelin-forming glial cell of the central nervous system, express high levels of neurofibromin, especially oligodendrocytes in the spinal cord *(148,149)*. In contrast, astrocytes lack detectable levels of neurofibromin expression *in situ (83,148,149)*. However, after injury involving cerebral ischemia, neurofibromin expression can be induced in astrocytes *(166)*.

7. ANIMAL MODELS OF NF1

7.1. Mouse Models of CNS Dysfunction in NF1

An important experimental model used to study the effect of loss of neurofibromin is cells and tissues from mice mutant at *Nf1*. Jacks and colleagues *(167)* and Brannan et al. *(168)* generated mouse *Nf1* knockouts by homologous recombination. Mice with homozygous *Nf1* mutations can be studied only as early embryos, as they die *in utero* before embryonic d 14 *(167,168)*. Heterozygous *Nf1* mouse mutants live to adulthood, breed normally, and can be studied throughout their lives.

Mice heterozygous for a mutation in the *Nf1* gene ($Nf1^{+/-}$) show hyperplasia of some neuronal populations *(168)*, as well as behavioral abnormalities that bear striking similarity to the learning disability observed in humans with NF1 *(169)*. Similar to the case in humans, this phenotype is variably penetrant in $Nf1^{+/-}$ mice. Adult mice do not have focal neurological deficits. However, a subset of mice (50–60%) show impaired performance in the spatial version of the Morris water maze test compared to unaffected littermates, but are able to learn tasks with extended training. Other cognitive functions such as associative learning are unaffected. Mouse brains also demonstrate astrogliosis similar to that observed in humans *(170,171)*.

To define the mechanism underlying the learning deficits in mice heterozygous for a mutation in the *Nf1* gene, Costa et al. *(164)* tested if Ras signaling during hippocampal-dependent learning was relevant. By breeding $Nf1^{+/-}$ mice to mice deficient in Ras ($K\text{-}Ras^{+/-}$) they rescued the NF1 learning defects. A drug that reduces Ras signaling by blocking farnesylation (a posttranslational modification necessary for Ras membrane localization and thus function) also blocked the $Nf1^{+/-}$ learning defect. Physiology studies in slice preparations indicate that the defects are caused by defects in long-term potentiation (LTP) via an increase in γ-aminobutyric acid (GABA)-mediated inhibition. Thus, it appears that Ras modulation by neurofibromin is essential for learning and memory in the mouse. Further evidence supporting a key role for Ras regulation in the NF1 phenotype comes from mutant mice lacking exon 23a of the *Nf1* gene, resulting in modifications of the GAP domain of neurofibromin. These mice show specific learning deficits *(164)*. The fact that brief drug treatment reverses spatial learning defects in *Nf1*$^{+/-}$ mice gives hope that human NF1 learning problems might also be sensitive to drug therapy.

Neither malignant brain tumors nor UBOs have been reported in *Nf1* hemizygous mice. Breeding of *Nf1*$^{+/-}$ mice to *p53*$^{+/-}$ mice, however, resulted in malignant brain tumors in all mice, especially on specific genetic backgrounds *(172)*. This reinforces the view that *NF1* mutation can predispose to malignant brain tumors, and the new model system should allow identification of modifier loci relevant to brain tumor formation.

7.2. Cell Autonomous and Non-Cell-Autonomous Defects Caused by Nf1 Mutations in Mice

In principle, defects in neurons, glial cells, or both cell types could underlie CNS pathology and learning disabilities in NF1. To begin to test effects of neurofibromin loss on specific cell types, neurons and astrocytes have been cultured from *Nf1* mutant mice. Both show defects. Vogel et al. *(173)* demonstrated that neurons isolated from neurofibromin-deficient mouse embryos (*Nf1*$^{-/-}$) survive in the absence of neurotrophic factors, suggesting that neurofibromin may act as a negative regulator of neurotrophin-mediated signaling, and that abnormal expression of neurofibromin may affect signal transduction within the nervous system. These effects are mediated through Ras, working through one of its effectors, PI3kinase *(174)*. Furthermore, cooperativity between mutations in *Nf1* and *p53* prolongs superior cervical ganglion (SCG) neuron proliferation and increases the incidence of neural tube defects in compound-mutant embryos *(175)*. Other findings suggest that neurofibromin could be important for astrocyte development and/ or maintenance. Neurofibromin is expressed in astrocytic tumors *(176)* and neurofibromin expression can be induced in cultured rat astrocytes under conditions that mimic reactive gliosis *(177)* to injury. Cultured neurofibromin-deficient astrocytes show subtle increases in cell proliferation *(170)*. In vivo, astrocyte number in the brain is increased in mice hemizygous for *Nf1* mutation, and overexpressing N-Ras in the mutant background potentiates the effect *(178)*. These data might suggest that the gliosos and/or white matter defects in NF1 patients might be caused by cell autonomous defects in astrocytes. However, when Zhu et al. *(179)* circumvented the problem of embryonic lethality in homozygous *Nf1* knockouts by using Cre/*loxP* technology to generate a conditional *Nf1* knockout in most differentiated neurons, but not astrocytes, mice had abnormal development of the cerebral cortex, and astrogliosis in the absence of conspicuous neurodegeneration or microgliosis. The ability to use cell type specific promoters to cause loss of function mutations in the *Nf1* gene in mice, followed by learning and memory tests, should allow better understanding of whether neurons, astrocytes, or both, contribute to learning defects.

No studies have addressed the role of neurofibromin in oligodendrocytes. It is of some interest that similar to their sporadic counterparts, NF1-associated JPA strongly expressed PEN5, a marker of post-O2A stage oligodendroglial precursor cells *(180)*. The cell of origin of the astrocytomas/gliomatoses in NF1 may be an oligodendrocyte or astrocyte, or a precursor of these cell types.

7.3. Drosophila *Models of* NF1

Drosophila (fruit flies) provide another important model system in which to study neurofibromin function. Flies homozygous for null mutations of the *NF1* gene are small in size and behaviorally "sluggish" compared to wild type *(144)*. *NF1* is necessary for activation of adenylyl cyclase in response to a neuropeptide (PACAP38) at the neuromuscular junction. Moreover, the *NF1* defect was rescued by exposure to pharmacological treatment that increased concentrations of cAMP *(142)*. The misregulation of cAMP involves the rutabaga adenylyl cyclase. The flies also have defects in learning (olfactory associative learning) that involve the cAMP pathway *(143)*. This defect can be rescued by reexpressing neurofibromin in adult flies, indicating that the learning defect is independent of its developmental effects.

Flies also require neurofibromin for appropriate Ras-mediated signals, as the dNF1 mutant flies have lost normal circadian rhythms that can be rescued by loss-of-function mutations in the Ras pathway *(181)*. The relevance of these findings to the pathophysiology of NF1 in humans is not known. Nonetheless, it is notable that learning defects are observed in flies and in mouse, as they are in human NF1 patients.

8. FUTURE DIRECTIONS

Over the past decade, we have achieved a much greater understanding of the NF1 cognitive phenotype, and identified possible radiological and pathological markers for cognitive deficits. However, many important issues remain to be addressed. These include better definition of specific neuropsychological deficits in attention, perceptual skills and executive function, the natural history of cognitive deficits, and clarification of the association between radiological findings and cognitive impairment. In terms of pathogenesis, it is not known if the neuropathology of NF1 is due to a GAP-related function of neurofibromin and/or to other functions of the protein. Does mutation in the NF1 gene result in aberrant myelination and astrocytic proliferation, and if so, how? Are abnormalities due to altered phenotypes of neurons, glial cells, or their progenitors? Are the CNS abnormalities in NF1 a static/ "developmental" problem or a dynamic process, that is, is there potential for intervention?

NF1 provides a unique opportunity to begin to uncover a molecular basis for cognitive impairment. If we can determine the mechanisms by which abnormalities in neurofibromin affect the function of the brain and neuronal pathways, these mechanisms should provide insight into the pathogenesis of cognitive impairment and learning disabilities in the general population. Understanding the etiology of cognitive deficits in NF1 should lead to development of therapies that go beyond symptomatic educational intervention.

ACKNOWLEDGMENTS

We gratefully acknowledge Maryellen Daston for editorial support, and E. Marigney and W. Weber for assistance with referencing, and Elizabeth Schorrey for manuscript review. NR is supported by NIH-NS28840, the National Multiple Sclerosis Society, and the DAMD Program on Neurofibromatosis. KN is supported by the DAMD Program on Neurofibromatosis A-9478.

REFERENCES

1. Crowe FW, Schull WJ, Neel JV. A clinical, pathological and genetic study of multiple neurofibromatosis. Springfield, IL: Charles C Thomas 1956;1181.
2. Huson SM, Harper PS, Compston DAS. Von Recklinghausen neurofibromatosis: a clinical and population study in south east Wales. Brain 1988;111:1355–81.
3. Rasmussen SA, Friedman JM. NF1 gene and neurofibromatosis 1. Am J Epidemiol 2000;151:33–40.
4. Mulvihill JJ, Parry DM, Sherman JL, Pikus A, Kaiser-Kupfer MI, Eldridge R. NIH conference. Neurofibromatosis 1 (Recklinghausen disease) and neurofibromatosis 2 (bilateral acoustic neurofibromatosis). An update. Ann Intern Med 1990;113:39–52.
5. Gutmann DH, Aylsworth A, Carey JC, et al. The diagnostic evaluation and multidisciplinary management of neurofibromatosis 1 and neurofibromatosis 2. JAMA 1997;278:51–7.

6. Huson SM, Compston DA, Harper PS. A genetic study of von Recklinghausen neurofibromatosis in south east Wales. II. Guidelines for genetic counseling. J Med Genet 1989;26:712–21.
7. Riccardi VM. Neurofibromatosis. Phenotype, natural history and pathogenesis. Baltimore: John Hopkins University Press, 2nd ed. 1992;88–85.
8. North, K. Neurofibromatosis type 1: review of the first 200 patients in an Australian clinic. J Child Neurol 1993;8:395–402.
9. Friedman JM, Birch PH. Type I neurofibromatosis: a descriptive analysis of the disorder in 1,728 patients. Am J Med Genet 1997;70:138–43.
10. Sorensen SA, Mulvihill JJ, Nielsen. A long-term follow-up of von Recklinghausen neurofibromatosis. Survival and malignant neoplasms. N Engl J Med 1986;314:1010–5.
11. Neerup Jensen L, Fenger K, Olsen JH, Mulvihill JJ, Sørensen SA (1998) Cancer and mortality in neurofibromatosis 1 (NF1): a 54-year follow-up of a nationwide cohort in Denmark. Am J Hum Genet 63:A114.
12. Zoller M, Rembeck B, Akesson HO, Angervall L. Life expectancy, mortality and prognostic factors in neurofibromatosis type 1. A twelve-year follow-up of an epidemiological study in Goteborg, Sweden. Acta Derm Venereol 1995;75:136–40.
13. Rasmussen SA, Yang Q, Friedman JM. Mortality in neurofibromatosis 1: an analysis using U.S. death certificates. Am J Hum Genet 2001;68:1110–8.
14. Airewele GE, Sigurdson AJ, Wiley KJ, et al. Neoplasms in neurofibromatosis 1 are related to gender but not to family history of cancer. Genet Epidemiol 2001;20:75–86.
15. Wallace MR, Marchuk DA, Andersen LB, et al. Type 1 neurofibromatosis gene: identification of a large transcript disrupted in three NF1 patients. Science 1990;249:181–6.
16. Cawthon RM, O'Connell P, Buchberg AM, et al. Identification and characterization of transcripts from the neurofibromatosis 1 region: the sequence and genomic structure of EVI2 and mapping of other transcripts. Genomics 1990;7:555–65.
17. Xu G, O'Connell P, Viskochil D, et al. The neurofibromatosis type 1 gene encodes a protein related to GAP. Cell 1990;62:599–608.
18. Viskochil D, White R, Cawthon R. The neurofibromatosis type 1 gene. Annu Rev Neurosci 1993;16:183–205.
19. Cummings LM, Trent JM, Marchuk DA. Identification and mapping of type 1 neurofibromatosis (NF1) homologous loci. Cytogenet Cell Genet 1996; 73:334–40.
20. Fahsold R, Hoffmeyer S, Mischung C. Minor lesion mutational spectrum of the entire NF1 gene does not explain its high mutability but points to a functional domain upstream of the GAP-related domain. Am J Hum Genet 2000;66:790–818.
21. Li Y, O'Connell P, Breidenbach HH, et al. Genomic organization of the neurofibromatosis 1 gene (NF1). Genomics 1995;25:9–18.
22. Shen MH, Harper PS, Upadhyaya M. Molecular genetics of neurofibromatosis type 1 (NF1). J Med Genet 1996;33:2–17.

23. Park VM, Pivnick EK Neurofibromatosis type 1 (NF1): a protein truncation assay yielding identification of mutations in 73% of patients. J Med Genet 1998;35:813–20.
24. Messiaen LM, Callens T, Roux KJ, et al. Exon 10b of the NF1 gene represents a mutational hotspot and harbors a recurrent missense mutation Y489C associated with aberrant splicing. Genet Med 1999;1:248–53.
25. Messiaen LM, Callens T, Mortier G, et al. Exhaustive mutation analysis of the NF1 gene allows identification of 95% of mutations and reveals a high frequency of unusual splicing defects. Hum Mutat 2000;15:541–55.
26. Upadhyaya M, Osborn MJ, Maynard J, Kim MR, Tamanoi F, Cooper DN. Mutational and functional analysis of the neurofibromatosis type 1 (NF1) gene. Hum Genet 1997;99:88–92.
27. Legius E, Marchuk DA, Collins FS, Glover TW. Somatic deletion of neurofibromatosis type 1 gene in a neurofibrosarcoma supports a tumor suppressor gene hypothesis. Nat Genet 1993;3:122–6.
28. Shannon KM, O'Connell P, Martin GA, et al. Loss of the normal NF1 allele from the bone marrow of children with type 1 neurofibromatosis and malignant myeloid disorders. N Engl J Med 1994;330:597–601.
29. Colman SD, Williams CA, Wallace MR. Benign neurofibromas in type 1 neurofibromatosis (NF1) show somatic deletions of the *NF1* gene. Nat Genet 1995;11:90–2.
30. Serra E, Rosenbaum T, Winner U, Aledo R, Ars E, Estivill X, Lenard HG, Lazaro C Schwann cells harbor the somatic NF1 mutation in neurofibromas: evidence of two different Schwann cell subpopulations. Hum Mol Genet 2000;9:3055–64.
31. Costa RM, Yang T, Huynh DP, et al. Learning deficits, but normal development and tumor predisposition, in mice lacking exon 23a of Nf1. Nat Genet 2001;27:399–405.
32. Easton DF, Ponder MA, Huson SM, Ponder BAJ. An analysis of variation in expression of neurofibromatosis (NF) type 1 (NF1): evidence for modifying genes. Am J Hum Genet 1993;53:305–13.
33. Bahuau M, Pelet A, Vidaud D, et al. GDNF as a candidate modifier in a type 1 neurofibromatosis (NF1) enteric phenotype. J Med Genet 2001;38:638–43.
34. Wang Q, Lasset C, Desseigne F, et al. Neurofibromatosis and early onset of cancers in hMLH1-deficient children. Cancer Res 1999;59:294–7.
35. Ricciardone MD, Ozcelik T, Cevher B, et al. Human MLH1 deficiency predisposes to hematological malignancy and neurofibromatosis type 1. Cancer Res 1999; 59(2):290–3.
36. Riva P, Corrado L, Natacci F, et al. NF1 microdeletion syndrome: refined FISH characterization of sporadic and familial deletions with locus-specific probes. Am J Hum Genet 2000;66:100–9.
37. Jenne DE, Tinschert S, Reimann H, et al. Molecular characterization and gene content of breakpoint boundaries in patients with neurofibromatosis type 1 with 17q11.2 microdeletions. Am J Hum Genet 2001;69:516–27.

38. Kayes LM, Riccardi VM, Burke W, Bennett RL, Stephens K. Large de novo DNA deletion in a patient with sporadic neurofibromatosis, mental retardation and dysmorphism. J Med Genet 1992;29:686.

39. Kayes LM, Burke W, Riccardi VM, et al. Deletions spanning the neurofibromatosis 1 gene: identification and phenotype of five patients. Am J Hum Genet 1994;54:424–36.

40. Upadhyaya M, Ruggieri M, Maynard J, et al. Gross deletions of the neurofibromatosis type 1 (NF1) gene are predominantly of maternal origin and commonly associated with a learning disability, dysmorphic features and developmental delay. Hum Genet 1998;102:591–7.

41. Tonsgard JH, Yelavarthi KK, Cushner S, Short MP, Lindgren V. Do NF1 gene deletions result in a characteristic phenotype? Am J Med Genet 1997;3:80–6.

42. North KN, Riccardi V, Samango-Sprouse C, et al. Cognitve function and academic performance in neurofibromatosis 1: Consensus statement from the NF1 Cognitive Disorders Task Force. Neurology 1997;48:1121–7.

43. Ozonoff S. Cognitive impairment in neurofibromatosis type 1. Am J Med Genet 1999;89:45–52.

44. Kayl AE, Moore BD. Behavioural phenotype of neurofibromatosis type 1. Mental retardation and developmental disabilities. Ment Retard Dev Disab 2000;6:117–24.

45. North K, Joy P, Yuille D, et al. Learning difficulties in neurofibromatosis type 1: the significance of MRI abnormalities. Neurology 1994;44:878–83.

46. North K, Joy P, Yuille D, Cocks N, Hutchins P. Cognitive function and academic performance in children with neurofibromatosis type 1. Dev Med Child Neurol 1995;37:427–36.

47. Wadsby M, Lindenhammer H, Eeg-Olofsson O. Neurofibromatosis in childhood: neuropsychological aspects. Neurofibromatosis 1989;2:251–60.

48. Eliason MJ. Neurofibromatosis: implications for learning and behaviour. J Dev Behav Pediatr 1986;7:175–9.

49. Varnhagen CK, Lewin S, Das JP, Bowen P, Ma K, Klimek M. Neurofibromatosis and psychological processes. J Dev Behav Pediatr 1988;9:257–65.

50. Stine SB, Adams WV. Learning problems in neurofibromatosis patients. Clin Orthop 1989;245:43–8.

51. Moore BD, Ater JL, Needle MN, Slopis J, Copeland DR. Neuropsychological profile of children with neurofibromatosis, brain tumor or both. J Child Neurol 1994;9:368–77.

52. Legius E, Descheemaeker MJ, Spaepen A, Casaer P, Fryns JP. Neurofibromatosis type 1 in childhood: a study of the neuropsychological profile in 45 children. Genet Couns 1994;5:51–60.

53. Ferner RE, Hughes RAC, Wenman J. Intellectual impairment in neurofibromatosis 1. J Neurol Sci 1996;138:125–33.

54. Steen RG, Taylor JS, Langston JW, et al. Prospective evaluation of the brain in asymptomatic children with neurofibromatosis type 1: relationship of mac-

rocephaly to T1 relaxation changes and structural brain abnormalities. Am J Neuroradiol 2001;22:810–7.

55. Hofman KJ, Harris EL, Bryan RN, Denckla MB. Neurofibromatosis type 1: the cognitive phenotype. J Pediatr 1994;124:S1–8.

56. Dilts CV, Carey JC, Kircher JC, et al. Children and adolescents with neurofibromatosis 1: a behavioral phenotype. Dev Behav Pediatr 1996;17:229–39.

57. Cutting LE, Koth CW, Burnette CP, Abrams MT, Kaufmann WE, Denckla MB. Relationship of cognitive functioning, whole brain volumes, and T2-weighted hyperintensities in neurofibromatosis-1. J Child Neurol 2000a; 15:157–60.

58. Cutting LE, Koth CW, Denckla MB. How children with neurofibromatosis type 1 differ from "typical" learning disabled clinic attenders: nonverbal learning disabilities revisited. Dev Neuropsychol 2000b;17:29–47.

59. Brewer VR, Moore BD, Hiscock M. Learning disability subtypes in children with neurofibromatosis. J Learn Disabil 1997;30:521–33.

60. Kayl AE, Moore BD 3rd, Slopis JM, Jackson EF, Leeds NE. Quantitative morphology of the corpus callosum in children with neurofibromatosis and attention-deficit hyperactivity disorder. J Child Neurol 2000;15:90–6.

61. Vogel SA. Gender differences in intelligence, language, visual–motor abilities and academic achievement in males and females with learning disabilities: a review of the literature. J Learn Disabil 1990;23:44–52.

62. Eliason MJ. Neuropsychological patterns: neurofibromatosis compared to developmental learning disorders. Neurofibromatosis 1988;1:17–25.

63. Benton A, Varney N, Hamsher K. Judgement of Line Orientation. Department of Neurology, University of Iowa, 1976.

64. Eldridge R, Denckla MB, Bien E, et al. Neurofibromatosis type 1 [Recklinghausen's disease]: neurologic and cognitive assessment with sibling controls. Am J Dis Child 1989;143:833–7.

65. Mazzocco MMM, Turner JE, Denckla MB, Hofman KJ, Scanlon DC, Vellutino FR. Language and reading deficits associated with neurofibromatosis type 1: evidence for not-so-nonverbal learning disability. Dev Neuropsychol 1995;11:503–22.

66. Joy P, Roberts C, North K, De Silva M. Neuropsychological function and MRI abnormalities in neurofibromatosis type 1. Dev Med Child Neurol 1995;37:906–14.

67. Zoller MET, Rembeck B, Backman L. Neuropsychological deficits in adults with neurofibromatosis type 1. Acta Neurol Scand 1997;95:225–32.

68. Bawden H, Dooley J, Buckley D, et al. MRI and nonverbal cognitive deficits in children with neurofibromatosis 1. J Clin Exp Neuropsychol 1996; 18:784–92.

69. DeWinter, AE, Moore, BD, Slopis J, et al. Quantitative morphology of the corpus callosum in children with neurofibromatosis and attention-deficit hyperactivity disorder. J Child Neurol 2000;15:90–6.

70. Koth CW, Cutting LE, Denckla MB. The association of neurofibromatosis type 1 and attention deficit hyperactivity disorder. Neuropsychol Dev Cogn C Child Neuropsychol 2000;6:185–94.

71. Samango-Sprouse C, Vezina LG, Brasseux C, Tillman, Tifft CJ. Cranial magnetic resonance findings and the neurodevelopmental performance in the young child with neurofibromatosis 1. Am J Hum Genet 1997;61:A35.
72. Lorch M, Ferner R, Golding J, Whurl R. The nature of speech and language impairments in adults with neurofibromatosis 1. J Neurolinguist 1999; 12:157–65.
73. Riccardi VM, Eichner JE. Neurofibromatosis. Phenotype, natural history and pathogenesis. Baltimore: Johns Hopkins University Press, 1986.
74. Moore BD, Slopis JM, Schomer D, Jackson EF, Levy B. Neuropsychological significance of areas of high signal intensity on brain magnetic resonance imaging scans of children with neurofibromatosis. Neurology 1996;46:1660–8.
75. Moore BD, Slopis, JM, Jackson, EF, De Winter AE. Brain volume in children with neurofibromatosis type 1: Relation to neuropsychological status. Neurology 2000;54:914–26.
76. Benjamin CM, Colley A, Donnai D, Kingston H, Harris R, Kerzin-Storrar L. Neurofibromatosis type 1 (NF1): knowledge, experience, and reproductive decisions of affected patients and families. J Med Genet 1993;30:567–74.
77. Porter Counterman A, Saylor CF, Pai S. Psychological adjustment of children and adolescents with neurofibromatosis. Child Health Care 1995;24;4:223–34.
78. Achenbach TM, Edelbrock CS. Achenbach child behaviour checklist. J Consult Clin Psychol 1979;47:223–33.
79. Johnson NS, Saal HM, Lovell AM, Schorry EK. Social and emotional problems in children with neurofibromatosis type 1: evidence and proposed interventions J Pediatr 1999;134:767–72.
80. Wolkenstein P, Zeller J, Revuz J, Ecosse E, Leplege A. Quality-of-life impairment in neurofibromatosis type 1: a cross-sectional study of 128 Cases. Arch Dermatol 2001;137:1421–5.
81. Rosman NP, Pearce J. The brain in multiple neurofibromatosis (von Recklinghausen's disease): a suggested neuropathological basis for the associated mental defect. Brain 1967;90:829–38.
82. Rubinstein LJ. The malformative central nervous system lesions in the central and peripheral forms of neurofibromatosis: a neuropathological study of 22 cases. Ann NY Acad Sci 1986;486:14–29.
83. Nordlund ML, Rizvi TA, Brannan CI, Ratner N. Neurofibromin expression and astrogliosis in neurofibromatosis (type 1) brains. J Neuropathol Exp Neurol 1995;54:588–600.
84. Korf BR, Schneider G, Poussaint TY. Structural anomalies revealed by neuroimaging studies in the brains of patients with neurofibromatosis type 1 and large deletions. Genet Med 1999;1:136–40.
85. Bognanno JR, Edwards MK, Lee TA, Dunn DW, Roos KL, Klatte EC. Cranial MR imaging in neurofibromatosis. Am J Neuroradiol 1988;9:461–8.
86. Dunn DW, Roos KL. MRI evaluation of learning difficulties and incoordination in neurofibromatosis type 1. Neurofibromatosis 1989;2:1–5.
87. Pont MS, Elster AD. Lesions of skin and brain: modern imaging of the neurocutaneous syndromes. Am J Radiol 1992;158:1193–1203.

88. Sevick RJ, Barkovich AJ, Edwards MSB, Koch T, Berg B, Lempert T. Evolution of white matter lesions in neurofibromatosis type 1: MR findings. Am J Radiol 1992;159:171–5.
89. Van Es S, North K, McHugh K, de Silva M . MRI abnormalities in children with NF1. Paediatr Radiol 1996;26:478–87.
90. Duffner PK, Cohen ME, Seidel FG, Shucard DW. The significance of MRI abnormalities in children with neurofibromatosis. Neurology 1989; 39:373–8.
91. North KN, Riccardi V, Samango-Sprouse C, et al. Cognitive function and academic performance in neurofibromatosis 1: Consensus statement from the NF1 Cognitive Disorders Task Force. Neurology 1997;48:1121–7.
92. Aoki S, Barkovich AJ, Nishimura K, et al. Neurofibromatosis types 1 and 2: cranial MR findings. Radiology 1989;172:527–34.
93. Itoh T, Magnaldi S, White RM, et al. Neurofibromatosis type 1: the evolution of deep gray and white matter MR abnormalities. Am J Neuroradiol 1994;15:1513–9.
94. Menor F, Marti-Bonmati L, Arana E, Poyatos C, Cortina H. Neurofibromatosis type 1 in children: MR imaging and follow-up studies of central nervous system findings. Eur J Radiol 1998;26:121–31.
95. Terada H, Barkovich AJ, Edwards MS, Ciricillo SM. Evolution of high-intensity basal ganglia lesions on T1-weighted MR in neurofibromatosis type 1. Am J Neuroradiol 1996;17:755–60.
96. DiPaolo DP, Zimmerman RA, Rorke LB, Zackai EH, Bilaniuk LT, Yachnis AT. Neurofibromatosis type 1: pathologic substrate of high-signal intensity foci in the brain. Radiology 1995;195:721–4.
97. Ferner RE, Chaudhuri R, Bingham J, Cox T, Hughes RAC. MRI in neurofibromatosis 1. The nature and evolution of increased intensity T2 weighted lesions and their relationship to intellectual impairment. J Neurol Neurosurg Psychiatry 1993;56:492–5.
98. Denckla MB, Hofman K, Bryan N, et al. Evidence that cognitive deficits in NF-1 are related to T2-weighted hyperintensities on MRI. Neurology 1994;(Suppl 2):A381–2.
99. Mott S, Kkryja PB, Baumgardner T, Abrams M, Reiss A, Denckla M. Neurofibromatosis type I (NF1): association between volumes of T2-weighted high intensity signals (UBOs) on magnetic resonance imaging (MRI) and impaired performance on the Judgement of Line Orientation (JLO). ASHA 1994;24:945.
100. Denckla MD, Hofman K, Mazzocco MMM, et al. Relationship between T2-weighted hyperintensities (unidentified bright objects) and lower IQs in children with neurofibromatosis-1. Am J Med Genet 1996;67:98–102.
101. Legius E, Descheemaeker MJ, Steyaert J, et al. Neurofibromatosis type 1 in childhood: correlation of MRI findings with intelligence. J Neurol Neurosurg Psychiatry 1995;59:638–40.
102. Moore BD. NF1, cognition and MRI. Neurology 1995;45:1029.
103. Chapman CA, Waber DP, Bassett N, Urion DK, KOrk BR. Neurobehavioral profiles of children with neurofibromatosis 1 referred for learning disabilities are sex-specific. Am J Med Genet 1996;67:127–32.

104. Said SMA, Yeh T, Greenwood RS, et al. MRI morphometric analysis and neuropsychological function in patients with neurofibromatosis. NeuroReport 1996;7:1941–4.
105. Dubovsky EC, Booth TN, Vezina G, Samango-Sprouse CA, Palmer KM, Brasseux CO. MR imaging of the corpus callosum in pediatric patients with neurofibromatosis type 1. Am J Neuroradiol 2001;22:190–5.
106. Kaplan AM, Lawson MA, Bonstelle CT, Wodrich DL. Positron emission tomography (PET) in children with NF1. Abstract 607, International Child Neurology Association Conference, San Francisco 1994.
107. Balestri P, Lucignani G, Fois A, et al. Cerebral glucose metabolism in neurofibromatosis type 1 assessed with [18F]-2-fluoro-2-deoxy-D-glucose and PET. J Neurol Neurosurg Psychiatry 1994;57:1479–83.
108. Gonen O, Wang ZJ, Viswanathan AK, Molloy PT, Zimmerman RA. Three-dimensional multivoxel proton MR spectroscopy of the brain in children with neurofibromatosis type 1. Am J Neuroradiol. 1999;20:1333–41.
109. Castillo M, Green C, Kwock L, et al. Proton MR spectroscopy in patients with neurofibromatosis type 1: evolution of hamartomas and clinical correlation. Am J Neuroradiol 1995;16:141–7.
110. Jones AP, Gunawardena WJ, Coutinho CM. 1H MR spectroscopy evidence for the varied nature of asymptomatic focal brain lesions in neurofibromatosis type 1. Neuroradiology 2001;43:62–7.
111. Wilkinson ID, Griffiths PD, Wales JK. Proton magnetic resonance spectroscopy of brain lesions in children with neurofibromatosis type 1. Magn Reson Imaging 2001;19:1081–9.
112. Wang PY, Kaufmann WE, Koth CW, Denckla MB, Barker PB. Thalamic involvement in neurofibromatosis type 1: evaluation with proton magnetic resonance spectroscopic imaging. Ann Neurol 2000;47:477–84.
113. Eastwood JD, Fiorella DJ, MacFall JF, Delong DM, Provenzale JM, Greenwood RS. Increased brain apparent diffusion coefficient in children with neurofibromatosis type 1. Radiology 2001;219:354–8.
114. Listernick R, Louis DN, Packer RJ, Gutmann, DH. Optic pathway gliomas in children with neurofibromatosis 1: consensus statement from the NF1 Optic Pathway Glioma Task Force. Ann Neurol 1997;41:143–9.
115. Sippel KC. Ocular findings in neurofibromatosis type 1. Int Ophthalmol Clin 2001;41:25–40.
116. Balcer LJ, Liu GT, Heller G, et al. Visual loss in children with neurofibromatosis type 1 and optic pathway gliomas: relation to tumor location by magnetic resonance imaging. Am J Ophthalmol 2001;131:442–5.
117. Gayre GS, Scott IU, Feuer W, Saunders TG, Siatkowski RM. Long-term visual outcome in patients with anterior visual pathway gliomas. J Neuroophthalmol 2001;21:1–7.
118. Parsa CF, Hoyt CS, Lesser RL, et al. Spontaneous regression of optic gliomas: thirteen cases documented by serial neuroimaging. Arch Ophthalmol 2001;119:516–29.
119. Grill J, Laithier V, Rodriguez D, Raquin MA, Pierre-Kahn A, Kalifa C. When do children with optic pathway tumors need treatment? An oncological perspective in 106 patients treated in a single centre. Eur J Pediatr 2000;159:692–6.

120. Sigorini M, Zuccoli G, Ferrozzi F, Bacchini E, Street ME, Piazza P, Rossi M, Virdis R Magnetic resonance findings and ophthalmologic abnormalities are correlated in patients with neurofibromatosis type 1 (NF1). Am J Med Genet 2000;93:269–72.

121. Ng YT, North KN. Visual-evoked potentials in the assessment of optic gliomas. Pediatr Neurol 2001;24:44–8.

122. Li J, Perry A, James CD, Gutmann DH. Cancer-related gene expression profiles in NF1-associated pilocytic astrocytomas. Neurology 2001;56:885–90.

123. Kluwe L, Hagel C, Tatagiba M, et al. Loss of NF1 alleles distinguish sporadic from NF1-associated pilocytic astrocytomas. J Neuropathol Exp Neurol 2001;60:917–20.

124. Gutmann DH, Donahoe J, Brown T, James CD, Perry A. Loss of neurofibromatosis 1 (NF1) gene expression in NF1-associated pilocytic astrocytomas. Neuropathol Appl Neurobio 2000;l26:361–7.

125. Stern J, Jakobiec FA, Housepian EM.The architecture of optic nerve gliomas with and without neurofibromatosis. Arch Ophthalmol 1980;98:505–11.

126. Griffiths PD, Blaser S, Mukonoweshuro W, Armstrong D, Milo-Mason G, Cheung S Neurofibromatosis bright objects in children with neurofibromatosis type 1: a proliferative potential? Pediatrics 1999;104:e49.

127. Raininko R, Thelin L, Eeg-Olofsson O. Atypical focal non-neoplastic brain changes in neurofibromatosis type 1: mass effect and contrast enhancement. Neuroradiology 2001;43:586–90.

128. Chateil JF, Soussotte C, Pedespan JM, Brun M, Le Manh C, Diard F. MRI and clinical differences between optic pathway tumors in children with and without neurofibromatosis. Br J Radiol 2001;74:24–31.

129. Marchuk DA, Collins FS. Molecular genetics of neurofibromatosis 1. In: Huson SM, Hughes RAC, eds. The neurofibromatoses. A pathogenetic and clinical overview. London: Chapman and Hall 1994;23–49.

130. Izawa I, Tamaki N, Saya H. Phosphorylation of neurofibromatosis type 1 gene product (neurofibromin) by cAMP-dependent protein kinase. FEBS Lett 1996;382:53–9.

131. McCormick F. Ras signaling and NF1. Curr Opin Genet Dev 1995;5:51–55.

132. Anderson SB, Ballester R, Marchuk DA, et al. A conserved alternative splice in the von Recklinghausen neurofibromatosis (NF1) gene produces two neurofibromin isoforms, both of which have GTPase-activating protein activity. Mol Cell Biol 1993;13:487–95.

133. Martin GA, Viskochil D, Bollag G, et al. The GAP-related domain of the neurofibromatosis type 1 gene product interacts with ras p21. Cell 1990; 63:843–9.

134. Klose A, Ahmadian MR, Schuelke M, et al. Selective disactivation of neurofibromin GAP activity in neurofibromatosis type 1. Hum Mol Genet 1998;7:1261–8.

135. Graham SM, Vojtek AB, Huff SY, et al. TC21 causes transformation by Raf-independent signaling pathways. Mol Cell Biol 1996;16:6132–40.

136. Rey I, Taylor-Harris P, van Erp H, Hall A. R-ras interacts with rasGAP, neurofibromin and c-raf but does not regulate cell growth or differentiation. Oncogene 1994;9(3):685–92.
137. Ohba Y, Mochizuki N, Yamashita S, et al. Regulatory proteins of R-Ras, TC21/R-Ras2, and M-Ras/R-Ras3. J Biol Chem 2000;275:20,020–36.
138. Hiatt KK, Ingram DA, Zhang Y, Bollag G, Clapp DW. Neurofibromin GTPase-activating protein-related domains restore normal growth in nf1–/– cells. J Biol Chem 2001;276:7240–5.
139. Bollag G, McCormick F, Clark R. Characterization of full-length neurofibromin: tubulin inhibits Ras GAP activity. EMBO J 1993;12:1923–27.
140. Xu H, Gutmann DH. Mutations in the GAP-related domain impair the ability of neurofibromin to associate with microtubules. Brain Res 1997; 759:149–52.
141. Hsueh YP, Roberts AM, Volta M, Sheng M, Roberts RG. Bipartite interaction between neurofibromatosis type I protein (neurofibromin) and syndecan transmembrane heparan sulfate proteoglycans. J Neurosci 2001;21:3764–70.
142. Guo HF, The I, Hannan F, Bernards A, Zhong Y. Requirement of *Drosophila* NF1 for activation of adenylyl cyclase by PACAP38-like neuropeptides. Science 1997;276:795–8.
143. Guo HF, Tong J, Hannan F, Luo L, Zhong Y. A neurofibromatosis-1-regulated pathway is required for learning in *Drosophila*. Nature 2000;403:946–7.
144. The I, Hannigan GE, Cowley GS, et al. Rescue of a *Drosophila* NF1 mutant phenotype by protein kinase A. Science 1997;276:791–4.
145. Tong J, Hannan F, Zhu Y, Bernards A, Zhong Y. Neurofibromin regulates G protein-stimulated adenylyl cyclase activity. Nat Neurosci 2002;5:95–6.
146. Kim HA, Ratner N, Roberts TM, Stiles CD. Schwann cell proliferative responses to cAMP and Nf1 are mediated by cyclin D1. J Neurosci 2001; 21:1110–6.
147. Tokuo H, Yunoue S, Feng L, et al. Phosphorylation of neurofibromin by cAMP-dependent protein kinase is regulated via a cellular association of N(G), N(G)-dimethylarginine dimethylaminohydrolase. FEBS Lett 2001;494:48–53.
148. Daston MM, Scrable H, Norlund M, Sturbaum AK, Nissen LM, Ratner N. The protein product of the neurofibromatosis type 1 gene is expressed at highest abundance in neurons, Schwann cells and oligodendrocytes. Neuron 1992;8:415–28.
149. Daston MM, Ratner N. Neurofibromin, a predominantly neuronal GTPase activating protein in the adult, is ubiquitously expressed during development. Dev Dynamics 1992;195:216–26.
150. Huynh DP, Nechiporuk T, Pulst SM. Differential expression and tissue distribution of type I and type II neurofibromins during mouse fetal development. Dev Biol 1994;161:538–51.
151. Gutmann DH, Cole JL, Collins FS. Expression of the neurofibromatosis type 1 (NF1) gene during mouse embryonic development. Prog Brain Res 1995a;105:327–35.

152. Gutmann DH, Geist RT, Wright DE, Snider WD. Expression of the neurofibromatosis 1 (NF1) isoforms in developing and adult rat tissues. Cell Growth Dev 1995b;6:315–22.
153. Nordlund M, Gu X, Shipley MT, Ratner N. Neurofibromin is enriched in the endoplasmic reticulum of CNS neurons. J Neurosci 1993;13:1588–1600.
154. Schafer GL, Ciment G, Stocker KM, Baizer L. Analysis of the sequence and embryonic expression of chicken neurofibromin mRNA. Mol Chem Neuropathol 1993;18:267–78.
155. Stocker KM, Baizer L, Coston T, Sherman L, Ciment G. Regulated expression of neurofibromin in migrating neural crest cells of avian embryos. J Neurobiol 1995;27:535–52.
156. Malhotra R, Ratner N. Localization of neurofibromin to keratinocytes and melanocytes in developing rat and human skin. J Invest Dermatol 1994; 102:812–8.
157. Boyer M, Gutmann DH, Collins FS, Bar-Sagi D. Crosslinking of the surface immunoglobulin receptor in B lymphocytes induces a redistribution of neurofibromin but not p120-GAP. Oncogene 1994; 9(2): 349–357.
158. Gregory PE, Gutmann DH, Boguski M, et al. The neurofibromatosis type 1 gene product, neurofibromin, associates with microtubules. Somat Cell Mol Genet 1993;19:265–74.
159. Roudebush M, Slabe T, Sundaram V, Hoppel CL, Golubic M, Stacey DW. Neurofibromin colocalizes with mitochondria in cultured cells. Exp Cell Res 1997;236:161–72.
160. DeClue JE, Cohen BD, Lowy DR. Identification and characterization of the neurofibromatosis type 1 gene product. Proc Natl Acad Sci USA 1991;88: 9914–8.
161. Danglot G, Regnier V, Fauvet D, Vassal G, Kujas M, Bernheim A. Neurofibromatosis 1 (NF1) mRNAs expressed in the central nervous system are differentially spliced in the 5' part of the gene. Hum Mol Genet 1995;4:915–20.
162. Nishi T, Lee PSY, Oka K, et al. Differential expression of two types of the neurofibromatosis type 1 (NF1) gene transcripts related to neuronal differentiation. Oncogene 1991;7:553–61.
163. Suzuki H, Takahashi K, Kubota Y, Fuse N, Shibahara S. Molecular cloning of a cDNA coding for neurofibromatosis type 1 protein isoform lacking the domain related to ras GTPase-activating protein. Biochem Biophys Res Commun 1992;187:984–92.
164. Costa RM, Federov NB, Kogan JH, et al. Mechanism for the learning deficits in a mouse model of neurofibromatosis type 1. Nature 2002;526–30.
165. Geist RT, Gutmann DH. Expression of a developmentally-regulated neuron-specific isoform of the neurofibromatosis 1 (NF1) gene. Neurosci Lett 1996;211:85–8.
166. Giordano MJ, Mahadeo DK, He YY, Geist RT, Hsu C, Gutmann DH. Increased expression of the neurofibromatosis 1 (NF1) gene product, neurofibromin, in astrocytes in response to cerebral ischemia. J Neurosci Res 1996;43:246–53.

167. Jacks T, Shih TS, Schmitt EM, Bronson RT, Bernards A, Weinberg RA. Tumor predisposition in mice heterozygous for a targeted mutation in NF1. Nat Genet 1994;7:353–61.
168. Brannan CI, Perkins AS, Vogel KS, et al. Targeted disruption of the neurofibromatosis type-1 gene leads to developmental abnormalities in heart and various neural crest-derived tissues. Genes Dev 1994;8:1019–29.
169. Silva AJ, Frankland PW, Marowitz Z, et al. A mouse model for the learning and memory deficits associated with neurofibromatosis type 1. Nat Genet 1997;15:281–4.
170. Gutmann DH, Loehr A, Zhang Y, Kim J, Henkemeyer M, Cashen A. Haploinsufficiency for the neurofibromatosis 1 (NF1) tumor suppressor results in increased astrocyte proliferation. Oncogene 1999;18:4450–9.
171. Rizvi TA, Akunuru S, de Courten-Myers G, Switzer RC 3rd, Nordlund ML, Ratner N Region-specific astrogliosis in brains of mice heterozygous for mutations in the neurofibromatosis type 1 (Nf1) tumor suppressor. Brain Res 1999;816:111–23.
172. Reilly KM, Loisel DA, Bronson RT, McLaughlin ME, Jacks T. Nf1;Trp53 mutant mice develop glioblastoma with evidence of strain-specific effects. Nat Genet 2000;26:109–13.
173. Vogel KS, Brannan CI, Jenkins NA, Copeland NG, Parada LF. Loss of neurofibromin results is neurotrophin-independent survival of embryonic sensory and sympathetic neurons. Cell 1995;82:733–42.
174. Klesse LJ, Parada LF. p21 ras and phosphatidylinositol-3 kinase are required for survival of wild-type and NF1 mutant sensory neurons. J Neurosci 1998;18:10,420–8.
175. Vogel KS, Parada LF. Sympathetic neuron survival and proliferation are prolonged by loss of p53 and neurofibromin. Mol Cell Neurosci 1998;11:19–28.
176. Gutmann DH, Giordano MJ, Mahadeo DK, Lau N, Silbergeld D, Guha A. Increased neurofibromatosis 1 gene expression in astrocytic tumors: positive regulation by p21-ras. Oncogene 1996;12:2121–7.
177. Hewett SJ, Choi DW, Gutmann DH. Expression of the neurofibromatosis 1 (NF1) gene in reactive astrocytes in vitro. NeuroReport 1995;6:1565–1568.
178. Bajenaru ML, Donahoe J, Corral T, et al. Neurofibromatosis 1 (NF1) heterozygosity results in a cell-autonomous growth advantage for astrocytes. Glia 2001;33:314–23.
179. Zhu Y, Romero MI, Ghosh P, et al. Ablation of NF1 function in neurons induces abnormal development of cerebral cortex and reactive gliosis in the brain. Genes Dev 2001;15:859–76.
180. Li C, Cheng Y, Gutmann DA, Mangoura D. Differential localization of the neurofibromatosis 1 (NF1) gene product, neurofibromin, with the F-actin or microtubule cytoskeleton during differentiation of telencephalic neurons. Brain Res Dev Brain Res 2001; 130:231–48.
181. Williams JA, Su HS, Bernards A, Field J, Sehgal A. A circadian output in *Drosophila* mediated by neurofibromatosis-1 and Ras/MAPK. Science 2001;293:2251–6.

6

Prader–Willi and Angelman Syndromes

Cognitive and Behavioral Phenotypes

Elisabeth M. Dykens and Suzanne B. Cassidy

1. INTRODUCTION

Although Prader–Willi and Angelman syndromes are genetically related, they are as different as one might imagine in their associated behavioral and physical features. First identified 45 years ago, Prader–Willi syndrome (PWS) *(1)* is characterized by infantile hypotonia, hypogonadism, short stature, characteristic facial features, mild levels of cognitive delay, hyperphagia, increased risks of obesity, and obsessive–compulsive and other behavioral problems. Table 1 summarizes some of the associated facial and physical features of PWS, as agreed on by the consensus clinical diagnostic criteria for this syndrome *(2)*. Of these, PWS is perhaps most famous for its characteristic hyperphagia and food-seeking behaviors. Indeed, even with today's improved early detection and intervention, complications of obesity remain the leading cause of death associated with this syndrome.

In contrast, Angelman syndrome (AS) *(3)* is characterized by microcephaly; severe levels of developmental delay; absence of expressive speech; seizure disorders; bouts of spontaneous laughter; a happy demeanor; and an ataxic, jerky gait. Table 2 summarizes common physical and behavioral features of AS. As a result of a series of discoveries, these two dramatically different syndromes have made molecular genetic history as the first known human genetic disorders associated with genomic imprinting.

In this chapter we first briefly review the genetic features of PWS and AS. We then describe in more detail the cognitive, linguistic, and behavioral phenotypes of these two syndromes, which are increasingly well understood. Whenever possible, we hypothesize about possible mechanisms that might be associated with the within-syndrome variability that is often observed in

From: *Contemporary Clinical Neuroscience:*
Genetics and Genomics of Neurobehavioral Disorders
Edited by: G. S. Fisch © Humana Press Inc., Totowa, NJ

Table 1
Summary of the Clinical Diagnostic Criteria for Prader–Willi Syndrome

Major criteria (1 point each):

Infantile central hypotonia
Rapid weight gain between 1 and 6 years
Characteristic facial features
Hypogonadism: genital hypoplasia, pubertal deficiency
Developmental delay/mental retardation

Minor criteria (1/2 point each):

Decreased fetal movement and infantile lethargy Infantile feeding problems/ failure to thrive
Typical behavior problems
Sleep disturbance\sleep apnea
Short stature for the family by age 15 years
Hypopigmentation
Small hands and feet for height age
Narrow hands with straight ulnar border
Esotropia, myopia
Thick, viscous saliva
Speech articulation difficulties
Skin picking

Supportive criteria (no points):

High pain threshold
Decreased vomiting
Temperature control problems
Scoliosis and/or kyphosis
Early adrenarche
Osteoporosis
Unusual skill with jigsaw puzzles
Normal neuromuscular studies

Note: The diagnosis should be strongly suspected in children <3 years of age with 5 points, 3 from major criteria; or in those above 3 years with 8 points, 4 from major criteria. The original diagnostic criteria included a major criterion of chromosome 15 deletion or other chromosome 15 anomaly.

Adapted from Holm et al., 1993.

both PWS and AS. These mechanisms include recent data that link molecular genetic status in each syndrome to physical features, cognition, and behavior. Throughout, we identify areas in need of further study, especially research that pushes forward current understandings of gene–brain–behavior relationships.

Table 2
Common Features of Persons with Angelman Syndrome

Characteristic	Percent
Ataxic movements	100
Severe mental retardation	100
Absent expressive language	100
Normal birth weight	100
Frequent smiling	96–100
Grabs things or people	100
Normal head circumference at birth	100
Abnormal EEG	92–100
Seizures	96
Large, wide mouth, large chin	92
Protruding tongue	81
Bouts of inappropriate laughter	77–91
Excessive mouthing	75–100
Hypopigmentation	73
Hyperactivity	64–100
Microcephaly	63
Sleeping problems	57–100
Eating problems	45–64

Data from Clayton-Smith, 1993 *(101)*; Laan, Boer, Hennekan, Reinera, and Brouwer, 1996 *(107)*; Smith et al., 1996 *(26)*; Summers, Allison, Lynch, and Feldman, 1995 *(102)*; Zori et al., 1992 *(105)*.

2. GENETICS OF PRADER–WILLI SYNDROME

PWS is caused by the absence of the normally active paternally inherited genes in the q11–q13 region of chromosome 15. The majority of cases (approx 70%) are due to a paternally derived deletion, or missing piece, of chromosome 15q11–q13 *(4,5)*. In most persons, the deletion is *de novo* in the affected individual, and generally the same size across individuals, with mostly identical breakpoints on the chromosome. Most others with PWS have maternal uniparental disomy (UPD), that is, when both members of the chromosome 15 pair are inherited from the mother, instead of the usual situation in which one is inherited from each parent *(6)*. In UPD, the chromosomes are themselves normal, but the inheritance pattern is amiss. UPD usually affects the whole chromosome, but it is only the small region of imprinted genes related to PWS in which it matters from whom the chromosome is inherited. PWS is actually the first recognized human disorder to exhibit genomic imprinting, that is, when genes are modified and expressed differently, depending on the sex of the parent *(7)*.

In addition to paternal deletions or maternal UPD, a few cases with PWS (from 1% to 5%) have an abnormality in the genomic imprinting process, called an imprinting defect. In some of these, a very small deletion can be detected in the center controlling the imprinting process within 15q11–13 *(8,9)*. Although small, this last group includes all known cases in which there has been a recurrence of PWS in the family.

Several genes that exhibit maternal imprinting have now been mapped to the Prader–Willi critical region, including the candidate gene, small nuclear ribonucleoprotein N (SNRPN). SNRPN is involved in alternative gene splicing, is found abundantly in brain, and is expressed from the paternally inherited chromosome only *(10,11)*. However, based on data from animal knockouts and rare cases in humans, the Prader–Willi phenotype does not appear to be the direct result of loss of SNRPN expression. Other candidate genes include the neuronal protein (NDN), a growth suppressor that in knockout mice leads to variable postnatal lethality. Surviving mice have reduction in oxytocin- and leutinizing hormone releasing hormone-secreting neurons *(12)*. As with many other deletion syndromes, it is likely that several genes contribute to the classic PWS physical and behavioral phenotype.

2.1. Genotype-Phenotype Findings: Physical Features

More detailed analyses of the genetics of PWS have led researchers to examine possible phenotypic differences across the various genetic subtypes of the disorder (*see* Table 3). Physically, those with paternal deletions seem more apt to show the syndrome's typical facial features, as well as hypopigmentation *(13–16)*. Hypopigmentation, or fair complexion or coloring, is attributed to deletion of a gene (P) for tyrosinase positive albinoidism in the Prader–Willi critical region *(17)*. Compared to those with deletions, people with UPD may have greater birth weight, a shorter course of gavage feeding in infancy, and later onset of hyperphagia *(15,16)*. Some of these features, however, are not consistently observed *(18)*. Advanced maternal age in UPD cases is also seen. More subtle physical features in cases with maternal UPD may lead to a later age of diagnosis in these individuals *(18)*. Observations about physical features have led to a series of new studies on possible behavioral differences across deleted vs UPD cases that are reviewed later in this chapter.

3. GENETICS OF ANGELMAN SYNDROME

Whereas Prader–Willi syndrome is associated with lack of expression of paternally derived imprinted information on chromosome 15q11–13,

Table 3
Preliminary Comparisons of Physical and Behavioral Features in Persons with Prader–Willi Syndrome Due to Paternal Deletion vs Maternal UPD

Deletion	UPD
Physical	
Hypopogmentation	More subtle facial features
Classic facial features	Increased birth weight
	Later onset hyperphagia (?)
	Complexion more typical of family
	Shorter course gavage feeding in infancy (?)
	Later age at diagnosis
Cognitive	
Somewhat lower Verbal IQs	Higher Verbal IQs
Possible splinter skills in	Poorer performances on visual–spatial tasks
jigsaw puzzles	Poorer performances on jigsaw puzzles
Maladaptive behavior	
More frequent or severe	Slight sparing, including skin-picking,
problems	hoarding, aggression
	Increased risk of autism, or adult-onset
	psychosis

Angelman syndrome is associated with the opposite pattern. That is, individuals with AS are lacking maternally derived imprinted information to this same region of the genome. A small percentage of AS cases—between 2% and 5%—are attributed to paternal uniparental disomy (UPD), that is, when both copies of chromosome 15 are inherited from the father *(19)*. Either through maternal deletion or paternal UPD, imprinted information is missing from the mother in the critical region for AS.

About 2– 3% of AS cases are due to imprinting defects, including some with deletions of the "imprinting center" on chromosome 15 *(8,9)*. A few cases (1%) have other, unusual chromosomal rearrangements involving chromosome 15 *(20)*. The remaining 22–25% of AS cases show none of these anomalies, and for a long time their genetic underpinnings were an enigma to researchers. In recent breakthroughs, however, about half of these cases were shown to have specific mutations in one of the genes in the Angelman/Prader–Willi critical region called *UBE3A (21,22)*. *UBE3A* appears to be specifically expressed in the brain *(23)*, yet it is unknown how the absence of *UBE3A*—which encodes for a protein ligase involved in intracellular protein processing—leads to the AS clinical phenotype.

In addition to *UBE3A*, newly developed animal models point to other candidate genes that appear to play a role in the AS phenotype. The Angelman/Prader–Willi deletion region contains a gene called *GABRA3*, a subunit of γ-aminobutyric acid A (GABA$_A$) receptors, which is implicated in epilepsy and is the target of certain anticonvulsive medications *(24)*. Using knockout mice, DeLorey and colleagues *(25)* recently found that disrupting the *GABRA3* gene in mice caused EEG abnormalities and seizures. Other key features of AS were also observed, such as poor learning and motor coordination, hyperactivity, and disrupted rest-activity patterns. Disruptions of both the *GABA3* and *UBE3A* genes are thus implicated in AS, although the relative contributions of each of these or other genes remain unknown.

3.1. Genotype-Phenotype Findings: Angelman Syndrome

Several phenotypic differences have now been identified across these genetic subtypes. Those with the deletion show most of the "classic" features of AS. Having examined 27 individuals with confirmed deletions, Smith and colleagues *(26)* found that all were severely mentally retarded, exhibited ataxic movements, absent speech, abnormal EEG, a happy disposition, normal birth weight and head circumference at birth, and a large, wide mouth. These and other clinical features of persons with paternal deletions are summarized in Table 2.

In contrast, milder phenotypic features are found among the relatively few known cases with AS due to paternal UPD *(27–30)*. Compared to their counterparts with deletions, individuals with paternal UPD often have better growth parameters, more subtle facial features, walk at earlier ages, have less severe or frequent seizure disorders, less ataxia, and a greater facility with rudimentary communication such as signing or gesturing. Those with imprinting center mutations are less apt to show microcephaly or hypopigmentation, and they also appear to have fewer severe seizure disorders *(9,31,32)*. Milder epilepsy is also noted among those AS cases with *UBE3A* abnormalities *(32)*. Further studies are needed that assess a wider range of behavior across these genetic subtypes, a challenge considering the rarity of some of these cases.

Many genetic advances have thus been made in both PWS and AS, and researchers continue to examine the function of known genes deleted or altered in this critical region of chromosome 15. In the meantime, behavioral studies have also progressed, albeit at a slower rate. However, behavioral studies have moved forward faster in PWS, PWS being the focus of more intensive behavioral and developmental research than AS. One aim of this chapter is to spark increased interest in basic developmental research in AS, as well as to fine-tune current understandings of behavior in PWS.

4. PRADER–WILLI SYNDROME: *COGNITION AND BEHAVIOR*

4.1. Range of Cognitive Functioning

Compared to persons with other genetic mental retardation syndromes, most individuals with PWS have relatively high IQ scores; the average IQ is approx 65–70 *(33)*. Aggregating IQ data from 575 subjects in 57 published studies, Curfs *(34)* found that 34% showed mild mental retardation, 27% had moderate delays, and 6% showed severe to profound levels of impairment. A surprisingly large proportion (32%) exhibited IQ scores above 70. Of these, 27% were in the borderline range (70–84), and 5% were average IQ scores (85 and above). Even among high-functioning individuals, however, adaptive behaviors rarely function at a level commensurate with IQ scores, owing to interference from food-related and other behavioral problems.

4.2. Cognitive Profiles

Many persons with PWS appear to have relative strengths in tasks assessing visual and visual–spatial processing. Although global evidence for this strength is found in some individuals who have elevated Performance over Verbal IQ scores *(35)*, profiles are more striking when specific cognitive tasks are examined. Compared to obese controls with mental retardation, for example, persons with PWS have significantly higher scores on the Wechsler-based Block design task, which assesses visual–motor integration *(36)*. Curfs et al. *(35)* also found that 9 of 13 children with PWS had relative strengths in Block Design. Similarly, compared to age- and IQ-matched persons with mixed mental retardation, Dykens *(37)* found that children and adolescents with PWS had significantly higher scores on the Triangles subtest of the Kaufman Assessment Battery for Children *(38)*, as well as on a written task assessing visual–motor integration. Assessing 15 children with PWS, Gabel et al. *(39)* found relative strengths in visual attention and visual recall tasks of the Detroit Tests of Learning Aptitude *(40)*. Dykens et al. *(33)* examined 21 adolescents and adults with PWS and found relative strengths in K-ABC tasks assessing perceptual closure, spatial organization, and attention to visual detail. Collectively, these studies point to relative strengths in visual and/or visual–spatial processing among many individuals with PWS.

Consistent with these strengths, many people with PWS have been reported by families to show an unusual facility with jigsaw puzzles. Although based on anecdotal impressions, Holm and colleagues *(2)* included jigsaw puzzle skills as a supportive finding in the consensus diagnostic criteria for PWS. Recently, Dykens *(37)* followed up these impressions with three studies of jigsaw puzzle skills in children and adults with PWS.

Compared to others with mental retardation, children and adolescents with PWS scored significantly higher on standardized visual–spatial tests, and on 40-piece jigsaw puzzles. Indeed, youngsters with PWS placed, on average, more than 15 times as many puzzle pieces as their counterparts. Compared to age-matched normal children, children with PWS scored lower on the standardized tasks (e.g., Block Design, Triangles, VMI). However, they far *outperformed* them on the jigsaw puzzles, correctly placing more than twice as many pieces as the normal group with average IQs *(37)*.

Jigsaw puzzle findings resemble so-called "splinter-skills," that is, skills that are outside the person's general intellectual level, but would not be considered remarkable or extraordinary in the absence of mental retardation *(41)*. Many splinter skills are seen in persons with autism, especially in their elevated performances on visual–spatial and pattern recognition tasks, for example, Block Design, Object Assembly, and Imbedded Familiar Figures *(42,43)*. Although formal studies are lacking, many persons with autism also reportedly excel at jigsaw puzzles. Such observations are particularly intriguing in light of recent connections between autism and chromosome 15 anomalies, including maternally derived cases of isodicentric 15, which includes the Prader–Willi region at 15q11 *(44,45)*.

4.3. Genotype-Phenotype Relations: Cognitive Functioning

Although further studies are needed, some of the cognitive features in PWS appear to differ across cases with paternal deletions compared to those with maternal UPD. Comparing 23 persons with 15q11–13 deletions and 23 age- and gender-matched individuals with UPD, Dykens, Cassidy, and King *(46)* found significantly higher overall IQ scores in the UPD group (mean IQ score of 71 vs 63, respectively). Roof et al. *(47)* found elevated Verbal IQ scores in a group of 14 persons with UPD compared to 24 with deletions. However, they found no difference in Performance IQ scores between the two groups. Further, many individuals with UPD showed a reduced capacity to discriminate forms that required the use of stereoscopic vision *(48)*.

Such findings are consistent with preliminary data showing poor performances on standardized visual–spatial tasks and jigsaw puzzles in persons with UPD as opposed to those with deletions *(37)*. Specifically, individuals with deletions scored significantly higher on standardized visual–spatial tasks such as Object Assembly and the Visual–Motor Integration Task, as well as on jigsaw puzzles. Indeed those with deletions correctly placed an average of 30 pieces in a 3-min time period, compared with an average of four puzzle pieces by those with UPD.

Thus, compared to those with paternal deletions, those with maternal UPD may have poorer visual and/or visual–spatial processing abilities, albeit slightly spared verbal skills (*see* Table 3). The genetic mechanisms for these phenotypic differences across subtypes remain unknown. Possible explanations include incomplete or leaky imprinting (leading to a partial or low level of genes in two doses in UPD cases but only one dose in deletion cases); haploinsufficiency of nonimprinted genes in cases with paternal deletions; or an overexpression of some gene(s) in persons with maternal UPD (*19*).

4.4. Cognitive Trajectories

An early study of eight children with PWS reported that IQ declines in early childhood (*50*). It was unclear, however, if these declined were assessed by formal IQ tests or by a failure to achieve developmental milestones. Using standardized IQ scores, Dykens et al. (*33*) conducted both cross-sectional and longitudinal analyses of IQ change in children and adults. IQ scores were cross-sectionally examined in 21 adolescents and adults, and longitudinal analyses included 31 subjects aged 5–30 years who had been given the same IQ test twice. IQ scores showed nonsignificant fluctuations in both cross-sectional and longitudinal analyses, with no evidence of IQ declines in childhood or early adulthood. We again found stable IQ scores in 20 children tested 2 years apart (Dykens, *unpublished data*) with the Kaufman Brief Intelligence Test (*51*). At an average age of 10.83 years, these children evidenced an average initial IQ score of 63. At 12.97 years, their mean retest IQ score was 65.

Although longitudinal studies of very young children or older adults have yet to be done, overall IQ scores appear relatively stable in school-age children and young adults with PWS. Further longitudinal work is needed to corroborate whether the trajectory is, in fact, stable, as it differs from the trajectories of intelligence seen in some other genetic syndromes, such as Down syndrome (*52*) or fragile X syndrome (*52–54*).

4.5. Linguistic Functioning

Language is a relatively unexplored aspect of the PWS behavioral phenotype. However, studies to date find no distinctive linguistic profile. Branson (*55*) found no common features in the language profiles of 21 children with PWS. On the other hand, although Kleppe et al. (*56*) found a variety of linguistic profiles in 18 children, they did find some common speech–language characteristics. These included hypernasality, errors with certain speech sounds and complex syntax, and reduced vocabulary skills relative to age expectations. More recent work validates these early observations, underscoring the high-pitched, nasal speech qualities of many with the syndrome, as well as the lack of strengths or weaknesses in grammar, vocabulary, or language comprehension *(57)*.

Lewis et al. *(58)* studied 55 people with PWS 0.5–42 years of age using standardized testing and spontaneous speech sample analysis. Although great variability was noted in speech and language abilities, most subjects presented with speech sound errors characterized by imprecise articulation (85%) and oral–motor difficulties (91%). Hypernasality was noted in 62% and hyponasality in 14%. Other speech characteristics included a slow speaking rate, flat intonation patterns, abnormal pitch of the voice, and harsh/hoarse voice quality. Narrative retelling abilities were poor, with specific deficits in sequencing of story events.

Speech and articulation difficulties are likely associated with hypotonia, and perhaps thick, viscous saliva *(56)*. Speech problems, primarily those associated with articulation and intelligibility, were also noted by 33 out of 43 parents of children with PWS aged 4–19 years *(59)*. In addition, parents report that individuals with PWS often talk excessively and perseverate verbally on a narrow range of topics *(60)*. It remains unknown, however, how preservation relates to linguistic features such as pragmatics, discourse, and the social uses of language.

4.6. Range and Severity of Maladaptive Behavior

Behavioral problems associated with PWS are so salient that they earned a place as a minor diagnostic criterion in the consensus clinical criteria for the disorder *(2)*. These behaviors reach clinically significant levels in as many as 72–85% of children and adolescents *(59,61)*. Table 4 depicts salient problems in 100 persons with PWS aged 4–46 years, as assessed by the Child Behavior Checklist *(62)*. In addition to food-related difficulties, we find high rates of tantrums, impulsivity, stubbornness, arguing with others, disobedience, stealing food or money to buy food, lability, skin-picking, compulsions, withdrawal, and anxiety. Other groups also find a similar range and frequency of behavior problems in persons with PWS *(63)*. From these and other studies, behavior problems can generally be clustered into three groups: overeating and food issues; obsessive–compulsive symptoms; and other psychopathologies such as lack of impulse control, affective disorders, and psychosis.

4.6.1. Overeating and Food Issues

Hyperphagia in PWS appears to stem from an impaired satiety response *(64)*. Although its etiology is unknown, recent data implicate anomalies in a

Table 4
Percentage of 100 Subjects with Prader–Willi Syndrome aged 4–46 years Showing Salient Maladaptive Behaviors on the Child Behavior Checklist

Overeats	98
Skin-picking	97
Stubborn	95
Obsessions	94
Tantrums	88
Disobedient	78
Impulsive	76
Labile	76
Excessive sleep	75
Talks too much	74
Compulsions	71
Anxious, worried	70
Prefers being alone	67
Gets teased a lot	65
Peers don't like	60
Hoards	55
Steals (food, money for food)	54
Withdrawn	53
Unhappy, sad	51

specific set of oxytocin-secreting neurons in the paraventicular nucleus of the hypothalamus. It is thought that these neurons are related to satiety *(65)*.

More specifically, persons with PWS seem to have significant delays in their satiety responses. Holland et al. *(64)* found that when given free access to food, most of the 13 adult subjects they studied eventually indicated that they were full, but at a much later time than controls, and only after eating very large amounts of food. In addition, these subjects with PWS stated that they were hungry again much sooner than normal controls.

Such observations have led to questions of whether persons with PWS are so hungry that they eat indiscriminately. As with others in the general population, however, people with PWS have distinct food preferences. Although early studies found a preference for sweet foods *(66,67)*, more recent investigations find that persons with PWS prefer high-carbohydrate foods. This preference is distinct from normal or obese controls *(68)*. Morever, although some individuals with the syndrome "just eat," others have certain rituals or rules that govern their eating *(60)*. Examples of rituals include eating all of one food type before moving onto the next, based on color (e.g., all green food first, then brown); texture (e.g., hardest to softest); caloric content (e.g., highest to lowest); type (e.g., meat followed by vegetables); or desirability (most to least preferred). Some individuals need to have their food cut or served in particular ways, or their utensils arranged in "just the right spot" before eating.

Yet food preferences or rituals do not necessarily prevent many with the syndrome from making poor food choices, such as eating food from the floor or garbage can, or eating unusual or unpalatable items, such as frozen meat or pet food. Dykens *(69)* recently administered food choice pictures and tasks to 50 adults with PWS and to controls with and without mental retardation. Most adults with PWS had similar understanding as normal controls about the fate and purpose of food. Despite these well developed perceptions, subjects with PWS were more likely than either comparison group to endorse eating contaminated food (e.g., cake with bug), or unusual food combinations (e.g., pizza with chocolate sauce). All subjects rejected non-food substances when they were presented alone, but some were willing to eat inedible substances when they were paired with a desired food. To date, medications have not been successful in curbing the drive for food in persons with PWS, especially over the long term. As such, treatment regimens emphasize behavioral interventions, for example, low-calorie diets, exercise, restricted access to food, and close supervision around food and spending money *(70)*. These interventions meet with variable but generally good success.

4.6.2. Obsessions and Compulsions

Most people with PWS are "obsessed" about food to varying degrees, but the majority also show a host of compulsive behaviors related to activities other than food. Having examined 91 children and adults, Dykens et al. *(60)* found high rates of specific symptoms on the Yale–Brown Obsessive–Compulsive Scale *(71)*. These included hoarding (e.g., toiletries, paper, pens); ordering and arranging items by color, shape, or size, or until they were "just right"; needing to tell or say things (e.g., repeated questioning); and being concerned with symmetry or exactness. Other obsessive–compulsive disorder (OCD)-related activities involve repeating tasks over and over (e.g., tying and untying shoes, rewriting homework, recutting coupons until the lines were perfect). For 45–80% of the sample, these symptoms were time consuming, distressful, or caused adaptive impairment, suggesting high rates of full-blown OCD. Although the exact prevalence of OCD in the Prader–Willi population is unknown, rates are likely to be many times higher than the 1–3% of persons with heterogeneous mental retardation and comorbid OCD *(72,73)*. Indeed, compared to nonretarded patients with OCD, adults with PWS had similar numbers of compulsions, as well as levels of severity of compulsive symptoms *(74)*.

Compulsive features in PWS are elevated compared to others with mental retardation, as shown in Table 5. Compared to those with Down syndrome, Smith-Magenis syndrome, Williams syndrome, or nonsyndromal mental retardation, individuals with PWS show higher rates of compulsive symptoms such as hoarding, repetitive rituals, talking too much, and skin picking *(59,75)*. Of these, skin picking seems the most prevalent. This behavior typically starts in early childhood *(76)*, and can be severe, with the face and legs the most common targets *(77)*.

Skin-picking and compulsivity are also elevated in PWS relative to a particularly powerful contrast group of "Prader–Willi-like patients" *(78)*. These individuals had clinical diagnoses of PWS, including mental retardation, obesity, food preoccupations, and salient behavioral problems. However, on DNA testing, they failed to show the Prader–Willi genotype. When eight "Prader–Willi-like" individuals were compared to age- and sex-matched patients with PWS due to paternal deletion, both groups exhibited similar IQ scores, degrees of obesity, and maladaptive behavior scores. On the other hand, subjects with PWS expressed an average of 6.25 symptoms on the Y-BOCS, while the Prader–Willi-like cases had a mean of 1.37 symptoms. Similar patterns were found in Y-BOCS symptom severity scores. Obsessive–compulsive symptoms cannot therefore be explained by mental retardation, obesity, or behavioral disturbance. Instead, they appear to be intrinsic to the Prader–Willi genotype.

The pathogenesis of PWS thus appears to predispose many individuals to obsessive–compulsive behavior, if not full-blown OCD. It may be that the Prader–Willi critical region on chromosome 15 is associated with some forms of OCD in the general population, especially those cases characterized by hoarding, and concerns with symmetry or exactness. Findings also bring advances in understanding and treating OCD to PWS. For example, as with those who are diagnosed with OCD, several case studies report that specific serotonin reuptake inhibitors (SSRIs) have helped some individuals with PWS gain better control of compulsive symptoms, including skin-picking *(79–82)*. Others, however, find that medications do not generally help with skin-picking over the long term *(83)*. Although SSRI usage is currently popular in the PWS community, controlled studies have not been published.

Understandings of the possible mechanisms in OCD may also prove helpful in PWS. Patients with non-tic-related OCD, for example, show elevated levels of cerebrospinal fluid oxytocin compared to normal controls *(84)*. Oxytocin is a neuropeptide implicated in a host of normative behaviors, such as grooming, aggression, appetite regulation, attachment, and reproduction

Table 5
Compulsive Symptoms on the Y-BOCS in Persons with PWS and Various Comparison Groups

Y-BOCS	PWS		Williams		Down		Mixed MR		PWS-Like		Normal	
	M	SD	M	SD	M	SD	M	SD	M	SD	M	SD
Number	6.14	(5.14)	2.02	(1.91)	1.27	(1.90)	2.08	(1.20)	1.37	(1.41)	1.27	(1.20)
Severity	3.89	(2.83)	1.63	(1.65)	1.16	(1.36)	1.80	(1.21)	1.87	(2.29)	.39	(.85)

PWS $n = 43$; Williams syndrome $n = 61$; Down syndrome $n = 43$; mixed mental retardation $n = 43$; PWS-Like $n = 8$; normal $n = 22$. PWS scored significantly higher than all comparison groups.

(84). Decreased oxytocin secreting neurons have been identified in the hypothalamic paraventricular nucleus of several Prader–Willi patients *(65)*, as well as in mice deficient in one of the imprinted genes in the Prader–Willi critical region, *Necdin (12)*. Compared to normal controls, high levels of cerebrospinal fluid oxytocin were recently found in five individuals with PWS *(85)*. Although the mechanisms are unclear, aberrant levels of oxytocin were seen in both studies. These anomalies may possibly mediate some of the compulsive features in PWS, and perhaps other behaviors as well.

4.6.3. Other Maladaptive and Psychiatric Vulnerabilities

In addition to food-related and obsessive–compulsive behaviors, other problems may also occur with increased frequency in persons with PWS. These include impulse control, psychotic, and affective disorders. Although temper tantrums, aggression, and stubbornness are common, their severity levels vary widely. We found temper tantrums in 88% of 100 individuals with PWS *(see* Table 4), while 42% engaged in property destruction and 34% physically attacked others. Some parents thus report mild tantrums and a "stubborn streak," while others report extreme rage reactions and property destruction. Often, the more extreme of these symptoms decline with age, but temper tantrums and stubbornness may not *(86)*. Further research needs to examine the extent to tantrums are associated with the beginning of hyperphagia in childhood, as well as the possible reasons for such wide variability in aggressive symptoms.

Many recent reports suggest a stronger than expected association between PWS and atypical psychosis. There are now published case studies of young adults with PWS and acute psychotic episodes *(87–91)*. Many of these episodes occurred suddenly, and were characterized more by depression than schizophrenia. Although many individuals responded well to pharmacotherapy and hospitalization, several showed vulnerabilities for disorganized thinking or behavior that persisted for years.

Many reports of single cases may be misleading in that collectively they convey an overall impression of a stronger association than may actually be observed *(92)*. Case reports notwithstanding, Clarke *(93)* administered a checklist to parents of 95 adults with PWS and found that 6.3% showed psychotic symptoms in the previous month. Stein and colleagues *(94)* also administered a parental report and noted visual or auditory hallucinations in 12.1% of 347 persons with PWS. These rates are high even relative to other persons with mental retardation, and underscore the need for future research on possible associations between PWS and psychosis, especially in young adulthood.

Finally, depressive features such as sadness and low self-esteem, as well as anxiety and worries, have been noted in various behavioral studies in PWS *(61,86,94,95)*. Examining Table 4, for example, 51–53% were unhappy, sad, or withdrawn, and 67% preferred being alone. Dykens and Cassidy *(61)* found that advancing age in children with PWS aged 4–12 years was correlated with heightened internal distress and features of depression, including withdrawal, isolation, negative self-image, and pessimism. Among adults with PWS, Beardsmore et al. *(87)* found that 17.4% of 25 young adults residing in the same county in the United Kingdom met formal criteria for affective disorders, all with psychotic components. Symptoms of sadness and withdrawal seem more prevalent than full-blown affective disorder, and future work is needed to identify those factors that predispose some individuals to develop more severe psychopathology.

In contrast to increased risks of OCD, impulse control, and perhaps psychotic and affective disorders, certain psychiatric disorders seem relatively infrequent in those with PWS. Even though many people with PWS steal food and are impulsive and distractible, rates for full-blown conduct disorder or ADHD seem low. In contrast to those with other disorders, for example, Williams syndrome, fears or phobic disorders are infrequent in PWS *(87)*. Although formal studies are lacking, we have yet to clinically observe persons with PWS with co-morbid tic disorders or dementia.

4.6.4. Genotype–Phenotype Relationships: Maladaptive Behavior

Individuals with PWS due to maternal UPD vs paternal deletion may show differences in the frequency or severity of some maladaptive behaviors (*see* Table 3). One set of findings suggest that persons with maternal UPD are somewhat spared, showing less frequent or severe problems than deleted cases. Dykens et al. *(46)* compared 23 age and gender matched persons with UPD to 23 cases with deletions. Compared to persons with UPD, those with paternal deletions showed higher maladaptive behavior scores on the CBCL, more clinically significant levels of CBCL maladaptive behavior, and more distress related to compulsive symptoms on the Y-BOCS. We observed many more individuals with deletions were withdrawn and overate, hoarded, bit their nails, sulked, and picked their skin. Symons et al. *(77)* also found that skin picking was more frequent among those with deletions as opposed to UPD.

In contrast, other data suggest increased risks of more severe psychopathology in persons with maternal UPD. In particular, findings from a population-based study in the United Kingdom, *(96)* and a longitudinal project in Belgium *(97)* suggest that increased rates of psychosis are found in cases with maternal UPD as opposed to those individuals with deletions. Holland et al. *(96)* screened eight counties in the United Kingdom and found five cases of young adults with psychosis, all of whom were diagnosed with maternal UPD. Similarly, Descheemaeker et al. *(97)* did a retrospective chart review of 59 persons followed over 15 years, and found that 6 developed psychosis; 5 had maternal UPD and 1 had an imprinting center mutation. Four of these six persons had autistic spectrum diagnoses in their childhood years. Although rates of autism or autistic traits in PWS are unknown, such diagnoses need further evaluation, especially in light recent connections between autism and maternally derived inverted duplications that involve the 15q11 region *(45,98)*.

Although contradictory, both sets of findings regarding maternal UPD cases may be accurate. Persons with PWS due to maternal UPD may, as a group, show fewer or less severe behavioral problems. However, there may also be a subgroup of those with maternal UPD who show more severe psychopathology, including autistic traits in childhood, and/or are prone to psychosis in young adulthood. It remains unknown why a subgroup of those with UPD might be prone to more serious psychopathology.

5. ANGELMAN SYNDROME: *COGNITION AND BEHAVIOR*

5.1. Cognition and Language

Persons with AS typically show severe levels of delay. However, studies have not documented these delays using standardized psychological testing. Indeed, many individuals are deemed "untestable," in part owing to their inattention and lack of speech. Recently, several psychometrically sound measures have been developed that can assess nonverbal intelligence and prelinguistic communication. Penner et al. *(99)* administered some of these measures to seven institutionalized adults with AS. Using a series of Piagetian tasks, they found that four subjects scored at sensory–motor stage 2, two at stage 3, and one at stage 5–6. For all subjects, their use of objects or means ends were better developed than their vocal and gestural imitation skills. None of these seven individuals engaged in imitative vocalizations or spontaneous speech-like babbling, as would be expected at this stage of development, and instead produced single-sound, open-mouth vowel-like sounds. As participants were also unable to imitate mouth motor acts, the researchers suggested that AS involves an oral–motor or developmental verbal dyspraxia. Further, six of seven subjects did not show joint attention, joint action on an object, or turn-taking; all of these are prerequisite skills for successful social interaction.

Additional developmental studies are needed, especially with children who have received benefit of early intervention, which may have not been the case with Penner et al.'s *(99)* older, institutionalized sample. Although many individuals seem to show unfocused, non-goal-related actions, and a lack of sustained attention to others, others show some babbling, use of gestures, turn-taking, and relatively well developed receptive language skills *(100,101)*. For example, 73 of 82 persons (90%) with AS used some type of signing or gesturing, but only 20% could be taught standardized sign language *(100,101)*. While 30% had no expressive vocabulary, most subjects had from one to three words. It is unknown how or if variations in developmental levels or skills are associated with age, early intervention, or genetic subtypes of this disorder.

5.2. Maladaptive Behavior and Neurological Findings

Beginning with Harry Angelman's first observations, data have been remarkably consistent in describing the behavior of persons with AS (*see* Table 2). Speech delays are salient, as are inappropriate laughter or bouts of laughter unrelated to context; mouthing objects; problems falling or staying asleep; feeding problems during infancy; motoric hyperactivity and inattention; and stereotypies such as hand-flapping or twirling *(102,103)*.

Although temper tantrums were noted in 45% of 11 children with AS *(102)*, tantrums and irritability were significantly lower among 27 children with AS compared to age- and IQ-matched controls *(103)*. Children with AS in this study were also less likely than controls to show social withdrawal; such findings are consistent with long-noted clinical observations of a happy disposition, marked by frequent smiling.

Anecdotally, family reports of persons with the AS indicate that they love to play with water, as well as with shiny objects such as mirrors or plastic, and musical toys or objects that make loud sounds *(101)*. These preoccupations are also seen in others with mental retardation, including those with autism and 5p- syndrome, but it is not known if they occur more frequently in individuals with AS compared to these or other groups.

The seizure disorder associated with AS is fairly well described. Many persons with the disorder show a similar pattern of abnormal EEG findings involving large amplitude slow-spike waves *(104)*. Seizures are not typically seen before 1 year of age, with most persons showing onset after age 3 years *(105)*. For many children with AS, seizures are initially severe and hard to control, but they often become less severe and more manageable over the course of development *(105)*. Many individuals who show improvement in their seizure disorders exhibit less frequent or severe involvement, and a subsiding of abnormal EEG patterns *(106)*. Laan and colleagues *(107)*, however, found that 82% of their sample of 28 adults with AS still manifested regular seizure activity. Others have identified patients who have a more variable course, showing periods of inactivity or "silence," followed by a sudden reemergence of hard-to-control seizure *(106,108)*. Diagnosis and treatment of seizures may be complicated by the ataxic gait and tremulous arm and leg movements shown by most individuals with the disorder.

Some of the syndrome's characteristic behavioral and neurological features may change over time. Hyperactivity may diminish with age, and persons may also calm down and show less sleep disturbance as they get older *(101,106)*. Unsteady gait, happy demeanor, bouts of laughter, and smiling seem to persist, yet adults may have a less excitable overall presentation, including fewer bouts of laughter *(107,108)*.

Seizures notwithstanding, most adults enjoy good general physical health, suggesting the possibility of near-normal life expectancies *(106)*. Compared to children, however, adults with AS may show increased risks of scoliosis, as well as decreased motility and greater need for wheelchair use *(106,107)*. To avoid contractures and other problems, many recommend that adults with AS be kept active and mobile for as along as possible *(101,105,106,108)*. In this vein, many adults perform basic dressing, toileting, and feeding tasks. As many as 85% of 28 institutionalized adults in Laan et al.'s *(107)* study used a fork and spoon and made their wants and needs known, 80% used gestures and followed simple commands, and 50–60% undressed themselves and had achieved daytime continence. Though rates of these skills may vary among younger or noninstitutionalized persons, most persons with the disorder require close, long-term supervision and care.

6. FUTURE RESEARCH DIRECTIONS

Mouse models of PWS and AS may provide important clues concerning the involvement of specific genes within the 15q11–13 region that cause specific components of these two disorders. In addition, they may serve an important role in identifying effective treatments. Yet even as researchers aim to understand better the function of specific genes in the Prader–Willi/Angelman critical region, families of affected individuals are clamoring for an additional and equally demanding research agenda that focuses on treatment outcomes. Parents and practitioners alike are asking for improved intervention and outcome studies. In PWS these include studies that evaluate the efficacy of psychotropic medications, appetite suppressants, and behavioral programming. Further, while behavioral researchers in PWS have understandably focused on urgent behavioral and emotional problems, of equal importance are studies that assess the relative strengths of affected individuals in personality and cognition, and how such strengths might offset elevated risks for specific problems.

In AS, the treatment of certain problems such as seizure disorders has received considerable attention. Yet virtually no studies have been done that carefully assess profiles of strength and weakness in cognitive or linguistic functioning using newly developed tools. For example, studies might assess how persons with AS fare on certain tasks assessing nonverbal prerequisites of communication, such as joint attention or gesturing. These data, in turn, might lead to treatment studies on how persons fare in intervention programs designed to augment and teach joint attention and other skills. Further, such findings may differ across genetic subtypes of AS. In both PWS and AS, then, studies are sorely needed that link genetic and behavioral findings, and that use such findings to optimize the day-to-day life for persons with these syndromes and their families.

REFERENCES

1. Prader A, Labhart A, Willi A. Ein syndrom von aidositas, kleinwuchs, kryptorchismus und oligophrenie nach myotonieartigem zustand im neugeborenenalter. Schweiz Med Wochenschr 1956;86:1260–1.
2. Holm VA, Cassidy SB, Butler MG, et al. Prader–Willi syndrome: consensus diagnostic criteria. Pediatrics 1993;91:398–402.
3. Angelman H. "Puppet" children: a report of three cases. Dev Med Child Neurol 1965;7:681–8.
4. Ledbetter DH, Riccardi VM, Airhart SD, Strobel RJ, Keenen SB, Crawford JD. Deletion of chromosome 15 as a cause of PWS. N Engl J Med 1981;304:325–9.
5. Butler MG. Prader–Willi syndrome: current understanding of cause and diagnosis. Am J Med Genet 1990;35:319–32.
6. Nicholls RD, Knoll JH, Butler MG, Karam S, Lalande M. Genetic imprinting suggested by maternal heterodisomy in nondeletion Prader–Willi syndrome. Nature 1989;16:281–5.
7. Nicholls RD. Genomic imprinting and uniparental disomy in Angelman and Prader–Willi syndrome: a review. Am J Med Genet 1993;46:16–25.
8. Buiting K, Saitoh S, Gross S, et al. Inherited microdeletions in the Angelman and Prader–Willi syndromes define an imprinting centre on human chromosome 15. Nat Genet 1994;9:395–400.
9. Saitoh S, Buiting K, Cassidy SB, et al. Clinical spectrum and molecular diagnosis of Angelman and Prader–Willi syndrome imprinting mutation patients. Am J Med Genet 1997;68:195–206.
10. Glenn CC, Saitoh S, Jong MT, et al. Gene structure, DNA methylation and imprinted expression of the SRNPN gene. Am J Hum Genet 1996;58:225–346.
11. Ozcelik T, Leff S, Robinson W, et al. Small nuclear ribonucleoprotein polypeptide N (SNRPN), an expressed gene in the PWS critical region. Nat Genet 1992;2:265–9.

12. Muscatelli F, Abrous DN, Massacrier A, et al. Disruption of the mouse Necdin gene results in hypothalamic and behavioral alterations reminiscent of the human Prader–Willi syndrome. Hum Mol Genet 2000;9:3101–10.

13. Butler MG. Hypopigmentation: a common features of Prader–Willi syndrome. Am J Hum Genet 1989;45:140–6.

14. Cassidy SB, Forsythe M, Heeger S, et al. Comparison of phenotype between patients with Prader–Willi syndrome due to deletion 15q and uniparental disomy 15. Am J Med Genet 1997;68:433–40.

15. Gillessen-Kaesbach G, Robinson W, Lohmann D, Kaya Westerloh S, Passarge E, Horsthemke B. Genotype–phenotype correlation in a series of 167 deletion and non-deletion patients with Prader–Willi syndrome. Hum Genet 1995;96:638–43.

16. Mitchell J, Schinzel A, Langlois S, et al. Comparison of phenotype in uniparental disomy and deletion Prader–Willi syndrome: sex specific differences. Am J Med Genet 1996;65:133–6.

17. Rinchik EMK, Bultman SJ, Horsthemke B, et al. A gene for the mouse pinkeye dilution locus and for human type II oculocuteaneous albinism. Nature 1993;361:72–6.

18. Gunay-Aygun M, Heeger S, Schwartz S, Cassidy SB. Delayed diagnosis in Prader–Willi syndrome due to uniparental disomy. Am J Med Genet 1997;71:106–10.

19. Robinson WP, Bernasconi F, Mutiranguara A, et al. Non-disjunction of chromosome 15: Origin and recombination. Am J Hum Genet 1993;53:740–51.

20. Chan CT, Clayton-Smith J, Cheng XJ, et al. Molecular mechanisms in the Angelman syndrome: a survey of 93 patients. J Med Genet 1993;30:895–902.

21. Kishino T, Lalande M, Wagstaff J. UBE3A/E6-AP mutations cause Angelman syndrome. Nat Genet 1997;15:70–3.

22. Matsuura T, Sutcliffe JS, Fang P, et al. De novo truncation mutations in E6-AP ubinquitin-protein ligase gene (UBE3A) in Angelman syndrome. Nat Genet 1997;15:74–7.

23. Albrecht U, Sutcliffe JS, Cattanach BM, et al. Imprinted expression of the murine Angelman syndrome gene, ube3a, in hippocampal and Purkinje neurons. Nat Genet 1997;17:75–8.

24. Olsen RW, Avoli M. GABA and epileptogenesis. Epilepsia 1997;38:399–407.

25. DeLorey TM, Handforth A, Anagnostaras SG, et al. Mice lacking the B_3 subunit of the $GABA_A$ receptor have the epilepsy phenotype and many of the behavioral characteristics of Angelman syndrome. J Neurosci 1998;18:8505–14.

26. Smith A, Wiles C, Haan E, et al. Clinical features in 27 patients with Angelman syndrome resulting from DNA deletion. J Med Genet 1996;22:107–12.

27. Bottani A, Robinson WP, DeLozier-Blanchet CD, et al. Angelman syndrome due to paternal uniparental disomy of chromosome 15: a milder phenotype? Am J Med Genet 1994;51:35–40.

28. Gillessen-Kaesbach G, Albrecht B, Passarge E, Horsthemke B. Further patient with Angelman syndrome due to paternal disomy of chromosome 15 and a milder phenotype (letter). Am J Med Genet 1995;56:328–9.

29. Smith A, Marks R, Haan E, Dixon J, Trent RJ. Clinical features in four patients with Angelman syndrome resulting from paternal uinparental disomy. J Med Genet 1997;34:426–9.
30. Smith A, Robson L, Buchholz B. Normal growth in Angelman syndrome due to paternal UPD. Clin Genet 1998;53:223–5.
31. Burger J, Kunze J, Sperliing K, Reis A. Phenotypic differences in Angelman syndrome patients: imprinting mutations show less frequently microcephaly and hypopigmentation than deletions. Am J Med Genet 1996;66:221–6.
32. Minassian BA, Delorey TM, Olsen RW, et al. Angelman syndrome: correlations between epilepsy phenotypes and genotypes. Ann Neurol 1998;43:485–93.
33. Dykens EM, Hodapp RM, Walsh KK, Nash L. Profiles, correlates, and trajectories of intelligence in Prader–Willi syndrome. J Acad Child Adolesc Psychiatry 1992;31:1125–30.
34. Curfs LMG. Psychological profile and behavioral characteristics in Prader–Willi syndrome. In: Cassidy SB, ed. Prader–Willi syndrome and other 15q deletion disorders. Berlin: Springer-Verlag, 1992;211–222.
35. Curfs LG, Wiegers AM, Sommers JR, Borghgraef M, Fryns JP. Strengths and weaknesses in the cognitive profile of youngsters with Prader–Willi syndrome. Clin Genet 1991;40:430–4.
36. Taylor RL. Cognitive and behavioral features. In: Caldwell ML., Taylor RL, eds. Prader–Willi syndrome: selected research and management issues. New York: Springer-Verlag, 1988;29–42.
37. Dykens EM. Are jigsaw puzzle skills "spared" in persons with Prader–Willi syndrome? J Child Psychol Psychiatry Allied Discip 2002;43:343–52.
38. Kaufman AS, Kaufman NL. Kaufman Assessment Battery for Children. Circle Pines, MN: American Guidance Service, 1983.
39. Gabel S, Tarter RE, Gavaler J, Golden W, Hegedus AM, Mair B. Neuropsychological capacity of Prader–Willi children: general and specific aspects of impairment. App Res Ment Retard 1986;7:459–66.
40. Baker HJ, Leland B. Detroit Tests of Learning Aptitude. Indianapolis, IN: Bobbs-Merrill, 1967.
41. Nettelbeck T. Savant syndrome-rhyme without reason. In: Anderson M, ed. The development of intelligence. East Sussex: Psychology Press, 1999; 247–274.
42. Shah, A, Frith U. An islet of ability in autistic children: a research note. J Child Psychol Psychiatry, 1983;24:613–20.
43. Jolliffe T, Baron-Cohen S. Are people with Asperger syndrome faster that normal on the Imbedded Figures Test? J Child Psychol Psychiatry 1997; 38:527–34.
44. Martin ER, Menold MM, Wolpert CM, et al. Analysis of linkage disequilibrium in gamma-amniobutyric acid receptor subunit genes in autistic disorder. Am J Med Genet 2000;96:43–8.
45. Wolpert, C, Menold, MM, Bass, MP, et al. Three probands with autistic disorder and isodicentric chromosome 15. Am J Med Genet 2000;96:365–72.
46. Dykens EM, Cassidy SB, King BH. Maladaptive behavior differences in Prader–Willi syndrome due to paternal deletion versus maternal uniparental disomy. Am J Ment Retard 1999;104:67–77.

47. Roof E, Stone W, MacLean W, Feurer ID, Thompson T, Butler MG. Intellectual characteristics of Prader–Willi syndrome: comparison of genetic subtypes. J Intell Disab Res 2000;44:25–30.

48. Roof E, Fox R, Feurer ID, et al. Visual perception in Prader–Willi syndrome. Paper presented to the 14th Annual Prader–Willi Syndrome Conference, San Diego, CA, July, 1999.

49. Cassidy SB, Dykens EM, Williams CA. Prader–Willi and Angelman syndromes: sister imprinted disorders. Am J Med Genet 2000;97:136–46.

50. Dunn HG. The Prader–Labhart–Willi syndrome: review of the literature and report of nine cases. Acta Paediatr Scand 1968;186:1–38.

51. Kaufman AS, Kaufman NL. Kaufman Brief Intelligence Test. Circle Pines, MN: American Guidance Service, 1990.

52. Hodapp RM, Zigler E. Applying the developmental perspective to children with Down syndrome. In: Cicchetti D, Beeghly M, eds. Children with Down syndrome: a developmental perspective. New York: Cambridge University Press, 1990;1–28.

53. Dykens EM, Hodapp RM, Leckman JF. Behavior and development in fragile X syndrome. Thousand Oaks, CA: Sage, 1994.

54. Fisch GS, Simensen R, Tarleton J, et al. Longitudinal study of cognitive abilities and adaptive behavior levels in fragile X males: a prospective multicenter analysis. Am J Med Genet 1996;64:356–61.

55. Branson, C. (1981). Speech and language characteristics of children with PWS. In: Holm VA, Sulzbacher S, Pipes P, eds. The Prader–Willi syndrome. Baltimore, MD: University Park Press, 1981;179–83.

56. Kleppe SA, Katayama KM, Shipley KG, Foushee DR. The speech and language characteristics of children with Prader–Willi syndrome. J Speech Hear Disord 1990;55, 300–9.

57. Akefeldt A, Akefeldt B, Gillberg C. Voice, speech and language characteristic of children with Prader–Willi syndrome. J Intell Disab Res 1997;41:302–11.

58. Lewis BA, Freebairn L, Heeger S, Cassidy SB. Speech and language skills of individuals with Prader–Willi syndrome. Am J Speech Lang Pathol, 2002;11:285–94.

59. Dykens EM, Kasari C. Maladaptive behavior in children with Prader–Willi syndrome, Down syndrome, and non-specific mental retardation. Am J Ment Retard 1997;102:228–37.

60. Dykens EM, Leckman JF, Cassidy SB. Obsessions and compulsions in Prader–Willi syndrome. J Child Psychol Psychiatry 1996;37:995–1002.

61. Dykens EM, Cassidy SB. Correlates of maladaptive behavior in children and adults with Prader–Willi syndrome. Am J Med Genet 1995;60:546–9.

62. Achenbach TM. Manual for the Child Behavior Checklist/4-18 and 1991 Profile. Burlington, VT: University of Vermont Department of Psychiatry, 1991.

63. Clarke DJ, Boer H, Chung MC, Sturmey P, Web, T. Maladaptive behavior in PWS in adult life. J Intell Disab Res 1996;40:159–165.

64. Holland AJ, Treasure J, Coskeran P, Dallow J. Characteristics of the eating disorder in Prader–Willi syndrome: implications for treatment. J Intell Disab Res 1995;39:373–81.

65. Swaab DF, Purba JS, Hofman MA. Alterations in the hypothalamic paraventricular nucleus and its oxytocin neurons (putative satiety cells) in Prader–Willi syndrome: A study of 5 cases. J Clin Endocrinol Metab 1995; 80:573–9.

66. Caldwell ML, Taylor RL. A clinical note on the food preference of individuals with Prader–Willi syndrome: the need for empirical research. J Ment Defic 1983;27:45–9.

67 Taylor RL, Caldwell ML. Type and strength of food preferences of individuals with Prader–Willi symndrome. Am J Ment Defic 1985;29:109–12.

68. Fieldstone A, Zipf WB, Schwartz HC, Berntson GG. Food preferences in Prader–Willi syndrome, normal weight, and obese controls. Int J Obes Relat Metab Dis 1997;21:1–7.

69. Dykens EM. Contaminated and unusual food combinations: what do people with Prader–Willi syndrome choose? Ment Retard 2000;38:163–71.

70. Dykens EM, Hodapp RM, Finucane BM. Genetics and mental retardation syndromes: A new look at behavior and interventions. Baltimore, MD: Brookes, 2000.

71. Goodman WK, Price LH, Rasmussen SA, et al. The Yale-Brown Obsessive-Compulsive Scale: development, use and reliability. Arch Gen Psychiatry 1989;46:1006–11.

72. Meyers BA. Psychiatric problems in adolescents with developmental disabilities. J Am Acad Child Adolesc Psychiatry 1987;26:74–9.

73. Vitiello B, Spreat S, Behar D. Obsessive–compulsive disorder in mentally retarded patients. J Nervous Ment Dis 1989;177:232–6.

74. Dykens E, Ort S, Cohen I, et al. Trajectories and profiles of adaptive behavior in males with fragile X syndrome: multicenter studies. J Autism Dev Disord 1996;26:287–301.

75. Dykens EM, Smith ACM. Distinctiveness and correlates of maladaptive behavior in children and adolescents with Smith–Magenis syndrome. J Intell Disab Res 1998;42:481–9.

76. Dimitropoulos A, Feurer I, Thompson T, Butler M. Compulsive behavior and tantrums in children with Prader–Willi syndrome, Down syndrome, and typical development. Presentation to the 14th Annual Prader–Willi Syndrome Scientific Conference, San Diego, CA, July, 1999.

77. Symons FJ, Butler MG, Sanders MD, Feurer ID, Thompson T. Self-injurious behavior and Prader–Willi syndrome: behavioral forms and body locations. Am J Ment Retard 1999;104:260–9.

78. State M, Dykens EM, Rosner B, Martin A, King BH. Obsessive–compulsive symptoms in Prader–Willi and "Prader–Willi-like" patients. J Am Acad Child Adolesc Psychiatry 1999;38:329–34.

79. Benjamin E, Buot-Smith T. Naltroxone and fluoxetinein Prader–Willi syndrome. J Am Acad Child Adolesc Psychiatry 1993;32:870–3.

80. Dech D, Budow L. The use of fluoxetine in an adolescent with Prader–Willi syndrome. J Am Acad Child Adolesc Psychiatry 1991;30:298–302.

81. Hellings JA, Warnock JK. Self-injurious behavior and serotonin in Prader–Willi syndrome. Psychopharmacol Bull 1994;30:245–50.

82. Warnock JK, Kestenbaum T. Pharmacologic treatment of severe skin-picking behaviors in Prader–Willi syndrome. Arch Dermatol 1992;128:1623–5.

83. Hanchett JM. Treatment of self-abusive behavior in Prader–Willi syndrome. Paper presented to the 20th Annual National Prader–Willi Syndrome Association Conference. Columbus, OH, July 1998.

84. Leckman JF, Goodman WK, North WJ, et al. The role of central oxytocin in obsessive compulsive disorder and related normal behavior. Psychoneuroendocrinology 1994;19:723–49.

85. Martin A, State M, Anderson GM, et al. Cerebrospinal fluid levels of oxytocin in PWS: a preliminary report. Biol Psychiatry 1998;44:1349–52.

86. Dykens EM, Hodapp RM, Walsh K, Nash LJ. Adaptive and maladaptive behavior in Prader–Willi syndrome. J Am Acad Child Adolesc Psychiatry 1992;31:1131–6.

87. Beardsmore A, Dorman T, Cooper SA, Webb T. Affective psychosis and Prader–Willi syndrome. J Intell Disab Res 1998;42:463–71.

88. Clarke DJ. Prader–Willi syndrome and psychoses. Br J Psychiatry 1993;163:680–4.

89. Clarke DJ, Boer H, Webb T, et al. Prader–Willi syndrome and psychotic symptoms: 1. Case descriptions and genetic studies. J Intell Disab Res 1998;42:440–50.

90. Clarke DJ, Webb T, Bachmann-Clarke JP. Prader–Willi syndrome and psychotic symptoms: report of a further case. Irish J Psychol Med 1995;12:27–9.

91. Verhoeven WMA, Curfs LMG, Tuinier S. Prader–Willi syndrome and cycloid psychoses. J Intell Disab Res 1998;42:455–62.

92. Rutter M, Bailey A, Bolton P, Le Couteur A. Autism and known medical conditions: myth and substance. J Child Psychol Psychiatry 1994;35:311–22.

93. Clarke DJ. PWS and psychotic symptoms 2. A preliminary study of prevalence using the Psychopathology Assessment Schedule for Adults with Developmental Disability Checklist. J Intell Disab Res 1998;42:451–4.

94. Stein DJ, Keating K, Zar HJ, Hollander E. A survey of the phenomenology and pharmacotherapy of compulsive and impulsive-aggressive symptoms in Prader–Willi syndrome. J Neuropsychiatry Clin Neurosci 6, 23–9.

95. Whitman BY, Accardo P. Emotional problems in Prader–Willi adolescents. Am J Med Genet 1987;28:897–905.

96. Holland T, Whittington J, Webb T, Butler J, Boer H, Clarke D. Findings from a population-based study of Prader–Willi syndrome. Paper presented to the Paper presented at the 4th Triennial International Prader–Willi Syndrome Organisation Scientific Conference, St. Paul, MN, July, 2001.

97. Descheemaeker MJ, Vogels A, Govers V, et al. Prader–Willi syndrome: new insights in the behavioural and psychiatric spectrum. J Intell Disab Res 2002;46:41–50.

98. Schroer RJ, Phelan MC, Michaelis RC, et al. Autism and maternally derived aberrations of chromosome 15. Am J Med Genet 1998;76:327–36.
99. Penner KA, Johnston J, Faircloth BH, Irish P, Williams CA. Communication, cognition, and social interaction in the Angelman syndrome. Am J Med Genet 1993;46:34–9.
100. Williams CA, Zori RT, Hendrickson J, et al. Angelman syndrome. Curr Prob Pediatr 1995;25:216–31.
101. Clayton-Smith J. Clinical research in Angelman syndrome in the United Kingdom: observations on 82 affected individuals. Am J Med Genet 1993;46:12–5.
102. Summers JA, Allison DB, Lynch PS, Sandler L. Behaviour problems in Angelman syndrome. J Intell Disab Res 1995;39:97–106.
103. Summers JA, Feldman MA. Distinctive pattern of behavioral functioning in Angelman syndrome. Am J Ment Retard 1999;104:376–84.
104. Boyd SG, Harden A, Patton MA. The EEG in early diagnosis of the Angelman (happy puppet) syndrome. Eur J Pediatr 1988;147:508–13.
105. Zori RT, Hendrickson J, Woolven S, Whidden EM, Gray B, Williams CA. Angelman syndrome: a clinical profile. J Child Neurol 1992;7:270–80.
106. Bunting IM, Hennekam RCM, Brouwer OF, et al. Clinical profiles of Angelman syndrome at different ages. Am J Med Genet 1995;56:176–83.
107. Laan LAEM, Boer ATD, Hennekam RCM, Reiner WO, Brouwer OF. Angelman syndrome in adulthood. Am J Med Genet 1996;66:356–60.
108. Buckley RH, Dinno N, Weber P. Angelman syndrome: are the estimates too low? Am J Med Genet 1998;80:385–90.

7

Tuberous Sclerosis

Julian R. Sampson and Julia C. Lewis

1. INTRODUCTION

Tuberous sclerosis (TSC) is an autosomal dominant disorder affecting approx 1:10,000 newborns and characterized by hamartias and hamartomas that affect many organs. Its manifestations are highly variable and include seizures, mental retardation, and a range of behavioral problems resulting from involvement of the central nervous system. Manifestations in the kidneys, heart, lungs, and skin are also of major clinical importance. Management should be directed toward early detection and intervention for the medical, developmental, and behavioral complications and the offer of genetic counseling. TSC is caused by mutations that inactivate both alleles of either the *TSC1* or *TSC2* gene by a "two-hit" mechanism. The proteins encoded by *TSC1* and *TSC2* are termed hamartin and tuberin. They interact together directly and play roles in regulating the cell cycle, cell size, and cell differentiation and migration.

2. PREVALENCE AND INHERITANCE

Geographically based surveys suggest that the minimum childhood prevalence of TSC is 1/10,000 to 1/15,000 *(1–3)*. Medical ascertainment is unlikely to be complete, however, and the true prevalence is certainly higher *(4)*. TSC is transmitted as an autosomal dominant trait with very high and probably complete penetrance *(5)*. Sixty to seventy percent of cases are sporadic and appear to represent new mutations, and the mutation rate has been estimated at 2.5×10^{-5} per gamete *(1)*. Even before identification of the *TSC1* and *TSC2* genes, reports of large families in which all affected members had particularly mild disease *(6)* or marked renal disease *(7)* suggested the possibility of genotype–phenotype correlation.

From: *Contemporary Clinical Neuroscience:*
Genetics and Genomics of Neurobehavioral Disorders
Edited by: G. S. Fisch © Humana Press Inc., Totowa, NJ

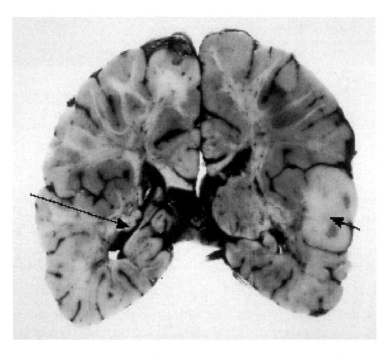

Fig. 1. Gross appearance of the brain in TSC. Coronal section of postmortem brain showing multiple subependymal nodules (*arrow on left*) and cortical tuber (*arrow on right*). (Photograph courtesy of Dr. A. Dean. Reproduced from Sampson JR, Tuberous Sclerosis. In: Scriver, Beaudet, Valle, et al., eds. The Metabolic and Molecular Bases of Inherited Disease, 8th ed. New York: McGraw-Hill. Used with permission.)

3. THE TUBEROUS SCLEROSIS PHENOTYPE

3.1. Central Nervous System

3.1.1. Pathologic and Radiographic Findings

The characteristic lesions in the central nervous system (CNS) are cortical tubers, subependymal nodules, and subependymal giant cell astrocytomas (Fig. 1) *(8)*. Abnormal white matter migration tracts may also be present, sometimes linking subependymal and cortical lesions. Spinal lesions appear to be extremely uncommon. Cranial magnetic nuclear resonance imaging (MRI) reveals a diagnostic combination of pathological changes in the brains of most patients with TSC. Fluid-attenuation inversion recovery (FLAIR) scanning increases sensitivity for the detection of tubers in myelinated brain tissue. A small proportion of patients has normal findings on cranial MRI.

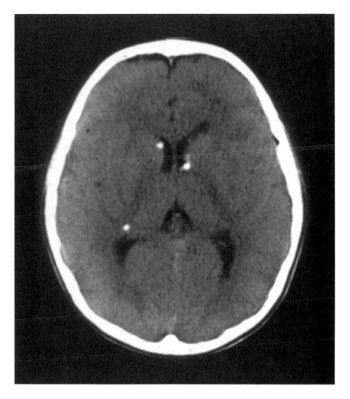

Fig. 2. Cranial computerized tomography in TSC. Axial section showing characteristic calcified subependymal nodules that are seen as three bright signals lying adjacent to the lateral walls of the ventricles.

Cortical tubers are discrete hamartias that exhibit macroscopic loss of normal sulcal and gyral morphology. In a severely affected brain, several dozen distinct lesions may be present, usually asymmetrically distributed. Large lesions may be several centimeters in diameter. Microscopically, tubers show disruption of normal hexalaminar cortical organization with abnormally oriented pyramidal neurons. The presence of abnormally large and dysplastic neuron-like cells and balloon cells is highly characteristic.

Subependymal nodules (SENs) are hamartomatous growths of less than 1 cm in diameter located in the lateral ventricles, or sometimes the aquaduct or fourth ventricle. They frequently calcify, leading to a very characteristic appearance on cranial computerized tomography (CT) scanning (Fig. 2). In some 5–6% of cases larger growths develop and these are classified as subependymal giant cell astrocytomas (SEGAs) (Fig. 3). They are potentially dangerous tumors that appear to arise in SENs, but the mechanism of

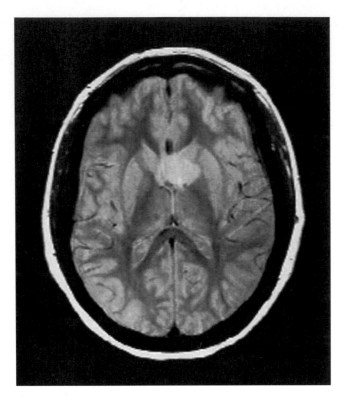

Fig. 3. Subependymal giant cell astrocytoma. T1-weighted magnetic resonance image of axial section of brain showing a hyperintense subependymal giant cell astrocyoma lying in the region of the foramen of Munro.

increased growth is unknown. SEGAs in the region of the foramen of Munro are likely to cause obstructive hydrocephalus and serious neurological problems. Surgical intervention is indicated for symptomatic or growing SEGAs. At a microscopic level, SENs and SEGAs frequently contain cells with heterogeneous morphologies, including spindle-shaped cells and abnormally large cells.

3.1.2. Epilepsy

More than 80% of those with recognized TSC experience seizures. Indeed, epilepsy is the most frequent presenting complaint in childhood. Although presentation with neonatal or even antenatal partial motor seizures is well recognized, onset of infantile spasms at 6 wk or more of age is typical. Initially, seizures may be very subtle and this frequently leads to delay in diagnosis. However, they usually become progressively more obvious and are frequently associated with changes in behavior, particularly loss of interest, failure to interact, reduced smiling, and increased irritability. Some cases have hypsarrhythmic EEGs. Infants and older children may develop partial seizures with or without secondary generalization or generalized seizures of any type except for classical petit mal. However, complex partial seizures are most common.

It is still unclear whether an early onset of seizures, particularly infantile spasms, actually causes CNS damage and contributes to poor neurodevelopmental outcome or whether the two manifestations are merely contemporaneous, each reflecting severe primary CNS involvement *(9,10)*. Because of the possibility of a causal link, prompt control of seizures is a priority. Vigabatrin is the favored drug for treatment of infantile spasms in TSC in Europe *(11,12)*. The association with visual field loss is a significant concern because of the impracticality of monitoring for field loss in the very young or severely handicapped child.

Many older patients with TSC develop several seizure types. Control is often problematic and polypharmacy is common. Exceptionally, intractable seizures can be attributed to one or more discrete epileptogenic foci and surgical treatment may then be considered *(13)*.

3.1.3. Psychological Manifestations

Mental retardation was noted in early descriptions of TSC *(14,15)*. Critchley and Earl *(16)* clearly described autistic symptoms in those with TSC but, as their report antedated the classical description of autism by Kanner *(17)*, the cases were labeled as a primitive form of catatonic schizophrenia. Individual case reports then described a variety of psychological manifestations, but systematic studies were not carried out for many years. Hunt *(18)* performed a postal survey of parents of children with TSC and found that behavioral problems including hyperactivity, aggression, screaming, and temper tantrums were reported in more than half of affected children and represented a major concern for their families. Psychoses *(19,20)*, mania *(21)*, anxiety disorder *(22)*, and sleep disorder *(23)* have all been reported among patients whose mental state could be properly examined (Table 1).

3.1.3.1. MENTAL RETARDATION

Mental retardation is the term favored for description of subnormal intellectual functioning (American Association of Mental Retardation). The term "learning disabilities" is often used in the United Kingdom, but does not have a consistent definition worldwide. The criteria for diagnosis of mental retardation, as specified in the Diagnostic and Statistical Manual of Mental

Table 1
Psychological Problems in TSC

Phenotype	Prevalence	Reference	Details
Intellectual handicap	38%	*24*	Related to early age at seizure onset, infantile spasms and seizure control
Autism	58% 33–86%	*19* *33*	More aloof, less gaze-avoidant and greater variation in IQ than is classical
Hyperactivity	59% (Hyperkinetic) 43% (ADHD)	*19* *41*	Associated with seizures and mental retardation
Anxiety	Unknown	Case reports only	Increased rates reported in individual families
Depression	Unknown	Case reports only	
Psychosis	Unknown	Case reports only	
Mania	Unknown	Case reports only	

Disorders, Fourth Edition (DSM IV), are: significant subaverage intelligence (IQ <70), significant limitations in adaptive functioning, and onset before the age of 18 years (American Psychiatric Association). The frequency of mental retardation in TSC has been estimated in a variety of settings that are likely to have lead to overestimation owing to ascertainment bias *(23)*. Furthermore, studies of intellectual function in TSC have usually not involved formal assessment via the use of well validated tools. Instead they have relied on retrospective data pertaining to educational attainment and the level of independent functioning in society. Attempts to study secondarily ascertained cases or to study geographically based populations suggest that some 40% of cases have mental retardation *(24)*. Two studies have reported a higher frequency of mental retardation in males than in females with TSC *(3,25)*.

Mental retardation in TSC has a well described relationship with seizures. Webb et al. *(3)* found that mental retardation in TSC was almost exclusively seen in patients with seizures and that its frequency was correlated with the age at first seizure, the type of seizure at onset (with the greatest risk for infantile spasms), and with seizure control. Although there is a relationship between infantile spasms and mental retardation in the general population, there appears to be an even stronger association when the infantile spasms occur as part of TSC. Riikonen and Simell *(26)* found that children with TSC and infantile spasms had a poorer long-term intellectual outlook than children with idiopathic infantile spasms or infantile spasms associated with other neurological disorders.

Neuroimaging studies have investigated whether there is a relationship between the number of cerebral lesions and the likelihood of mental retardation. Several MRI-based studies have reported a direct relationship between the number of tubers and the risk of mental retardation *(10,27,28)*. One study found an inverse relationship between the number of tubers and age at onset of seizures and that tuber number also predicted the likelihood of infantile spasms *(10)*. In contrast, others have not identified a relationship between the number of cerebral lesions and presence of mental retardation *(29–31)*. Limitations of study size, the inability of imaging to reveal all functionally significant TSC-associated pathology, and the importance of tuber location *(9,32)* may underlie the apparently conflicting findings of these studies.

3.1.3.2. AUTISM

Autism belongs to a group of disorders known collectively as the pervasive developmental disorders. It is characterized by abnormalities in social interaction, communication and play, and by restricted patterns of interest. Onset is before the age of 3 years. Although autism is associated with several specific diseases of childhood, the strongest association is with TSC. Estimates of the rate of autism in TSC vary considerably and reflect the range of assessment tools and ascertainment methods that have been used. Hunt and Shepherd *(33)* surveyed 300 individuals with TSC and identified a variety of pervasive developmental disorders with frequencies ranging from 33% to 86%.

Autism is associated with infantile spasms but its link with TSC does not appear to be simply a consequence of this. In 1981, Riikonen and Amnell *(34)* studied 192 children with a diagnosis of infantile spasms (from any cause) and, using well established criteria, found that 12.5% had autism. Using the same criteria Hunt and Dennis *(19)* found that 58% of children with TSC and a history of infantile spasms had autism. Hunt and Shepherd *(33)* suggested that the high frequency of autism in TSC pointed to a more fundamental relationship between the disorders. However, there appear to be differences in the symptom profile of autism in those with TSC compared with idiopathic autism. Those with TSC are reported to be more aloof, less gaze-avoidant, and to have a greater variation in IQ than others with autism and some cases have been noted to become less autistic with time *(35)*. It is clear that not all individuals with autism and TSC have mental retardation *(36)*, although it has been suggested that, in nonretarded cases, autistic-like behavior could be a manifestation of social anxiety *(22)*.

Studies of the neuroanatomical correlates of autism in TSC have been small and their findings inconsistent. Jambaqué et al. *(37)* suggested that involvement of the frontal lobe (either via the presence of tubers or epileptic foci) was crucial. They postulated that disruption of the connections between the areas involved in perception-related functions and the anterior cortex could explain the pattern of behavioral problems seen in autism. Others have highlighted the potential importance of lesions of the hippocampus and amygdala *(36,38)* but only on the basis of anecdotal observations. However, a study of 18 children with TSC found a significant association between tubers of the temporal lobe and the presence of autism *(39)*. The authors suggested that effects of the lesions on recognition of facial expression might be involved in development of autism in these cases. A study of brain stem auditory evoked response in patients with TSC and autism identified abnormalities of the N1 component to which temporal lobe pathways contribute *(40)*.

3.1.3.3. HYPERACTIVITY

In ICD10 (the classification system preferred in the United Kingdom), diagnosis of Attention Deficit Hyperactivity Disorder (ADHD) requires evidence of inattention, hyperactivity, and impulsivity. In the United States only evidence of inattention or hyperactivity/impulsivity is required. Here, the term ADHD is used only when referring to the condition as described in ICD 10, otherwise the less specific term "hyperactivity" is used.

Hyperactive behavior is commonly reported in young patients with TSC *(19,41)*. It appears to be associated with the presence of seizures, mental retardation, and possibly autism *(9,23,41)*. In a postal survey of 300 patients with TSC Hunt *(23)* found that 35% of those with mental retardation were reported to be hyperactive (compared to 2% of those with normal intelligence) and 30% of those with a history of seizures were hyperactive (compared to 5% of those without seizures). Curatolo et al. *(9)* studied 34 children with TSC and found hyperactivity in half of those with mental retardation (sample size 8). Gillberg et al. *(41)* studied 28 children with TSC. Twelve fulfilled criteria for a diagnosis of ADHD, of whom 11 also had autistic disorder. In population samples ADHD is characterized by a male excess of four- to sixfold *(42–44,46)*. However, in TSC no gender difference has been reported *(41)*.

Although methylphenidate is frequently used in the treatment of hyperactivity, its capacity to lower seizure threshold has led to caution in its use in TSC.

3.1.3.4. SLEEP DISORDER

In her questionnaire survey of 300 patients with TSC, Hunt *(23)* found that 58% had problems with sleep, often those who had seizures. A further questionnaire-based study of 40 children with TSC, their normal siblings, and a mixed group of children with mental retardation due to other causes found that sleep problems were significantly more common in children with TSC than in the control groups *(45)*. Within the TSC group, sleep disturbance was associated with current seizures and with daytime behavioral problems. No association was found between levels of sleep disturbance and either the presence of pervasive developmental disorders or high levels of parental stress. A polysomnography study of 10 children with TSC and partial epilepsy identified a range of sleep problems including reduced REM sleep, sleep instability, and sleep fragmentation by frequent awakenings *(46)*. These problems were more evident in subjects with large bifrontal and temporal tubers identified on MRI than in those with isolated parietal or posterior tubers. Melatonin has been evaluated for the treatment of sleep problems in TSC *(47)*. A small but significant improvement in total sleep time was found, although the sample size was small. Nighttime sedatives or behavioral techniques were reported to have met with little success in the TSC patient group.

3.1.3.5. ANXIETY DISORDER

Anecdotal evidence suggests that anxiety disorder may be frequent in patients of normal intellect with TSC. Significant association of psychiatric symptoms, particularly anxiety disorder, was found in affected members of a large kindred with TSC compared to relatives unaffected by TSC *(22)*. Instances of panic disorder, simple phobia, obsessive–compulsive disorder, separation anxiety disorder, and overanxious disorder were all found.

3.1.3.6. DEPRESSION, MANIA, AND PSYCHOSIS

Patients with neurological and neurogenetic disorders are at increased risk of depression. Bridges and Goldberg *(48)* found that 25% of a neurology in-patient sample had symptoms of depression. In a study of neurofibromatosis type 1, Samuelsson *(49)* found that 33% of patients had psychological problems, most commonly depression, alcoholism, and anxiety. There are many anecdotal reports of the co-occurrence of TSC and depression, mania, or psychosis *(19–21,50–52)*. However, systematic studies have not been performed.

3.1.3.7. OTHER PSYCHOLOGICAL PROBLEMS

Even among patients with TSC and normal intelligence there is evidence of a variety of neuropsychological deficits. Specific problems including speech delay, visual–spatial disturbances, dyspraxia, and memory impairment have been reported *(9,37)*. Other reported behavioral problems include aggression *(3,9,23)*, obsessive–compulsive disorder and bulimia *(9)*, temper tantrums *(23)*, and self mutilation *(3)*.

3.2. Ophthalmic Findings

Fundal hamartomas are astrocytic hamartomas, and histologically resemble SENs. They are reported to occur in approximately half of patients with TSC *(43)*, Achromic patches affecting the retinal pigment epithelium are also common *(53)*. The retinal lesions of TSC usually do not affect vision.

3.3. Dermatologic Findings

Identification of skin lesions frequently enables confident diagnosis of TSC (Fig. 4). Dermatologic manifestations include angiofibromas of the face (that are sometimes inaccurately termed adenoma sebaceum) and of the nail beds (subungual or periungual fibromas), fibromatous plaques of the forehead and scalp, shagreen patches (collagenous hamartomas of the dermis), hypopigmented macules (that are best visualized by Wood's light in fair-skinned individuals), and skin tags (molluscum fibrosum pendulum) *(43,54)*. Treatments for facial angiofibromas include laser obliteration and surgical excision. Camouflaging makeup can also be useful.

3.4. Renal Findings

Angiomyolipomas, cysts, and occasionally carcinoma and other kidney tumors are the renal manifestations of TSC (Fig. 5). Angiomyolipomas are seen on ultrasound scan in 50–80% of patients by 10 years of age *(55,56)*. Severe or symptomatic involvement appears to be more common in females and this may reflect hormonally promoted growth, as expression of estrogen and progesterone receptors has been demonstrated in angiomyolipomas *(57)*. Histological examination reveals fat, smooth muscle, and abnormal vessels *(58)*. Hemorrhage into the retroperitoneal space or collecting system is the most frequent serious complication. The risk of bleeding is related to lesion

---

Fig. 4. Dermatologic findings in TSC. **(A)** Facial angiofibromas. The nasolabial folds are particularly involved and the cheeks and chin also affected. The philtrum is relatively spared, as is typical. **(B)** Ungual fibroma affecting the lateral border of the right great toe nail bed. The groove in the nail is characteristic and may be seen

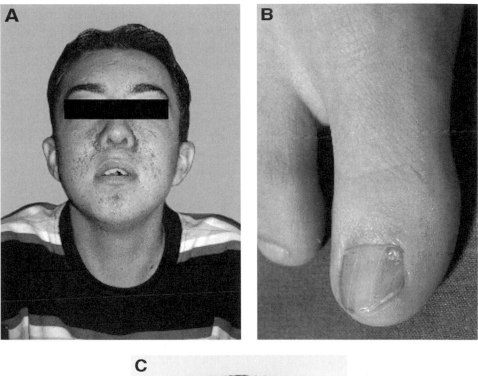

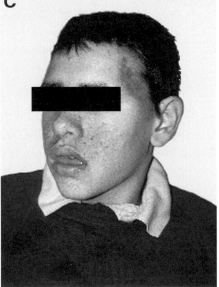

Fig. 4. (*continued*) in the absence of a visible nail bed fibroma. (**C**) Forehead plaque affecting the left temple. (**D**) Shagreen patch in the lumbar region. (*See* page 170.) (**E**) Hypopigmented macules with typical lance-ovate or "ash-leaf" morphology.

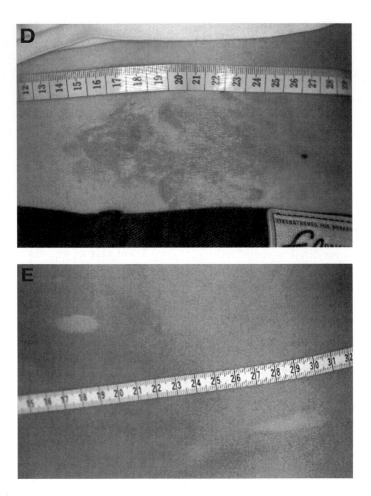

size *(59)* and may necessitate embolization or partial or total nephrectomy. Renal failure may occur if normal renal tissue is obliterated bilaterally *(60)*, but this is rare. Renal function should be monitored in patients with radiographically confirmed renal abnormalities.

Although renal cysts are commonly seen, severe polycystic kidney disease with hypertension and functional impairment occurs almost exclusively in patients with a contiguous gene deletion syndrome involving *TSC2* and the immediately adjacent *PKD1* gene (Fig. 6) *(61)*. These cases may present

---

Fig. 6. Polycystic kidney disease in TSC. Magnetic resonance image of transverse section of abdomen. Both kidneys are enlarged and contain numerous low signal intensity cysts that largely replace the renal parenchyma. Some have

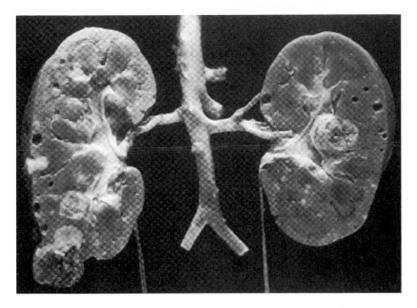

Fig. 5. Renal findings in TSC. Gross postmortem appearance of kidneys on coronal sectioning. There are several angiomyolipomas within and protruding from the renal parenchyma. Numerous cortical cysts of up to a few millimeters are also seen. (Reproduced from Gomez MR, ed. Tuberous Sclerosis, 2nd ed. New York: Raven Press, 1988. Used with permission).

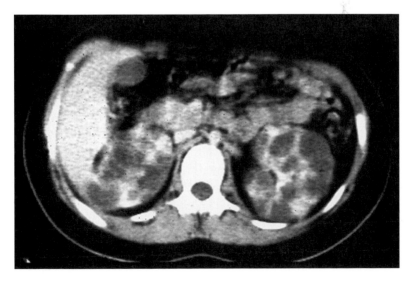

Fig. 6. (*continued*) variable signal intensity reflecting previous hemorrhage. The patient had a contiguous gene deletion of *TSC2* and *PKD1* and eventually required kidney transplantation for end stage renal disease.

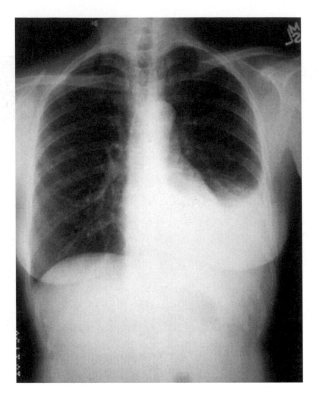

Fig. 7. Chylothorax complicating pulmonary TSC. Chest X-ray showing left-sided chylothorax in a female patient with TSC and lymphangioleimyomatosis. (Courtesy of Dr. F. McCormack.)

antenatally, in infancy, or later and progression to end-stage renal disease is common.

Reports of bilateral and multifocal renal cell carcinoma (RCC) occurring at an early age in patients with TSC suggest that some germline *TSC1* and/or *TSC2* mutations might act as RCC prediposition alleles *(62)*. Immunohistochemical positivity for HMB-45 does not appear to distinguish angiomyolipoma from carcinoma in patients with TSC, while sporadic RCC is normally HMB-45 negative *(63)*. An apparently distinct class of TSC associated malignant angiomyolipoma has also been suggested recently *(64)*.

3.5. Pulmonary Findings

Postpubertal females with TSC are at risk of developing lymphangioleiomyomatosis (LAM). This condition is characterized by obstructive infiltration of alveolar septa, bronchioles, lymphatics, and blood vessels by smooth-muscle-like cells, leading to cystic destruction of the lung parenchyma. Symptomatic LAM is recognized in a small proportion of females with TSC, although undiagnosed mild disease may be more common. Presentation usually includes pneumothorax, chylothorax (Fig. 7), or progres-

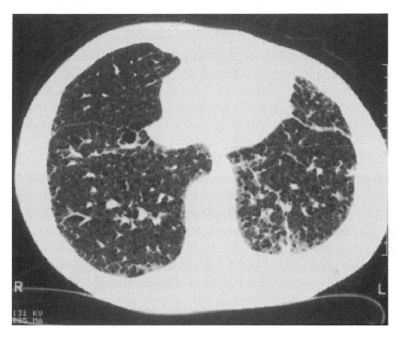

Fig. 8. Radiographic features of lymphangioleimyomatosis. Computed axial tomography, transverse section of chest, showing extensive cystic changes throughout both lungs. (Courtesy of Dr. F. McCormack.)

sive dyspnea on exertion with or without cough or hemoptysis. Progression may be relentless and lead to death *(43)*. High-resolution CT scan of the chest is a sensitive diagnostic test (Fig. 8). The smooth-muscle-like cells of LAM are HMB-45 positive, as are their counterparts in angiomyolipomas *(65)*. A sporadic form of LAM also occurs, but it is extremely rare *(66)*. It can be associated with extrapulmonary lymphatic involvement and with renal angiomyolipoma, but without cutaneous, brain, or other manifestations of TSC. Sproradic LAM has been shown to be caused by somatic inactivation of both alleles of one of the TSC genes in the proliferating clone of smooth-muscle-like cells *(67)*. Treatments for LAM are unsatisfactory. Hormonal manipulation has yet to be fully evaluated and lung transplantation may be indicated.

3.6. Cardiac Findings

Cardiac rhabdomyomas are seen on echocardiography in approx 60–80% of infants with TSC and are usually multiple *(68,69)*. They develop *in utero* and appear to regress postpartum. Identification of rhabdomyomas during routine antenatal ultrasound screening is increasingly leading to unexpected detection of possible TSC. Fetal scanning for cardiac rhabdomyomas has also been used as a prenatal test in pregnancies at high risk *(70)*. The prognosis of cardiac rhabdomyomas is good and they usually remain asymptomatic. Rarely, critically located tumors may compromise cardiac function, leading to intrauterine or neonatal death. Arrhythmia is the most frequent presentation in older children and adults. Conduction abnormalities may be present in the absence of echocardiographically demonstrable rhabdomyomas.

3.7. Other Systems

Areas of bony sclerosis, expansion or cystic change are frequent, but rarely symptomatic *(43)*. Enamel pits in the teeth are more frequent than in the general population *(71,72)*. Papillary adenoma of the thyroid, parathyroid hyperplasia, pancreatic islet cell tumors, pituitary adenomas, and adrenal angiomyolipoma have been reported in TSC *(43,73)*. Aneurysmal dilatation of major arteries is a recognized complication *(74,75)* and localized overgrowth resembling the Klippel–Trennaunay or Parkes–Weber syndromes appears to be an associated phenotype (author's unpublished observation).

4. DIAGNOSIS

Diagnosis is traditionally based on identification of manifestations by clinical examination and/or radiographic and histopathologic investigation. Criteria for diagnosis have been revised recently *(76)*. Under some circumstances a definitive clinical diagnosis cannot be made. Traditionally the signs or combinations of signs are then considered to warrant only a probable or possible diagnosis of TSC (Table 2).

Molecular genetic diagnosis is increasingly available for TSC. The sensitivity of assays for mutations of the *TSC1* and *TSC2* genes is increasing through the implementation of successive technical advances and refinements *(77)*. Molecular confirmation of the diagnosis is not required for most cases, as traditional approaches usually enable a definitive diagnosis to be made. However, molecular genetic testing can be helpful to clarify genetic status for relatives and for the provision of early prenatal diagnosis, once the specific mutation in a family has been identified.

5. GENETIC AND CELLULAR ASPECTS OF TUBEROUS SCLEROSIS

5.1. Identification and Characterization of TSC1 and TSC2

Linkage studies in multiplex families with TSC revealed evidence for two TSC determining loci, *TSC1* at 9q34 *(78)* and *TSC2* at 16p13.3 *(79)*. Among families large enough to permit linkage analysis, approximately half

Table 2
Diagnostic Criteria for Tuberous Sclerosis

Major features
    Facial angiofibromas or forehead plaques
    Nontraumatic ungual or periungual fibromas
    > Three hypomelanotic macules
    Shagreen patch (connective tissue nevus)
    Multiple retinal hamartomas
    Cortical tuber[a]
    Subependymal nodule
    Subependymal giant cell astrocytoma
    Cardiac rhabdomyoma
    Lymphangioleiomyomatosis[b]
    Renal angiomyolipoma[b]
Minor features
    Multiple randomly distributed pits in dental enamel
    Hamartomatous rectal polyps
    Bone cysts[c]
    Cerebral white matter "migration tracts"[a,c]
    Gingival fibromas
    Nonrenal hamartoma[c]
    Retinal achromic patch
    "Confetti" skin depigmentation
    Multiple renal cysts

Definite TSC: either two major features or one major plus two minor features

Probable TSC: one major feature plus one minor feature

Possible TSC: either one major feature or two or more minor features

[a]When cerebral cortical dysplasia and cerebral white matter migration tracts occur together, they should be counted as one feature of TSC.
[b]When both lymphangioleiomyomatosis and renal angiomyolipomas are present, other features of tuberous sclerosis should be present before a definite dignosis is made.
Adapted from Roach, Gomez, Northrup, 1998.
[c]Histological confirmation suggested.

show linkage to 9q34 and half to 16p13, and no conclusive evidence has been established to support a third locus *(80,81)*.

5.1.1. Positional Cloning of TSC2

Linkage studies originally defined an approx 1.5-Mb region of chromosome 16p as likely to contain the *TSC2* gene *(79,82)*. Although this region had already been more intensively mapped than many other parts of the genome, identification of *TSC2* still presented a daunting task. The process was unexpectedly simplified by the discovery of a family with both tuberous sclerosis and autosomal dominant polycystic kidney disease (family 77) that segregated a translocation between chromosomes 16p and 22q. In family 77, a mother and her daughter each carried a balanced translocation involving 16p13.3 (karyotypes 46,XX, t[16;22][p13.3;q11.21]). They had polycystic kidney disease but no evidence of tuberous sclerosis. The son (77-4) had inherited an unbalanced karyotype, 45, XY, −16,−22,+der(16) (16qter→16p13.3::22q11.21→22qter), and was hemizygous for the chromosomal regions 16p13.3→16pter and 22q11.21→22pter. He was severely mentally impaired, epileptic, and autistic and had clinical signs that were diagnostic of TSC, including facial angiofibromas, hypopigmented macules, renal cysts, and calcified SENs on brain CT scan. It was deduced that his TSC was likely to reflect loss of one copy of the *TSC2* gene within the deleted terminal segment of 16p. By contrast, a previously reported patient (BO) who had a *de novo* truncation of 16p *(83)* was reinvestigated and found to have no clinical or radiological features of tuberous sclerosis. Comparison of the breakpoints on 16p in patients 77-4 and BO showed that the deletion in patient 77-4 extended only approx 300-kb further centromerically, suggesting that this approx 300 kb region contained the *TSC2* gene. The region was cloned. Then, using pulsed field gel electrophoresis, a search for TSC-associated DNA rearrangements was undertaken in a panel of 255 unrelated patients. Five TSC-associated deletions were identified and mapped to a 120-kb interval from which four genes were isolated. One gene was disrupted by all five deletions, and its identity as *TSC2* was confirmed by the detection of intragenic deletions by conventional Southern analysis of patient DNA samples. The sequence of *TSC2* predicted a previously unknown protein product of approx 200 kDa that was subsequently named tuberin *(84,85)*.

5.1.2. Positional Cloning of TSC1

Following initial mapping of *TSC1* to 9q34 by linkage analysis, progress in refinement of its localization was hampered by a lack of meiotic recombination events in families that could be assigned with confidence to the *TSC1* locus. This difficulty reflected the small size of most families with TSC. Eventually a 1.5-Mb *TSC1* candidate region was defined by analysis of large families showing clear linkage to chromosome 9q34 *(86,87)*. The region was cloned and large deletions and rearrangements at the *TSC1* locus were sought using PFGE, but none were identified. Identification of *TSC1* was finally achieved by sequence analysis of clones spanning the candidate region through collaboration between TSC researchers and the Human Genome Project. As sequence was obtained it was analyzed *in silico* for known and novel genes and exons. Heteroduplex analysis of exons was initiated in a panel of 20 unrelated familial TSC cases linked to 9q34 and 40 sporadic TSC cases. Mutations were identified in an exon shown to correspond to an 8.6-kb cDNA encoding a novel predicted protein of 130-kDa protein that was called hamartin *(88)*.

5.1.3. Initial Characterization of TSC1 and TSC2

The *TSC2* gene comprises 41 coding exons and a noncoding leader exon (exon 1a) *(89,90)* distributed over an approx 44-kb genomic region. Exon 25 and the first 3 basepairs of exon 26, and exon 31 are alternatively spliced *(89,91)* and this is also the case in other species in which *TSC2* transcripts have been characterized, including mouse *(91,92)*, rat *(93)* and puffer fish *(89)*. Tuberin, the predicted 1807-amino-acid product of the *TSC2* gene product, contains an approx 200 amino-acid region of homology with the GTPase activating protein (GAP) rap1GAP *(94)*. *TSC2* missense mutations identified patients with TSC appear to show nonrandom clustering in the rap1GAP-related region *(89,95)* and the region is highly conserved in distantly related organisms, including human, puffer-fish, and fruit fly *(89,96)*. Although these observations suggest a critical functional role for the GAP-related domain, biochemical investigation has so far demonstrated only modest GAP activity toward the GTPases rap1 and rab5, the physiological relevance of which remains unclear *(97,98)*.

The *TSC1* gene comprises 23 exons, including two untranslated exons, distributed over (50 kb of genomic DNA) *(88)*. Exon 2 is alternatively spliced and exon 23 represents a 4.5-kb segment in the 3' untranslated region. Hamartin, the predicted protein product, comprises 1164 amino acids, is generally hydrophilic, and contains strongly predicted coiled-coil regions spanning amino acids 730–996. Initial database searches revealed a likely yeast *Schizosaccharomyces pombe* homolog of *TSC1* encoding a hypothetical 103-kDa protein, but no strong matches with known vertebrate proteins *(99)*.

5.1.4. TSC1 and TSC2 Are Inactivated by a "Two-Hit" Mechanism

The possibility that the TSC phenotype might result from two-step inactivation of both alleles of the causative gene(s) was recognized long before either *TSC1* or *TSC2* were identified. TSC is characterized by discrete multifocal hamartomas within an otherwise normal soma. This suggested that an additional local event (or events) was required for hamartoma development and that the additional event might be a somatic "second hit" mutation leading to inactivation of the second allele at the TSC locus in a susceptible cell. This two-hit mechanism of tumor suppressor gene action, suggested as a general phenomenon by Knudson *(99)*, had already been confirmed by molecular genetic analysis in a number of familial cancer and hamartoma predisposition syndromes. Experimental evidence that the two-hit mechanism also applied to TSC (Fig. 9) was rapidly forthcoming. Several reports demonstrated loss of heterozygosity across the *TSC1* or *TSC2* chromosomal regions at 9q34 and 16p13 in hamartomas from individuals with TSC *(100–103)*. Following identification of the TSC genes, somatic intragenic mutations of one allele of *TSC1* or *TSC2* together with a corresponding inherited germline mutation were reported, in a renal cell carcinoma and a pancreatic tumor respectively, in patients with TSC *(88,104)*.

In the largest study of loss of heterogygosity (LOH) in TSC-associated hamartomas yet reported, LOH was observed in 14 of 25 cases informative for markers at the *TSC2* locus, but in only 1 of 27 cases informative at the *TSC1* locus *(103)*. Smaller studies have also identified LOH at the *TSC2* locus more commonly than at *TSC1 (105,106)*, probably reflecting unequal representation of *TSC1* and *TSC2* germline mutations among patients with TSC.

5.1.5. Spectrum of Inherited Mutations in TSC1 and TSC2

Cheadle et al. *(95)* reviewed a total of 439 published constitutional mutations identified in individuals with TSC, 155 in *TSC1* and 284 in *TSC2*. They applied a standardized nomenclature system and used rigorous criteria when assessing evidence for pathogenicity. Listings of *TSC1* and *TSC2* sequence variations can also be found on the TSC Variation Database site at http://expmed.bwh.harvard.edu/ts.

Both *TSC1* and *TSC2* exhibit wide but distinct mutational spectra. Virtually all inherited mutations reported in *TSC1* are small truncating lesions. In the review by Cheadle et al. *(95)* 47% of *TSC1* mutations were single-base substitutions, 81% (59 of 73) of which were nonsense mutations. The other major category of single base changes in *TSC1* was mutations affecting splicing (12 of 73, 16%). The rest of the *TSC1* mutation spectrum was made up of small insertions of fewer than 28 basepairs (26 of 155, 17%) and small deletions of less than 23 basepairs (56 of 155, 36%). In-frame deletions and missense changes are exceptionally rare at the *TSC1* locus and some of those that have been reported lack conclusive evidence for pathogenicity. Large rearrangements (e.g., whole exon or multiexon deletions) are also uncommon at the *TSC1* locus, although a handful of well documented cases exist *(107)*. By contrast, Cheadle et al. *(95)* found that nonsense mutations and missense mutations had roughly equal frequencies at the *TSC2* locus, each accounting for ≈20% of mutations. *TSC2* deletions included more in-frame changes than were seen at the *TSC1* locus. Large deletions, of whole exons, multiple exons, the whole gene, or multiple genes were also prevalent at the *TSC2* locus and appeared to account for about 15% of all TSC mutations *(95,108)*.

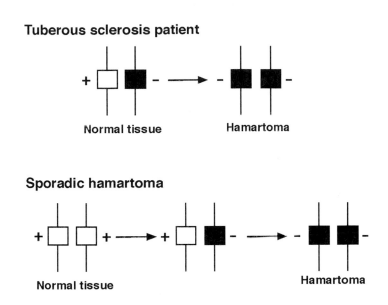

Fig. 9. Two-hit model for hamartoma development. Each somatic cell normally contains two alleles of each *TSC* gene. In nonmosaic patients with TSC the somatic cells initially contain one mutant allele (*filled box*, –) and one normal allele (*open box*, +). A single somatic mutation is sufficient to render the cell null at the *TSC* locus involved and initiate the pathway to hamartoma formation. Individuals without TSC initially have two normal of each *TSC* gene in each somatic cell. Two (independent) somatic mutations will be required to initiate hamartoma formation from a susceptible cell. Although possible, this will be a rare scenario and will lead to sporadic counterparts to TSC hamartomas in otherwise normal individuals.

5.1.6. Contiguous Deletions of TSC2 and PKD1

The *TSC2* gene and the autosomal dominant polycystic kidney disease type 1 (PKD1) gene are in extremely close proximity *(85)*. The polyadenylation signals at their 3' ends are only 60 basepairs apart. Therefore, large deletion mutations at this locus frequently involve both genes. Such mutations are associated with a distinct phenotype of tuberous sclerosis with very severe and early onset (usually prenatal) polycystic kidney disease *(61,109)*. The renal cystic disease often progresses to end-stage renal disease by late childhood or early adulthood *(61)*. A two-hit mechanism, similar to that for TSC, has been proposed for autosomal dominant polycystic kidney disease *(110)*. Large somatic deletion mutations at the *TSC2*/PKD1 locus will frequently inactivate alleles of both genes. Therefore, patients with the contiguous gene syndrome may develop early and severe renal cystic disease as a consequence of their susceptability to biallelic inactivation of *TSC2* and PKD1 in a single somatic mutational event.

5.1.7. Mosaicism for TSC1 and TSC2 Mutations

Both gonosomal and confined gonadal mosaicism for *TSC1* and *TSC2* mutations have been described in many patients, and mosaicism has important implications for gene testing and genetic counseling.

In a study of patients with the *TSC2* and PKD1 contiguous gene deletion syndrome, 7 of 27 index cases were shown to be mosaic by direct counting of deleted chromosomes using fluorescence *in situ* hybridization or by allelic quantification after Southern analysis *(61)*. However, patients who are mosaic for the contiguous gene deletion syndrome may be more likely to come to medical attention than individuals with other mosaic TSC mutations, as their renal disease is often severe. Among 62 families with *TSC1* or *TSC2* mutations, Verhoef et al. *(111,112)* identified 6 with mosaicism in the founding family member (5 gonosomal and 1 apparently confined gonadal). Reported patients who were mosaic for *TSC1* or *TSC2* mutations have often had mild disease. In several cases, minor asymptomatic manifestations of TSC were recognized only after initial diagnosis of TSC in their more severely affected nonmosaic offspring *(61,111,113)*. By contrast, Kwiatkowska et al. *(114)* reported surprisingly severe disease in a patient who was mosaic for a *TSC1* mutation. Because of the possibility of gonadal mosaicism, an empiric recurrence risk of 1–2% is considered prudent in genetic counseling for the apparently unaffected parents of a single child with TSC.

5.1.8. TSC2 Mutations Account for Most Sporadic TSC

TSC1 mutations have been identified in only 10–15% of sporadic TSC patients following comprehensive mutation analysis *(115)* while *TSC2* mutations have been identified in approx 60% *(108)*. In part this may be explained by a higher mutation rate at the *TSC2* than the *TSC1* locus. Although the mutation rates at the two loci have not been quantified independently, the *TSC2* coding region is larger and the gene's genomic structure is more complex and contains more repetitive sequences, providing potentially more opportunities for acquisition of pathogenic mutations.

5.1.9. Disease Appears Less Severe in TSC1 than TSC2 Cases

Although *TSC2* mutations are more common than *TSC1* mutations in sporadic TSC patients, this does not appear to be the case in multigenerational TSC families. Both genetic linkage analyses and direct mutation analysis indicate that mutations in the two genes are found with approximately equal frequency in the latter situation *(81,108)*. These observations suggest that patients with *TSC1* mutations may be less severely affected than those with *TSC2* mutations, and so more likely to found a family than a new *TSC2* patient. Several studies have provided evidence to support this hypothesis. Jones et al. *(115)* found that intellectual disability was significantly more frequent among sporadic cases with *TSC2* than with *TSC1* mutations. Dabora et al. *(116)* used a questionnaire to collect medical history data relating to a wide range of TSC organ involvement in a large cohort of TSC cases and found more severe disease in *TSC2* than in *TSC1* cases. Recently, we used validated measures to assess IQ and behavior more formally in a cohort of 98 sequentially ascertained TSC cases. Learning difficulties and autism were significantly more frequent in patients with *TSC2* than *TSC1* disease (Lewis and Sampson, *unpublished data*).

5.2. Animal Models for Tuberous Sclerosis

A number of animals with mutations of their orthologous *TSC1* and *TSC2* genes have been characterized, including the naturally occurring Eker (*TSC2* mutant) rat *(117,118)*, engineered *TSC1* and *TSC2* "knockout" mice *(119–121)*, and Drosophila mutant models for *TSC1* and *TSC2* *(96,122,123)*. Studies of these animals, and cell lines derived from them, are helping to provide insights into the roles of *TSC1* and *TSC2*.

5.2.1. The Eker Rat

The Eker rat is heterozygous for a mutation caused by a retrotransposed 6.3-kb intracisternal A particle that disrupts codon 1272 of rat *TSC2* (*TSC2EK*). The mutation appears to prevent protein production from the *EK* allele *(117,118)*. The Eker rat is predisposed to development of renal cysts, adenomas, and cancers that develop from proximal tubular and collecting duct epithelial cells *(124,125)*. Penetrance of the renal phenotype is virtually 100%. Pituitary adenomas (55% at 2 years), uterine leiomyomas and leiomyosarcomas (47–62% females at 14 mo–2 years), splenic hemangiomas (23–68% at 14 mo–2 years) *(126,127)*, and brain hamartomas resembling human TSC subependymal nodules *(128)* are also seen. However, seizures and behavioral changes have not been noted. A proportion of even the earliest renal tubular lesions show LOH involving the wild-type *TSC2* gene, consistent with two-step inactivation of *TSC2* being the initiating molecular step in tumor pathogenesis *(129)*. However, Eker tumors show organ-specific variation in the frequency with which LOH is identified as the second hit. LOH is seen in 40–60% of renal tumors, but appears rare in splenic hemangiomas and in subependymal and subcortical hamartomas *(128,130,131)*. Screening for intragenic mutations has shown that some tumors without LOH carry point mutations in the wild-type *TSC2* allele *(132)*. It is not yet known whether haploinsufficiency for *TSC1* or *TSC2* has effects on any cell type. *TSC2Ek/Ek* homozygosity is associated with death at embryonic age 10–12 d in a number of different genetic backgrounds. The cause has not been determined.

Analysis of carcinogen-induced renal tumors in non-Eker rats has revealed biallelic inactivating point mutations in *TSC2* is some cases *(133)*. However, rat renal carcinomas induced by ferric nitrilotriacetate do not display mutation or inactivation of the *TSC2* gene (or of the *VHL* gene) *(134)*. These observations suggest that the *TSC2* gene is a critical target in some, but not all, forms of rat renal cancers.

5.2.2. TSC2 *Knockout Mice*

Mice with targetted disruption of *TSC2* have been engineered and characterized *(119,120)*. Their phenotypes were similar to those of the Eker rat. Renal cystadenomas developed by 6 mo and appeared to grow progressively thereafter. Renal carcinoma and metastatic disease developed in 5–10% of mice by 18 months, suggesting a very low rate of malignant progression for the cystadenomas (approx 1 in 1000). Other phenotypic manifestations included liver hemangiomas (50% by 18 mo), lung adenomas (30%), and hemangiosarcomas (10%). Brain lesions have not been reported.

Strain-dependent differences in tumor development have been noted. For example, $TSC2^{+/-}$ N3 outbred Black Swiss mice had significantly ($p < 0.001$) fewer renal cystadenoma, but more renal carcinomas than F1 129/SvJae-BALB/cJ mice. LOH analysis and immunohistochemical studies support the expected two-hit mechanism of tumorigenesis in $TSC2^{+/-}$ mice. $TSC2^{-/-}$ embryos die at E10.5–12.5 with liver hypoplasia *(119)*.

5.2.3. TSC1 *Knockout Mice*

Mice with targetted disruption of *TSC1* have been developed and partially characterized *(121)*. Heterozygotes developed renal cystadenomas, liver hemangiomas, and tumors of the extremities, as seen in $TSC2^{+/-}$ mice. However, the tumors developed more slowly than in $TSC2^{+/-}$ mice of the same background strain. Dysplastic renal tubules were seen at 9–12 mo and cystadenomas of up to 2 mm at 15–18 mo. The apparent difference in natural history of $TSC1^{+/-}$ and $TSC2^{+/-}$ mice may be relevant to the disease severity differences suggested by studies of TSC in humans.

5.2.4. Drosophila TSC2 *and* TSC1 *Mutants*

In *Drosophila* the Tsc1 and Tsc2 proteins function together to regulate cell size and proliferation and hence organ size *(122,123)*. Mutations in the *Drosophila Tsc2* orthologue cause the *gigas* phenotype *(96,135)*. Mutant flies die during larval development but clones of *gigas* cells have been stud-

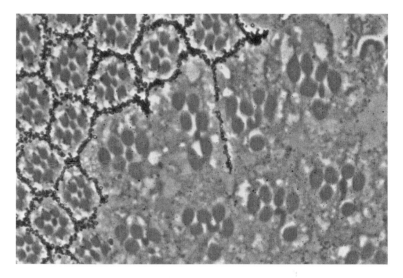

Fig. 10. Increased cell size in *Drosophila dtsc1* null cells. Section through retina of an adult mosaic *tsc1* mutant fly. Outlines of wild-type cells (*upper left*) are highlighted by pigment produced by the *mini-white* marker gene. Mutant cells (*lower right*) lack the pigment marker, are larger overall, and have enlarged rhabdomeres. (Courtesy of Dr. Naoto Ito.)

ied in vivo in mosaic flies. Mutant cells develop to an abnormally large size in the eye and wing, but retain normal morphology. Cells mutant for *Drosophila Tsc1* have similar properties (Fig. 10), but only co-overexpression of both Tsc1 and Tsc2 proteins appears to restrict cell size and number, and so organ size *(122)*.

5.3. Insights into Cellular Functions of Hamartin and Tuberin

When the *TSC1* and *TSC2* genes were identified by positional cloning in humans, hamartin and tuberin were unknown proteins. Other than the rap1GAP-related region of tuberin, the predicted protein sequences gave little clue as to their possible functions. Progress in elucidating their roles is being made, particularly through the analysis of *TSC1* and *TSC2* animal models, but few findings have yet been subject to independent confirmation.

5.3.1. Tuberin and Hamartin Are Widely Expressed Interacting Cytosolic Proteins

TSC1 and *TSC2* are widely expressed in embryonic and adult tissues in mouse and man *(88,92,136,137)*. Both hamartin and tuberin appear to be predominantly cytoplasmic proteins *(138–140)*. Evidence from assays in the yeast two-hybrid system, co-immunoprecipitation, and protein expression patterns in transfection experiments has shown that the proteins interact directly *(139,141–144)*. The domains that mediate the interaction have not been precisely defined, but the N-terminal regions of both proteins appear to be involved *(142,144)*. The interaction appears to be important for the physiological function of the proteins, as a number of nontruncating mutations that disrupt the interaction (directly or via changes in phosphorylation status) are associated with the TSC phenotype *(142,144,145)*. The hamartin–tuberin complex has been detected in all phases of the cell cycle *(146)* and appears to stabilize tuberin by preventing its ubiquitination and degradation *(143)*.

5.3.2. Hamartin and Tuberin Regulate Cell Size and Proliferation

In *Drosophila* the most marked phenotype associated with loss of *TSC1* or *TSC2* is increase in cell size *(96,122,123)*. Giant cells are also characteristic of a variety of TSC associated hamartomas in humans *(43)*. Deficiency of hamartin or tuberin in mammalian cells promotes those in G_0 to reenter the cell cycle and is associated with shortening of G_1 *(146,147)*. The *Tsc1* and *Tsc2* gene products appear to have similar cell cycle regulatory roles in the *Drosophila* imaginal disc *(96,122,123)*. Genetic epistasis data in *Drosophila* suggest that *Tsc1* and *Tsc2* may function downstream of *dPTEN* as negative regulators of the insulin signaling pathway in cell size and proliferation control *(122,123)*.

5.3.3. Other Reported Properties of Hamartin and Tuberin

Tsuchiya et al. *(148)* reported that regions comprising amino acids 1163–1359 and 1690–1743 of tuberin were both capable of GAL4-dependent *LacZ* activation in yeast, suggesting that tuberin might function in transcriptional activation. Similar results were obtained in CAT assays in Hela and NIH3T3 cells with a construct comprising amino acids 1163–1359. Henry et al. *(149)* reported that tuberin binds to and modulates transcription mediated by members of the steroid receptor superfamily of genes.

Soucek et al. *(150)* reported posttranslational up-regulation of tuberin expression when neuronal differentiation was induced in the neuroblastoma cell lines SK-N-SH and LAN-1, independent of proliferation status. Conversely, neuronal differentiation was blocked by antisense inhibition of tuberin. These observations suggest a role for tuberin in neuronal differentiation.

Lamb et al. *(151)* demonstrated that hamartin (amino acids 881–1084) binds ezrin and activates Rho (through amino acids 145–510) to regulate cell adhesion. The relationship between these observations and the growth suppressing properties of hamartin has yet to be fully characterized.

6. THE MOLECULAR AND CELLULAR BASES OF NEUROBEHAVIORAL ABNORMALITIES IN TSC: *A CHALLENGE FOR THE FUTURE*

The identification of the *TSC1* and *TSC2* genes and the initial characterization of their protein products and roles represent significant advances in the understanding of TSC that have been achieved over the last decade. However, progress in elucidating neurobehavioral aspects of TSC has been limited and there is still much scope for descriptive as well as experimental study in this area. The neurobehavioral phenotypes of TSC require better definition: their true frequencies need to be determined by systematic studies in large and well defined patient cohorts. The different risks of *TSC1* and *TSC2* associated disease need to be established, especially as decisions regarding prenatal diagnosis can now rest on these. Any differences in *TSC1* and *TSC2* disease severity will require explanation, as critical functions of hamartin and tuberin appear to require the interaction of both proteins. Perhaps disease severity is effectively determined by the somatic mutation rate at the two loci. If this is higher at the *TSC2* locus than at the *TSC1* locus one would expect a greater frequency of "second hits" at *TSC2* and the development of more hamartomas and hamartias in *TSC2* than *TSC1* cases.

A better understanding of the relationship between seizures and neurodevelopmental outcome is critically important. If poor outcome is in part a consequence of early seizures, particularly infantile spasms, might genetic testing and prophylactic antiepileptic therapy be indicated in newborns who are at risk because of their family history?

The link between TSC and autism demands detailed clinical and molecular genetic investigation. Are the autistic phenotypes associated with TSC qualitatively different from those associated with idiopathic autism? Could the *TSC1* or *TSC2* genes play a currently unrecognized wider role in determining idiopathic neurobehavioral phenotypes?

REFERENCES

1. Sampson JR, Scahill SJ, Stephenson JBP, Mann L, Connor JM. Genetic aspects of tuberous sclerosis in the West of Scotland. J Med Genet 1989;26:28–31.
2. Shepherd CW, Beard CM, Gomez MR, Kurland JT, Whisnant JP. Tuberous sclerosis complex in Olmstead county, Minnesota, 1950-1989. Arch Neurol 1991;48:400–1.
3. Webb DW, Fryer AE, Osborne JP. Morbidity associated with tuberous sclerosis: a population study. Dev Med Child Neurol 1996;338:146–55.
4. O'Callaghan FJK, Shiell AW, Osborne JP, Martyn C. Prevalence of tuberous sclerosis estimated by capture-recapture analysis. Lancet 1998;351:1490.

5. Young JM, Burley MW, Jeremiah SJ, et al. A mutation screen of the *TSC1* gene reveals 26 protein truncating mutations and 1 splice site mutation in a panel of 79 tuberous sclerosis patients. Ann Hum Genet 1998;62:203–13.

6. Fryer AE, Osborne JP, Tan R, Siggers DC. Tuberous sclerosis: a large family with no history of seizures or mental retardation. J Med Genet 1987;24:547–8.

7. O'Callaghan TJ, Edwards JA, Tobin M, Mookerjee BK. Tuberous sclerosis with striking renal involvement in a family. Arch Intern Med 1987; 135:1082–7.

8. Scheithauer BW. The neuropathology of tuberous sclerosis. J Dermatol 1992;19:897–903.

9. Curatolo P, Cusmai R, Cortesi F, Chiron C, Jambaqué I, Dulac O. Neuropsychiatric aspects of tuberous sclerosis. Ann NY Acad Sci 1991;615:8–16.

10. Shepherd CW, Houser OW, Gomez MR. MR findings in tuberous sclerosis complex and correlation with seizure development and mental impairment. Am J Neuroradiol 1995;16:149–55.

11. Chiron C, Dumas C, Jambaque I, Mumford J, Dulac O. Randomized trial comparing vigabatrin and hydrocortisone in infantile spasms due to tuberous sclerosis. Epilepsy Res 1997;26:389–95.

12. Hancock E, Osborne JP. Vigabatrin in the treatment of infantile spasms in tuberous sclerosis: literature review. J Child Neurol 1999;14:71–4.

13. Chugani HT, Da Silva E, Chugani DC. Infantile spasms: III. Prognostic implications of bitemporal hypometabolism on positron emission tomography. Ann Neurol 1996;39:643–9.

14. Bourneville D-M. Sclerose tubereuse des circoncolutions cerebraes: Idiote et epilepsie hemiplegique. Arch Neurol (Paris) 1880;1:81–91.

15. Vogt H. Zur diagnostik der tuberosen sklerose. Z. Erforsch Behandl Jugendl Schwachsinns 1908;2:1–12.

16. Critchley M, Earl CJC. Tuberose sclerosis and allied conditions. Brain 1932;55:311–46.

17. Kanner L. Autistic disturbance of affective contact. Nervous Child 1943;2:217–50.

18. Hunt A. Tuberous sclerosis: a survey of 97 cases. Dev Med Child Neurol 1983;25:346–57.

19. Hunt A, Dennis J. Psychiatric disorder among children with tuberous sclerosis. Dev Med Child Neurol 1987;29:190–8.

20. Holschneider DP, Szuba MP. Capgras syndrome and psychosis in a patient with tuberous sclerosis. J Neuropsychiatry Clin Neurosci 1982;4:353.

21. Khanna R, Borde M. Mania in a five-year-old child with tuberous sclerosis. Br J Psychiatry 1989;155:117–9.

22. Smalley SL, Burger F, Smith M. Phenotypic variation of tuberous sclerosis in a single extended kindred. J Med Genet 1994;31:761–5.

23. Hunt A. Development, behavior and seizures in 300 cases of tuberous sclerosis. J Intell Disab Res 1993;37:41–51.

24. Webb DW, Fryer AE, Osborne JP. On the incidence of fits and mental retardation in tuberous sclerosis. J Med Genet 1991;28:395–7.

25. Bundey S, Evans K. Tuberous sclerosis: a genetic study. J Neurol Neurosurg Psychiatry 1969;32:591–603.

26. Riikonen R, Simell O. Tuberous sclerosis and infantile spasms. Dev Med Child Neurol 1990;32:203–9.
27. Roach ES, Williams DP, Laster DW. Magnetic resonance imaging in tuberous sclerosis. Arch Neurol 1987;44:301–3.
28. Inoue Y, Nakajima S, Fukuda T, et al. Magnetic resonance images of tuberous sclerosis. Neuroradiology 1988; 30:379–84.
29. Kingsley DPE, Kendall BE, Fitz CR. Tuberous sclerosis: a clinicoradiological evaluation of 110 cases with particular reference to atypical presentation. Neuroradiology 1986;28:38–46.
30. Menor F, Martí-Bonmatí L, Mulas F, Poyatos C, Cortina H. Neuroimaging in tuberous sclerosis: a clinicoradiological evaluation in pediatric patients. Pediatr Radiol 1992;22:485–9.
31. Webb DW, Thomson JLG, Osborne JP. Cranial magnetic resonance imaging in patients with tuberous sclerosis and normal intellect. Arch Dis Child 1991;66:1375–7.
32. Clarke A, Cook P, Osborne JP. Cranial computed tomographic findings in tuberous sclerosis are not affected by sex. Dev Med Child Neurol 1996; 38:139–44.
33. Hunt A, Shepherd C. A prevalence study of autism in tuberous sclerosis. J Autism Dev Dis 1993;23:323–39.
34. Riikonen R, Amnell G. Psychiatric disorders in children with earlier infantile spasms. Dev Med Child Neurol 1981;23:747–60.
35. Gillberg C. Subgroups in autism: are there behavioral phenotypes typical of underlying medical conditions? J Intell Disab Res 1992;36:201–14.
36. Williamson DA, Bolton PF. Brief report: atypical autism and tuberous sclerosis in a sibling pair. J Autism Dev Dis 1995;25:435–42.
37. Jambaqué I, Cusmai R, Curatolo P, Cortesi F, Perrot C, Dulac O. Neuropsychological aspects of tuberous sclerosis in relation to epilepsy and MRI findings. Dev Med Child Neurol 1991;33:698–705.
38. Deonna T, Ziegler A, Moura-Serra J, Innocenti G. Autistic regression in relation to limbic pathology and epilepsy: report of two cases. Dev Med Child Neurol 1993;35:158–76.
39. Bolton PF, Griffiths PD. Association of tuberous sclerosis of temporal lobes with autism and atypical autism. Lancet 1997;349:392–5.
40. Seri S, Cerquiglini A, Pisani F, Curatolo P. Autism in tuberous sclerosis: evoked potential evidence for a deficit in auditory sensory processing. Clin Neurophysiol 1999;110:1825–30.
41. Gillberg IC, Gillberg C, Ahlsén G. Autistic behavior and attention deficits in tuberous sclerosis: a population based study. Dev Med Child Neurol 1994;36:50–6.
42. Gaub M, Carlson CL. Gender differences in ADHD: a meta-analysis and critical review. J Am Acad Child Adolesc Psychol 1997;36:1036–45.
43. Gomez MR, Sampson JR, Holets-Whittemore V. Tuberous sclerosis complex. Oxford: Oxford University Press, 1999.
44. Pine DS, Wasserman GA, Workman SB. Memory and anxiety in prepubertal boys at risk for delinquency. J Am Acad Child Adolesc Psychiatry 1999;38:1024–31.

45. Hunt A, Stores G. Sleep disorder and epilepsy in children with tuberous sclerosis: a questionnaire-based study. Dev Med Child Neurol 1994;36:108–15.
46. Bruni O, Cortesi F, Giannotti F, Curatolo P. Sleep disorders in tuberous sclerosis: a polysomnographic study. Brain Dev 1995;17:52–6.
47. O'Callaghan FJK, Clarke AA, Hancock E, Hunt A, Osborne JP. Use of melatonin to treat sleep disorders in tuberous sclerosis. Dev Med Child Neurol 1999;41:123–6.
48. Bridges KW, Goldberg DP. Psychiatric illness in inpatients with neurological disorders: patients' views on discussion of emotional problems with neurologists. Br Med J 1984;289:656–8.
49. Samuelsson B. Neurofibromatosis (von Recklinghausen's disease): a clinical psychiatric and genetic study. (Thesis) 1981.
50. Zlotlow M, Kleiner S. Catatonic schizophrenia associated with tuberous sclerosis. Psychiatr Q 1965;29:466–75.
51. Clarke DJ, Buckley ME, Burns BH. Epilepsy and psychosis—ask the family. Br J Psychiatry 1986;150:702–3.
52. Harvey KV, Mahr G, Balon R. Psychiatric manifestations of tuberous sclerosis. Psychosomatics 1995;36:314–5.
53. Northrup H, Kwiatkowski DJ, Roach ES, et al. Evidence for genetic heterogeneity in tuberous sclerosis: one locus on chromosome 9 and at least one locus elsewhere. Am J Hum Genet 1992;51:709–20.
54. Webb DW, Clarke A, Osborne JP. The cutaneous features of tuberous sclerosis: a population study. Br J Dermatol 1996;135:1–5.
55. Cook JA, Oliver K, Mueller RF, Sampson J. A cross sectional study of renal involvement in tuberous sclerosis. J Med Genet 1996;33:480–4.
56. Ewalt DE, Sheffield E, Sparagana SP, Delgada MR, Roach ES. Renal lesion growth in children with tuberous sclerosis complex. J Urol 1998;160:141–5.
57. Logginidou H, Ao X, Russo I, Henske EP. Frequent estrogen and progesterone receptor immunoreactivity in renal angiomyolipomas from women with pulmonary lymphangioleiomyomatosis. Chest 2000;117:25–30.
58. Elbe JN. Angiomyolipoma of the kidney. Semin Diagn Pathol 1998;15:21–40.
59. Hellstrom PA, Mehik A, Talja MT, Siniluoto TM, Perala JM, Leinonen SS. Spontaneous subcapsular or perirenal haemorrhage caused by renal tumors: a urological emergency. Scand J Urol Nephrol 1999;33:17–23.
60. Neumann HPH, Bruggen V, Berger DP, et al. Tuberous sclerosis complex with end stage renal failure. Nephrol Dial Transplant 1995;10:349–53.
61. Sampson JR, Maheshwar MM, Aspinwall R et al. Renal cystic disease in tuberous sclerosis: role of the polycystic kidney disease 1 gene. Am J Hum Genet 1997;61:843–51.
62. Sampson JR, Patel A, Mee AD. Multifocal renal cell carcinoma in sibs from a chromosome 9 linked (*TSC1*) tuberous sclerosis family. J Med Genet 1995;32:848–50.
63. Bjornsson J, Short MP, Kwiatkowski DJ, Henske EP. Tuberous sclerosis-associated renal cell carcinoma—clinical, pathological and genetic features. Am J Pathol 1996;149:1201–8.

64. Pea M, Bonetti G, Martignoni E, Henske E, Manfrin E, Colato C, Bernstein J. Apparent renal cell carcinomas in tuberous sclerosis are heterogeneous: the identification of malignant epithelioid angiomyolipoma. Am J Surg Pathol 1998;22:180–7.

65. Bonetti F, Chiodera PL, Pea M, et al. Transbronchial biopsy in lymphangiomyomatosis of the lung. HMB45 for diagnosis. Am J Surg Pathol 1993;17:1092–102.

66. Johnson SR, Tattersfield AE. Clinical experience of lymphangioleiomyomatosis in the UK. Thorax 2000;55:1052–7.

67. Carsillo T, Astrinidis A, Henske EP. Mutations in the tuberous sclerosis complex gene *TSC2* are a cause of sporadic pulmonary lymphangioleiomyomatosis. Proc Natl Acad Sci USA 2000;97:6085–90.

68. Smith HC, Watson GH, Patel RG, Super M. Cardiac rhabdomyomata in tuberous sclerosis: their course and diagnostic value. Arch Dis Child 1989;64:196–200.

69. Webb DW, Thomas RD, Osborne JP. Cardiac rhabdomyomas and their association with tuberous sclerosis. Arch Dis Child 1993;68:367–70.

70. Crawford DC, Garrett C, Tynan M, Neville B, Allan LD. Cardiac rhabdomyomata as a marker for the antenatal detection of tuberous sclerosis. J Med Genet 1983;20:303–12.

71. Mlynarczyk G. Enamel pitting: a common symptom of tuberous sclerosis. Oral Surg Oral Med Pathol 1991;71:63–7.

72. Sampson JR, Attwood D, Al Mughery AS, Reid JS. Pitted enamel hypoplasia in tuberous sclerosis. Clin Genet 1992;42:50–2.

73. Ilgren EB, Westmoreland D. Tuberous sclerosis: unusual associations in four cases. J Clin Pathol 1984;37:272–8.

74. van Reedt Dortland RWH, Bax NMA, Huber J. Aortic aneurysm in a 5 year old boy with tuberous sclerosis. J Paediatr Surg 1991;26:1420–2.

75. Hite SH, Kuo JS, Cheng EY. Axillary artery aneurysm in tuberous sclerosis: cross sectional imaging findings. Pediatr Radiol 1998;28:554–6.

76. Roach ES, Gomez MR, Northrup H. Tuberous sclerosis complex consensus conference: revised clinical diagnostic criteria. J Child Neurol 1998;13:624–8.

77. Jones AC, Sampson JR, Hoogendoorn B, Cohen D, Cheadle JP. Application and evaluation of denaturing HPLC for molecular genetic analysis in tuberous sclerosis. Hum Genet 2000;106:663–8.

78. Fryer AE, Chalmers A, Connor JM, et al. Evidence that the gene for tuberous sclerosis is on chromosome 9. Lancet 1987;i:659–61.

79. Kandt RS, Haines JL, Smith M, et al. Linkage of an important gene locus for tuberous sclerosis to a chromosome 16 marker for polycystic kidney disease. Nat Genet 1992;2:37–41.

80. Janssen B, Sampson JR, van der Est M, et al. Refined localization of *TSC1* by combined analysis of 9q34 and 16p13 data in 14 tuberous sclerosis families. Hum Genet 1994;94:437–40.

81. Povey S, Burley MW, Attwood J, et al. Two loci for tuberous sclerosis: one on 9q34 and one on 16p13. Ann Hum Genet 1994;58:107–27.

82. Kwiatkowski DJ, Armour J, Bale AE, et al. Report on the second international workshop on human chromosome 9. Cytogenet Cell Genet 1993;64:94–106.

83. Wilkie AOM, Buckle VJ, Harris PC, et al. Clinical features and molecular analysis of the α-thalassemia/mental retardation syndromes. 1. Cases due to deletions involving chromosome band 16p13.3. Am J Hum Genet 1990; 46:1112–26.

84. The European Chromosome 16 Tuberous Sclerosis Consortium. Identification and characterization of the tuberous sclerosis gene on chromosome 16. Cell 1993;75:1305–15.

85. The European Polycystic Kidney Disease Consortium. The polycystic kidney disease 1 gene encodes a 14kb transcript and lies within a duplicated region on chromosome 16. Cell 1994;77:881–94.

86. Haines JL, Short MP, Kwiatkowski DJ, et al. Localization of one gene for tuberous sclerosis within 9q32–9q34, and further evidence for heterogeneity. Am J Hum Genet 1991;49:764–72.

87. Nellist M, Brook-Carter PT, Connor JM, Kwiatkowski DJ, Johnson P, Sampson JR. Identification of markers flanking the tuberous sclerosis locus on chromosome 9 (*TSC1*). J Med Genet 1993;30:224–7.

88. van Slegtenhorst M, deHoogt R, Hermans C, et al. Identification of the tuberous sclerosis gene *TSC1* on chromosome 9q34. Science 1997;77:805–8.

89. Maheshwar MM, Sandford R, Nellist M, et al. Comparative analysis and genomic structure of the tuberous sclerosis 2 (*TSC2*) gene in human and pufferfish. Hum Mol Genet 1996;5:131–7.

90. Kobayashi T, Urakami S, Cheadle JP, et al. Identification of a leader exon and a core promoter for the rat tuberous sclerosis 2 (*TSC2*) gene and structural comparison with the human homolog. Mammal Genome 1997;8:554–8.

91. Xu L, Sterner C, Maheshwar MM, et al. Alternative splicing of the tuberous sclerosis 2 (*TSC2*) gene in human and mouse tissues. Genomics 27:475–80.

92. Olsson PG, Schofield JN, Edwards YH, Frischauf AM. Expression and differential splicing of the mouse *TSC2* homolog. Mammal Genome 1996; 7:212–15.

93. Kobayashi T, Nishizawa M, Hirayama Y, Kobayashi E, Hino O. cDNA structure, alternative splicing and exon–intron organization of the predisposing tuberous sclerosis (*TSC2*) gene of the Eker rat model. Nucleic Acids Res 1995;23:2608–13.

94. Maheshwar MM, Cheadle JP, Jones AC, et al. The GAP-related domain of tuberin, the product of the *TSC2* gene, is a target for missense mutations in tuberous sclerosis. Hum Mol Genet 1997;6:1991–6.

95. Cheadle JP, Reeve MP, Sampson JR, Kwiatkowski DJ. Molecular genetic advances in tuberous sclerosis. Hum Genet 2000;207:97–114.

96. Ito N, Rubin G. *gigas*, a *Drosophila* homolog of tuberous sclerosis gene product-2, regulates the cell cycle. Cell 1999;96:529–39.

97. Wienecke R, Konig A, DeClue JE. Identification of tuberin, the tuberous sclerosis-2 product—tuberin possesses specific rap1GAP activity. J Biol Chem 1995;270:16,409–14.

98. Xiao G-H, Shoarinejad F, Jin F, Golemis EA, Yeung RS. The tuberous sclerosis 2 gene product, tuberin, functions as a Rab5 GTPase activating protein (GAP) in modulating endocytosis. J Biol Chem 1997;272:6097–100.

99. Knudson AG. Mutation and cancer: statistical study of retinoblastoma. Proc Natl Acad Sci USA 1971;68:820–3.

100. Green AJ, Johnson PH, Yates JRW. The tuberous sclerosis gene on chromosome 9q34 acts as a growth suppressor. Hum Mol Genet 1994;3:1833–4.

101. Green AJ, Smith M, Yates JRW. Loss of heterozygosity on chromosome 16p13.3 in hamartomas from tuberous sclerosis patients. Nat Genet 1994; 6:193–6.

102. Carbonara C, Longa L, Grosso E, et al. 9q34 loss of heterozygosity in a tuberous sclerosis astrocytoma suggests a growth suppressor-like activity also for the *TSC1* gene. Hum Mol Genet 1994;3:1829–32.

103. Henske EP, Scheithauer BW, Short MP. Allelic loss is frequent in tuberous sclerosis kidney lesions but rare in brain lesions. Am J Hum Genet 1996;59:400–6.

104. Verhoef S, van Diemen-Steenvoorde R, Akkersdijk WL, et al. Malignant pancreatic tumor within the spectrum of tuberous sclerosis complex in childhood. Eur J Pediatr 1999;158:284–7.

105. Carbonara C, Longa L, Grosso E, et al. Apparent preferential loss of heterozygosity at *TSC2* over *TSC1* chromosomal regions in tuberous sclerosis hamartomas. Genes Chromosom Cancer 1996;15:18–25.

106. Sepp T, Green AJ, Yates JRW. Loss of heterozygosity in tuberous sclerosis hamartomas. J Med Genet 1996;33:962–4.

107. Longa L, Saluto A, Brusco A, et al. *TSC1* and *TSC2* deletions differ in size, preference for recombinatorial sequences, and location within the gene. Hum Genet 2001;108:156–66.

108. Jones AC, Shyamsundar MM, Thomas MW, et al. Comprehensive mutation analysis of *TSC1* and *TSC2* and phenotypic correlations in 150 families with tuberous sclerosis. Am J Hum Genet 1999;64:1305–15.

109. Brook-Carter PT, Peral B, Ward CJ, et al. Deletion of the *TSC2* and PKD1 genes associated with severe infantile polycystic kidney disease—a contiguous gene syndrome. Nat Genet 1994;8:328–32.

110. Qian F, Watnick TJ, Onuchic LF, Germino GG. The molecular basis of focal cyst formation in human autosomal dominant polycystic kidney disease type I. Cell 1996;87:979–87.

111. Verhoef S, Vrtel R, van Essen TV, et al. Somatic mosaicism and clinical variation in tuberous sclerosis complex. Lancet 1995;345:202.

112. Verhoef S, Bakker L, Tempelaars AMP, et al. High rate of mosaicism in tuberous sclerosis complex. Am J Hum Genet 1999;64:1632–7.

113. Jones AC, Sampson JR, Cheadle JP. Low level mosaicism detectable by DHPLC but not by direct sequencing. Hum Mutat 2001;17:233–4

114. Kwiatkowska J, Wigowska-Sowinska J, Napierala D, Slomski R, Kwiatkowski DJ. Mosaicism in tuberous sclerosis as a potential cause of the failure of molecular diagnosis. N Engl J Med 1999;340:703–7.

115. Jones AC, Daniells CE, Snell RG, et al. Molecular genetic and phenotypic analysis reveals differences between *TSC1* and *TSC2* associated familial and sporadic tuberous sclerosis. Hum Mol Genet 1997;6:2155–61.
116. Dabora SL, Jozwiak S, Franz DN, et al. Mutational analysis in a cohort of 224 tuberous sclerosis patients indicates increased severity of *TSC2*, compared with *TSC1*, disease in multiple organs. Am J Hum Genet 2001;68:64–80.
117. Yeung RS, Xiao GH, Jin F, Lee WC, Testa JR, Knudson AG. Predisposition to renal carcinoma in the Eker rat is determined by germ-line mutation of the tuberous sclerosis 2 (*TSC2*) gene. Proc Natl Acad Sci USA 1994;91:11,413–6.
118. Kobayashi T, Hirayama Y, Kobayashi E, Kubo Y, Hino O. A germline insertion in the tuberous sclerosis (*TSC2*) gene gives rise to the Eker rat model of dominantly inherited cancer [published erratum appears in Nat Genet 9:218]. Nat Genet 1995;9:70–4.
119. Onda H, Lueck A, Marks PW, Warren HB, Kwiatkowski DJ. *TSC2*(+/−) mice develop tumors in multiple sites that express gelsolin and are influenced by genetic background. J Clin Invest 1999;104:687–95.
120. Kobayashi T, Minowa O, Kuno J, Mitani H, Hino O, Noda T. Renal carcinogenesis, hepatic hemangiomatosis, and embryonic lethality caused by a germline *TSC2* mutation in mice. Cancer Res 1999;59:1206–11.
121. Kobayashi T, Minowa O, Sugitani Y, et al. A germ-line Tsc1 mutation causes tumor development and embryonic lethality that are similar, but not identical to, those caused by Tsc2 mutation in mice. Proc Natl Acad Sci USA 2001; 98:8762–7.
122. Potter CJ, Huang H, Xu T. *Drosophila* Tsc1 functions with Tsc2 to antagonize insulin signaling in regulating cell growth, cell proliferation, and organ size. Cell 2001;105:357–68.
123. Tapon, N, Ito N, Dickson BJ, Treisman JE, Hariharan IK. The *Drosophila* tuberous sclerosis complex gene homologs restrict cell growth and cell proliferation. Cell 2001;105:345–55.
124. Eker R. Familial renal adenomas in Wistar rats. Acta Pathol Microbiol Scand 1954;34:554–62.
125. Wolf DC, Whiteley HE, Everitt JI. Preneoplastic and neoplastic lesions of rat hereditary renal cell tumors express markers of proximal and distal nephron. Vet Pathol 1995;32:379–86.
126. Everitt JI, Goldsworthy TL, Wolf DC, Walker CL. Hereditary renal cell carcinoma in the Eker rat: a rodent familial cancer syndrome. J Urol 1992; 148:1932–6.
127. Hino O, Mitani H, Katsuyama H, Kubo Y. A novel cancer predisposition syndrome in the Eker rat model. Cancer Lett 1994;83:117–21.
128. Yeung RS, Katsetos CD, Klein-Szanto A. Subependymal astrocytic hamartomas in the Eker rat model of tuberous sclerosis. Am J Pathol 1997; 151:1477–86.
129. Kubo Y, Klimek F, Kikuchi Y, Bannasch P, Hino O. Early detection of Knudson's two-hits in preneoplastic renal cells of the Eker rat model by the laser microdissection procedure. Cancer Res 1995;55:989–90.

130. Yeung RS, Xiao GH, Everitt JI, Jin F, Walker CL. Allelic loss at the tuberous sclerosis 2 locus in spontaneous tumors in the Eker rat. Mol Carcinogen 1995;14:28–36.

131. Kubo Y, Kikuchi Y, Mitani H, Kobayashi E, Kobayashi T, Hino O. Allelic loss at the tuberous sclerosis (*TSC2*) gene locus in spontaneous uterine leiomyosarcomas and pituitary adenomas in the Eker rat model. Jpn J Cancer Res 1995;86:828–32.

132. Kobayashi T, Urakami S, Hirayama Y, et al. Intragenic *TSC2* somatic mutations as Knudson's second hit in spontaneous and chemically induced renal carcinomas in the Eker rat model. Jpn J Cancer Res 1997;88:254–61.

133. Satake N, Kobayashi T, Kobayashi E, Izumi K, Hino O. Isolation and characterization of a rat homologue of the human tuberous sclerosis 1 gene (*TSC1*) and analysis of its mutations in rat renal carcinomas. Cancer Res 1999;59:849–55.

134. Toyokuni S, Okada K, Kondo S, et al. Development of high-grade renal cell carcinomas in rats independently of somatic mutations in the *TSC2* and VHL tumor suppressor genes. Jpn J Cancer Res 1998;89:814–20.

135. Ferrus A, Garcia-Bellido A. Morphogenetic mutants detected in mitotic recombination clones. Nature 1976;260:425–6.

136. Geist RT, Gutmann DH. The tuberous sclerosis 2 gene is expressed at high levels in the cerebellum and developing spinal cord. Cell Growth Differ 1995;6:1477–83.

137. Wienecke R, Maize JC, Reed JA, de Gunzburg J, Yeung RS, DeClue JE. Expression of the *TSC2* product tuberin and its target rap1 in normal human tissues. Am J Pathol 1997;150:43–50.

138. Wienecke R, Maize JC, Shoarinejad F, et al. Co-localization of the *TSC2* product tuberin with its target Rap1 in the Golgi apparatus. Oncogene 1996;13:913–23.

139. Plank TL, Yeung RS, Henske EP. Hamartin, the product of the tuberous sclerosis 1 (*TSC1*) gene, interacts with tuberin and appears to be localized to cytoplasmic vesicles. Cancer Res 1998;58:4766–70.

140. Nellist M, van Slegtenhorst MA, Goedbloed M, van den Ouweland AMW, Halley DJJ, van der Sluijs P. Characterization of the cytosolic tuberin-hamartin complex: tuberin is a cytosolic chaperone for hamartin. J Biol Chem 1999;274:35,647–52.

141. van Slegtenhorst M, Nellist M, Nagelkerken B, et al. Interaction between hamartin and tuberin, the *TSC1* and *TSC2* gene products. Hum Mol Genet 1998;7:1053–7.

142. Nellist M, Verhaaf B, Goedbloed MA, Reuser AJ, van den Ouweland AM, Halley DJ. *TSC2* missense mutations inhibit tuberin phosphorylation and prevent formation of the tuberin–hamartin complex. Hum Mol Genet 2001;10:2889–98.

143. Benvenuto G, Li S, Brown S, et al. The tuberous sclerosis-1 (*TSC1*) gene product hamartin suppresses cell growth and augments the expression of the *TSC2* product tuberin by inhibiting its ubiquitination. Oncogene 2000;19:6306–16.

144. Hodges AK, Li S, Maynard J, et al. Pathological mutations in *TSC1* and *TSC2* disrupt the interaction between hamartin and tuberin. Hum Mol Genet 2001;10:2899–905.
145. Aicher LD, Campbell JS, Yeung RS. Tuberin phosphorylation regulates its interaction with hamartin. Two proteins involved in tuberous sclerosis. J Biol Chem 2001;276:21,017–21.
146. Miloloza A, Rosner M, Nellist M, Halley D, Bernaschek G, Hengstschlager M. The *TSC1* gene product, hamartin, negatively regulates cell proliferation. Hum Mol Genet 2000;9:1721–7.
147. Soucek T, Pusch O, Wienecke R, DeClue JE, Hengstschlager M. Role of the tuberous sclerosis gene-2 product in cell cycle control. J Biol Chem 1997;272:29,301–8.
148. Tsuchiya H, Orimoto K, Kobayashi T, Hino O. Presence of potent transcriptional activation domains in the predisposing tuberous sclerosis (*TSC2*) gene product of the Eker rat model. Cancer Res 1996;56:429–33.
149. Henry KW, Yuan X, Koszewski NJ, Onda H, Kwiatkowski DJ, Noonan DJ. Tuberous sclerosis gene 2 product modulates transcription mediated by steroid hormone receptor family members. J Biol Chem 1998;273:20,535–9.
150. Soucek T, Holzl G, Bernaschek, G, Hengstschlager M. A role of the tuberous sclerosis gene-2 product during neuronal differentiation. Oncogene 1998; 16:2197–2204.
151. Lamb RF, Roy C, Diefenbach TJ, et al. The *TSC1* tumor suppressor hamartin regulates cell adhesion through ERM proteins and the GTPase Rho. Nat Cell Biol 2000;2:281–7.

8
Behavioral Phenotype in Velo–Cardio–Facial Syndrome

Kieran C. Murphy

1. INTRODUCTION

Velo–cardio–facial syndrome (VCFS), the most frequent known interstitial deletion found in humans, occurs with an incidence of approx 1/4000 live births *(1)*. VCFS is associated with chromosomal microdeletions in the q11 band of chromosome 22 in over 90% of those with the disorder *(2)*. The VCFS phenotype is complex, with multiple congenital abnormalities affecting a wide range of tissues and organs, often occurring in different combinations and with widely differing severity. Although in excess of 100 phenotypic features have been described, the most common include characteristic dysmorphology, congenital heart disease, cleft palate, borderline learning disability, and psychiatric disorder (Fig. 1). Variability in phenotypic expression has resulted in the same deletion being linked to several syndromes including DiGeorge syndrome, conotruncal anomaly face syndrome, Cayler syndrome, and Opitz GBBB syndrome, and the term "22q11 deletion syndrome" has been proposed as a replacement term for these other designators.

2. PSYCHIATRIC DISORDER IN PEOPLE WITH VCFS

There have been surprisingly few studies of mental health and behavior in VCFS children or adults. Moreover, those that have been performed are confounded by methodological constraints including lack of operational criteria for psychiatric diagnosis, sample heterogeneity, small sample size, and lack of control groups. Nevertheless, several common temperamental features have been noted in studies of children and adolescents with VCFS. These include behavioral excitation, an exaggerated response to threatening

From: *Contemporary Clinical Neuroscience:*
Genetics and Genomics of Neurobehavioral Disorders
Edited by: G. S. Fisch © Humana Press Inc., Totowa, NJ

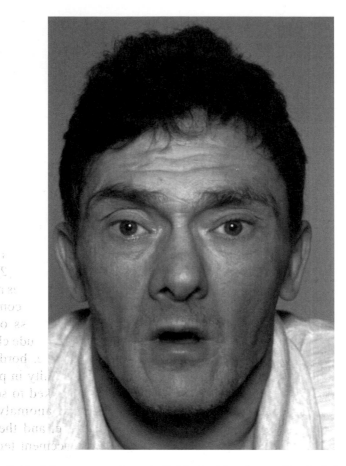

Fig. 1. Facial appearance in an individual with velo–cardio–facial syndrome and schizophrenia. (From Murphy KC, Jones RG, Griffiths E, Thompson PW, Owen MJ. Br J Psychiatry 1998;172:180–3. (Reprinted with permission of British Journal of Psychiatry.)

stimuli, and an enduring fearfulness of painful situations *(3)*. In addition, children with VCFS are reported to have poor social interaction skills, a flat affect with minimal facial expression, attentional difficulties, and high levels of anxiety and depression *(3,4)*. In a study of 15 children and adolescents, Papolos and colleagues reported that 47% (*n* = 7) were found to have bipolar disorder and 40% (*n* = 6) had attention deficit disorder (ADD/ ADHD) *(1)*. More recently, however, Arnold and colleagues reported that, although 60% (*n* = 12) of a series of 20 VCFS children and adolescents had a psychiatric disorder, none had bipolar disorder, and 35% (*n* = 7) had

ADHD *(5)*. Using a dimensional measure of psychopathology, these researchers also observed that subjects with VCFS had higher rates of ADHD, separation anxiety, and depression compared to (non-IQ-matched) sibling controls. Furthermore, subjects with VCFS achieved a significant lower academic level and required significantly more educational assistance than sibling controls. However, as sibling controls were likely to have significantly higher IQ levels than their VCFS siblings, these results are not unexpected.

What are we to make of the discrepancy between these two studies in the prevalence of bipolar disorder in VCFS children and adolescents? Arnold and colleagues suggest that the discrepancy may be related to the inherent difficulties in making the diagnosis of juvenile-onset bipolar disorder *(5)*. Difficulties include symptom pattern (e.g., typically irritable rather than euphoric mood), course (chronic rather than episodic), and overlap with common childhood disorders (e.g., ADHD) which distinguishes it from classic adult bipolar disorder *(6)*.

As the first cohort of children with VCFS was followed into adolescence and early adulthood, evidence also began to accumulate for a high prevalence of psychosis in these individuals. Shprintzen and colleagues suggested that more than 10% had developed psychiatric disorders that mostly resembled chronic schizophrenia with paranoid delusions, although operational criteria were not used *(7)*. Later, in a small study of adults with VCFS ($n = 14$), Pulver and colleagues found that 11 (79%) received a psychiatric diagnosis *(8)*. Using DSM-III-R criteria, four of those were diagnosed with schizophrenia or schizoaffective disorder. In a study of 10 adults with VCFS, Papolos and colleagues reported that four (40%) of their sample had psychotic symptoms while six (60%) met DSM-III-R criteria for a spectrum of bipolar affective disorders *(1)*. Interestingly, although no individual received a diagnosis of schizophrenia, the two oldest members of this group (aged 29 years and 34 years) were diagnosed with schizoaffective disorder. Similarly, follow-up data on two subjects in the series reported by Arnold and colleagues revealed that both had received a diagnosis of schizophrenia *(5)*.

In the largest study of its kind to date, Murphy and colleagues found that 18 (42%) of a sample of 50 adults with VCFS were diagnosed with a major psychiatric disorder; 15 (30%) were psychotic; 12 (24%) met DSM-IV criteria for schizophrenia, and another 6 (12%) exhibited major depression without psychotic features *(9)*. Individuals with schizophrenia presented with fewer negative symptoms and age at onset occurred relatively late (mean age = 26 years) compared to nondeleted schizophrenic controls. Using different ascertainment strategies however, Bassett and colleagues (1998) reported a relatively early age at onset (mean age = 19 years) in their sample of 10 individuals with VCFS and schizophrenia *(10)*. This discrepancy is likely to result from small sample sizes and differences in ascertainment between these studies. Consequently, although it is an attractive and plausible hypothesis that a clinical subtype of schizophrenia occurs in VCFS, future research with larger samples is required to confirm this hypothesis conclusively.

Many studies of individuals with VCFS have reported an association between VCFS and schizophrenia *(9–13)*. However, as we have noted, Papolos and colleagues have suggested that, in addition to increased rates of ADHD, the spectrum of severe psychiatric disorder seen in children with VCFS might also extend to include affective disorders such as bipolar disorder *(1)*. Longitudinal studies are required to test this hypothesis. It has been suggested that the psychiatric or behavioral phenotype observed in children and adolescents with VFCS might, in some cases, evolve into schizophrenia or schizoaffective disorder as these individuals age *(9)*.

Learning disability is a recognized but by no means invariable component of the VCFS phenotype. In addition, in a large study examining individuals with learning disability, Murphy and colleagues reported that 12% of people with mild learning disability were found to have a chromosome 22q11 deletion *(14)*. This raises the question of whether the high prevalence of schizophrenia in VCFS simply reflects a nonspecific association with learning disability. This appears unlikely, as it is generally estimated that the prevalence of schizophrenia in people with learning disability is only 3% *(15)* compared with a risk of 24% reported in VCFS *(9)*. Moreover, Murphy et al. found no correlation between the presence of psychosis and degree of intellectual impairment. The mean IQ of individuals with VCFS and schizophrenia was in the nonmentally retarded range (IQ > 70) *(9)*. Genetic evidence reviewed in the following paragraphs implicating 22q11 in psychosis in individuals without VCFS also suggests a more specific relationship between chromosome 22q11 and psychosis.

What is the true prevalence of schizophrenia in VCFS? Although we have reported that 12 of 50 adults (24%) with VCFS fulfilled DSM-IV criteria for schizophrenia, 80% were younger than 40 years and therefore remain within the age at risk *(9)*. In addition, there is an ascertainment bias implicit in any study of VCFS adults as they will have been selected for a less severe phenotype to have survived into adulthood. If this is the case, the true lifetime prevalence of schizophrenia in VCFS may be considerably higher than the 24% reported in this study. Consequently, longitudinal studies of VCFS children are required to determine the true lifetime prevalence of schizophrenia in VCFS individuals.

Over the past three decades, a major goal of schizophrenia research has been the identification of precursor symptoms and areas of dysfunction in children and adolescents that are a prelude to the later development of schizophrenia. Using a prospective, longitudinal research design, the high-risk method was developed to assess early social, psychological, and biological characteristics prior to onset of psychopathology in individuals with higher than average risk of psychiatric disorders, for example, schizophrenia. Several high-risk studies of children and adolescents have been performed and the majority selected children who are the offspring of parents with schizophrenia as their patient cohort *(16,17)*. Children with VCFS offer a unique opportunity to perform a novel high-risk study of schizophrenia susceptibility. In view of this, longitudinal studies of children with VCFS are also required to identify precursor symptoms and areas of dysfunction that precede the later development of schizophrenia in individuals with VCFS. Identification of such prodromal features in VCFS may have enormous implications for the clinical management of individuals with schizophrenia, with or without VCFS.

3. THE NEUROPSYCHOLOGICAL PROFILE IN VCFS

Early reports of children with VCFS described language abnormalities including immature language usage, poor development of numeric skills, and significant impairments in reading and spelling *(3,18)*. In a study of 37 children with VCFS, Swillen and colleagues reported a wide variability in intelligence ranging from moderate learning disability to average intelligence with a mean full-scale IQ (FSIQ) of approx 70 *(4)*. Forty-five percent of individuals ($n = 17$) were diagnosed with a learning disability, for whom the vast majority (82%) was mild. Similarly, Moss and colleagues reported that the mean FSIQ of their sample of 33 children and adults was 71, with 17 (52%) of their sample demonstrating learning disability *(19)*. There were no differences in mean FSIQ measures between children with additional symptoms, that is, congenital heart disease or palate anomalies, compared to those without. However, VCFS individuals with a familial deletion were found to have a lower mean FSIQ than individuals with a *de novo* deletion *(4,20)*.

A specific neuropsychological profile has been described in children with VCFS in which verbal IQ significantly exceeds performance IQ on tests of general intellectual functioning *(4,19,21,22)*. This discrepancy may relate to difficulties in planning ability, visual–spatial ability, and nonverbal reasoning in addition to deficits in novel reasoning and concept formation *(19)*. Unfortunately, however, these studies have been limited by small sample sizes and the absence of appropriately matched control groups.

In a recent study, Henry and colleagues examined the neuropsychological profile in 19 adults with VCFS compared with an age-, sex-, and IQ-matched control group *(23)*. Contrary to previous findings reported in children, Verbal IQ was not significantly higher than Performance IQ in these adults. Such a finding in adults suggests that: (1) previous reports of significant differences in Verbal/Performance IQ in children may be explained by methodological differences used in these studies; or (2) children with VCFS may significantly improve their Performance IQ as they get older. Longitudinal prospective studies of children with VCFS are therefore required to address these issues.

Henry and colleagues also reported that, compared to controls, adults with VCFS had significant impairments in visual–spatial ability, problem-solving and planning, and abstract and social thinking, features that have also been reported in children with VCFS *(23)*. It is unclear, however, whether the neuropsychological deficits observed in VCFS are associated with the presence of psychiatric disorder in these individuals. Future studies are needed to address this issue.

4. BRAIN STRUCTURAL ABNORMALITIES IN VCFS

It is now widely recognized that individuals with VCFS have severe neuropsychological deficits with high rates of major psychiatric disorder. Until recently, however, little was known about the neurobiology underlying these abnormalities. Most structural neuroimaging studies of individuals with VCFS have been qualitative. They report the presence of a small cerebellum (36%), white matter hyperintensities (27–90%), and developmental midline anomalies such as cavum septum pellucidum and cavum vergae (40–45%) *(24–26)*. The few quantitative neuroimaging studies that have been performed report relatively reduced volumes of total brain, left parietal lobe gray matter, and right cerebellar white matter volumes but increased volumes of both frontal lobes, midsagittal corpus callosum areas, and enlarged Sylvian fissures *(13,27,28)*. Furthermore, Eliez and colleagues have reported evidence for imprinting in children with VCFS, with greater cerebral volume reduction in children receiving a maternally derived deletion *(29)*. Unfortunately, these studies have been limited by small sample sizes and the absence of appropriately IQ-matched control groups, and studies have involved only children with VCFS. Recently, however, in a quantitative neuroimaging study of adults with VCFS, van Amelsvoort and colleagues compared adults with VCFS to an age- and IQ-matched control group *(26)*. They found that adults with VCFS exhibited widespread differences in white matter bilaterally and regional specific differences in gray matter in left cerebellum, insula, and frontal and right temporal lobes.

It remains unclear whether brain structural abnormalities reported in VCFS individuals relate to the neuropsychological deficits or major psychiatric disorder observed in such individuals. Previous structural neuroimaging studies of individuals with schizophrenia reported enlarged ventricles, reduced total brain volume, and midline brain abnormalities including cavum septum pellucidum and a hypoplastic vermis *(30–33)*, abnormalities that are also present in individuals with VCFS *(24–26,33,34)*. In addition, Eliez and colleagues reported that children with VCFS have significantly smaller temporal lobes and hippocampal volumes *(35)*, findings that have also previously been reported in people with schizophrenia *(36,37)*

5. MOLECULAR DISSECTION OF THE BEHAVIOURAL PHENOTYPE IN VCFS

The high rates of psychiatric dysfunction found among individuals with VCFS suggest that haploinsufficiency (reduced gene dosage) of a gene or genes mapping to the deleted region of chromosome 22 may be responsible for these disorders. In particular, the strong association between schizophrenia and VCFS suggests that a gene or genes mapping to chromosome 22q11 may play an etiological role in both. If so, what is the common pathogenetic mechanism? There is compelling evidence that a defect in early embryonic development is the cause of many of the abnormalities present in VCFS individuals. The importance of cephalic neural crest derived cells in the development of the conotruncal region of the heart, the thymus, the parathyroid glands, and the palate, all structures that are affected in VCFS, has been demonstrated by microablation and transplantation studies in avian embryos *(38)*. Based on these observations, it is therefore reasonable to hypothesize that a gene or gene located within the 22q11 deleted region is involved in the process of neuronal migration or differentiation in the pharyngeal arches. As a result haploinsufficiency of such a gene or genes would disrupt proper development of these systems, leading to multiple organ and tissue abnormalities.

There are at least three possible strategies that one can adopt to determine the role that single gene deletion plays in determining the high rates of schizophrenia in VCFS *(39)*. The first approach is to attempt to correlate variability in the VCFS phenotype with allelic variation in genes from the deleted region of the normal copy of chromosome 22. To prioritize genes for mutational analysis, this approach would be greatly facilitated by the identification of a critically deleted region in individuals with VCFS. Most individuals with VCFS have an interstitial deletion of approx 3 Mb, the typically deleted region (TDR). However, based on cases with deletions and unbalanced translocations, the shortest region of deletion overlap (SRDO) has been defined. Considerable excitement was generated when a breakpoint

in one case (patient ADU) carrying a chromosome 2:22 balanced translocation was found to map to this SRDO *(40)*. It was suggested that
haploinsufficiency of a single gene, disrupted by the ADU balanced translocation, resulted in the major clinical features found in VCFS. However, cloning of the balanced translocation breakpoint showed that transcripts
disrupted by the rearrangement appeared to belong to a pseudogene *(41)*. In
addition, Levy and colleagues reported a patient with VCFS who had an
interstitial deletion excluding the ADU breakpoint (the G deletion), suggesting that haploinsufficient gene or genes on 22q11 could be influenced
by position effects of genes mapping adjacent to the deletion *(42)*. More
recently, several other atypical deletions have been described in people with
VCFS. Some of these deletions do not overlap with the SRDO *(43,44)* and
one has no overlap with the TDR *(45)*. Consequently, it is difficult to draw a
definitive conclusion concerning the position of critical genes although one
might expect such genes to be within 1 Mb of DNA distal to the ADU
breakpoint *(46)*.

Besides attempting to identify a critically deleted region in VCFS, genes
for mutational analysis might also be prioritized on the basis of postulated
function and/or gene expression data. It is likely that haploinsufficiency of a
neurodevelopmental gene or genes mapping to chromosome 22q11, leading
to disturbed neural cell migration, underlies susceptibility to psychosis in
VCFS. Thus, clearly genes such as *UFD1L* and *GSCL*, which map to the
VCFS region and are plausibly involved in neural development, are candidate genes for the psychosis seen in VCFS *(47,48)*. On the other hand,
although schizophrenia is increasingly seen as a neurodevelopmental disorder, disturbances in catecholamine neurotransmission have also long been
postulated to play a key etiological role. Consequently, since the gene coding
for catechol-*O*-methyltransferase (*COMT*), an enzyme catalyzing the
O-methylation of catecholamine neurotransmitters (dopamine, adrenaline,
and noradrenaline), maps to the VCFS region of chromosome 22q11, this is
an outstanding candidate gene for schizophrenia. In particular, Dunham and
colleagues have postulated that VCFS individuals hemizygous for a low
activity allelic variant (Val-108-met) of this gene may be predisposed to the
development of schizophrenia as a result of increased brain dopamine levels
(49). Although we were unable to demonstrate an association between
the low-activity *COMT* allele and schizophrenia *(9)*, we recently found a
trend for association ($p = 0.08$) between a promoter polymorphism of the
COMT gene and psychosis in VCFS individuals *(50)*. Our preliminary finding will require replication in a larger sample.

A second approach towards ascertaining the role single gene deletion may play is to attempt to identify cases with the VCFS phenotype without detectable deletions of 22q11, in the hope of detecting cases in which point mutations disrupt the function of a single gene. However, cases of VCFS without 22q11 deletions are relatively uncommon and these cannot be guaranteed to result from point mutations in 22q11. In addition, nondeleted VCFS individuals are likely to represent an etiologically heterogeneous group comprising true cases of VCFS and other non-VCFS phenocopies. Furthermore, although it is possible that the entire syndrome is attributable to deletion of a single gene, it is also likely that VCFS may be a contiguous gene disorder, where haploinsufficiency of several genes results in varying manifestations of the clinical phenotype.

A third approach is to use gene targeting in experimental animals. Historically, animal models for psychiatric disorders have been difficult to construct as such disorders are still predominantly defined in terms of subjective experiences described by affected individuals. Recently, however, more objective measures, for example, subtle abnormalities of cell migration and sensorimotor gating abnormalities that include defects in prepulse inhibition, have also been described in individuals with schizophrenia *(51,52)*. In an interesting development, a mutation of the proline dehydrogenase gene, a candidate gene for schizophrenia that maps to the syntenic region of mouse chromosome 16, resulted in sensorimotor gating deficits in mice *(53)*. Such objectively measured abnormalities hold great promise as they can be measured in both humans and animals.

A mouse model deleted for the syntenic region of mouse chromosome 16 that corresponds to human chromosome 22q11 has been produced and congenital cardiac abnormalities similar to those in VCFS observed *(54)*. In a further development, three recent papers have implicated a putative neurodevelopmental gene, *Tbx1*, as a candidate gene for the cardiovascular phenotypes expressed in VCFS *(55–57)*. *Tbx1* is a member of the T-box transcription factor family and lies the commonly deleted region. When $Tbx1^{-/-}$ mice are engineered, they display a wide range of developmental anomalies including hypoplasia of the thymus and parathyroid glands, cardiac outflow tract abnormalities, abnormal facial structures, abnormal vertebrae and cleft palate, characteristic features of the physical phenotype in humans. Although the majority of the abnormalities were present only in –/– mice, +/– mice displayed a less severe phenotype that may be due to a species difference in gene dosage sensitivity resulting in altered penetrance of the phenotype. It is unknown whether polymorphism of this gene is associated with the presence of schizophrenia in VCFS or in the nondeleted population and studies are currently underway to examine the role of *Tbx1* in the etiology of schizophrenia in VCFS and in the wider population.

6. CONCLUSIONS

There is now clear evidence for a characteristic behavioral phenotype in VCFS. High rates of ADHD and mood disorder have been reported in VCFS children while high rates of schizophrenia are found in adults with VCFS. In addition, a characteristic neuropsychological profile has been described with significant impairments in visual–spatial ability, problem solving, planning, and abstract and social thinking. Neuroimaging studies of children and adults with VCFS report decrease brain volumes with regional specific differences in cerebral gray and white matter.

Apart from the offspring of a dual mating or the MZ co-twin of an affected individual, the presence or a chromosome 22q11 deletion represents the highest known risk factor for the development of schizophrenia identified to date. It is likely that haploinsufficiency of a moderately common allelic variant of a neurodevelopmental gene or genes mapping to chromosome 22q11, leading to disturbed neural cell migration, may be a common neurodevelopmental mechanism for the physical, psychiatric, neuropsychological, and brain structural abnormalities in VCFS.

While deletion of chromosome 22q11 may account for only a small proportion of risk to the development of schizophrenia in the general population, nondeletion mutations or polymorphisms in genes within the VCFS region may make a more general and widespread contribution to susceptibility to schizophrenia in the wider population. Experience with other complex diseases, for example, Alzheimer's disease, diabetes, and breast cancer, suggests that understanding the molecular basis for uncommon subtypes with high penetrance has been shown to be the most successful approach to understanding the genetics and underlying pathophysiology of complex diseases. As the entire sequence of chromosome 22 has recently been determined, the future identification of the genetic determinants of the psychiatric, neuropsychological and neuroanatomical phenotypes in VCFS individuals will have profound implications for our understanding of the molecular genetics and pathogenesis of schizophrenia in the wider population.

REFERENCES

1. Papolos DF, Faedda GL, Veit S, et al. Bipolar spectrum disorders in patients diagnosed with Velo-cardio-facial syndrome: Does a hemizygous deletion of

chromosome 22q11 result in bipolar affective disorder? Am J Psychiatry 1996;153:1541–7.

2. Driscoll DA, Spinner NB, Budarf ML, et al. Deletions and microdeletions of 22q11.2 in Velo-cardio-facial syndrome. Am J Med Genet 1992;44:261–8.

3. Golding-Kushner, KJ, Weller G, Shprintzen RJ. Velo-cardio-facial syndrome: language and psychological profiles. J Craniofac Genet 1985;5:259–66.

4. Swillen A, Devriendt K, Legius E, et al. Intelligence and psychological adjustment in velocardiofacial syndrome: a study of 37 children and adolescents with VCFS. J Med Genet 1997;34:453–8.

5. Arnold PD, Siegel-Bartelt J, Cytrynbaum C, Teshman I, Schachar R. Velo-cardio-facial syndrome: implications of microdeletion 22q11 for schizophrenia and mood disorders. Am J Med Genet (Neuropsych Genet), 2001; 105:354–62.

6. McClellan J, Werry J. Practice parameters for the assessment and treatment of children and adolescents with bipolar disorder. J Am Acad Child Adolesc Psychiatry 1997;36:138–57.

7. Shprintzen RJ, Goldberg R, Golding-Kushner KJ, Marion RW. Late-onset psychosis in the velo-cardio-facial syndrome. Am J Med Genet 1992;42:141–2.

8. Pulver AE, Nestadt G, Goldberg R, et al. Psychotic illness in patients diagnosed with Velo-cardio-facial syndrome and their relatives. J Nerv Ment Dis 1994;182:476–8.

9. Murphy KC, Jones LA, Owen .J. High rates of schizophrenia in adults with Velo-cardio-facial syndrome. Arch Gen Psychiatry 1999;56:940–5.

10. Bassett AS, Hodgkinson K, Chow EWC, Correia S, Scutt LE, Weksberg R. 22q11 deletion syndrome in adults with schizophrenia. Am J Med Genet 1998;81:328–37.

11. Karayiorgou M, Morris MA, Morrow B, et al. Schizophrenia susceptibility associated with interstitial deletions of chromosome 22q11. Proc Natl Acad Sci USA 1995;92:7612–6.

12. Gothelf D, Frisch A, Munitz H, et al. Velocardiofacial manifestations and microdeletions in schizophrenic inpatients. Am J Med Genet 1997;72:455–61.

13. Usiskin SI, Nicolson R, Krasnewich DM, et al. Velocardiofacial syndrome in childhood-onset schizophrenia. J Am Acad Child Adolesc Psychiatry 1999;38:1536–43.

14. Murphy KC, Jones RG, Griffiths E, Thompson PW, Owen MJ. Chromosome 22q11 deletions: an under-recognised cause of idiopathic learning disability. Br J Psychiatry 1998;172:180–3.

15. Fraser W, Nolan M. Psychiatric disorders in mental retardation. In: Bouras N, ed. Mental Health in Mental Retardation. Cambridge: Cambridge University Press, 1994;79–92.

16. Erlenmeyer-Kimling L, Rock D, Squires-Wheeler E, Roberts S, Yang J. Early life precursors of psychiatric outcomes in adulthood in subjects at risk for schizophrenia or affective disorders. Psychiatry Res 1991;39:239–56.

17. Cannon TD, Mednick SA. The schizophrenia high-risk project in Copenhagen: three decades of progress. Acta Psychiatr Scand 1993;87(Suppl. 370):33–47.

18. Goldberg R, Motzkin B, Marion R, Scambler PJ, Shprintzen RJ. Velo-cardio-facial syndrome: a review of 120 patients. Am J Med Genet 1993;45:313–9.
19. Moss EM, Batshaw ML, Solot CB, et al. Psychoeducational profile of the 22q11 microdeletion: a complex pattern. J Pediatr 1999;134:193–8.
20. Gerdes M, Solot C, Wang PP, et al. Cognitive and behaviour profile of pre-school children with chromosome 22q11.2 deletion. Am J Med Genet 1999;85:127–33.
21. Woodin M, Wnag PP, Aleman D, McDonald-McGinn D, Zackai E, Moss E. Neuropsychological profile of childrena nd adolescents with the 22q11.2 microdeletion. Genet Med 2001;3:34–9.
22. Swillen A, Vandeputte L, Cracco J, et al. Neuropsychological, learning and psychosocial profile of primary school aged children with the Velo-cardio-facial syndrome (22q11 deletion): evidence for a non-verbal learning disability? Child Neuropsychol 2000;6:1–12.
23. Henry JC, van Amelsvoort T, Morris RG, Owen MJ, Murphy DGM, Murphy KC. An investigation of the neuropsychological profile in adults with velo-cardio-facial syndrome (VCFS). Neuropsychologia 2002;40:471–8.
24. Mitnick RJ, Bello JA, Shprintzen RJ. Brain anomalies in Velo-cardio-facial syndrome. Am J Med Genet 1994;54:100–6.
25. Chow EWC, Mikulis DJ, Zipursky RB, Scutt LE, Weksberg R, Bassett AS. Qualitative MRI findings in adults with 22q11 deletion syndrome and schizophrenia. Biol Psychiatry 1999;46:1436–42.
26. van Amelsvoort T, Daly E, Robertson D, et al. (2001) Structural brain abnormalities associated with deletion of chromosome 22q11: a quantitative neuroimaging study of adults with velo-cardio-facial syndrome. Br J Psychiatry 2001;178:412–9.
27. Bingham PM, Zimmerman RA, McDonald-McGinn D, Driscoll D, Emanuel BS, Zackai E. Enlarged sylvian fissures in infants with interstitial deletion of chromosome 22q11. Am J Med Genet (Neuropsychiatr Genet), 1997;74:538–43.
28. Eliez S, Schmitt EJ, White CD, Reiss AL. Children and adolescents with Velo-cardio-facial syndrome: a volumetric MRI study. Am J Psychiatry 2000; 57:409–15.
29. Eliez S, Antonarakis SE, Morris MA, Dahoun SP, Reiss AL. Parental origin of the deletion 22q11.2 and brain development in velo-cardio-facial syndrome (VCFS): a preliminary study. Arch Gen Psychiatry 2001;58:64–8.
30. Lewis SW, Mezey GC. Clinical correlates of septum pellucidum cavities: an unusual association with psychosis. Psychol Med 1985;15:43–54.
31. Martin P, Albers M. Cerebellum and schizophrenia: a selective review. Schizophr Bull 1995;21:241–50.
32. Ward KE, Friedmanm L, Wise A. Meta-analysis of brain and cranial size in schizophrenia. Schizophr Res 1996;22, 197–213.
33. Lynch DR, McDonald-McGinn DM, Zackai EH, et al. Cerebellar atrophy in a patient with Velo-cardio-facial syndrome. J Med Genet 1995;32:561–3.
34. Vataja R, Elomaa E. Midline brain anomalies and schizophrenia in people with CATCH 22 syndrome. Br J Psychiatry 1998;172:518–20.

35. Eliez S, Blasey CM, Schmitt EJ, White CD, Hu D, Reiss AL. Velocardiofacial syndrome: are structural changes in the temporal and mesial temporal regions related to schizophrenia? Am J Psychiatry 2001;158:447–53.
36. Razi K, Greene KP, Sakuma M, Ge SM, Kushner M, DeLisi LE. Reduction of the parahippocampal gyrus and the hippocampus in patients with chronic schizophrenia. Br J Psych 1999;174:512–9.
37. Wright IC, Rabe-Hesketh S, Woodruff PWR, David AS, Murray RM, Bullmore ET. Meta-analysis of regional brain volumes in schizophrenia. Am J Psychiatry 2000;157:16–25.
38. Le Dourain NM, Zillei C, Couly GF. Patterning of neural crest derivatives in the avian embryo: in vivo and in vitro studies. Dev Biol 1993;159:24–49.
39. Murphy KC. Schizophrenia and velo-cardio-facial syndrome. Lancet 2002;359:426–30.
40. Augusseau S, Jouk S, Jalbert P, Prieur M. DiGeorge syndrome and 22q11 rearrangements. Hum Genet 1986;74:206.
41. Sutherland HF, Wadey R, McKie JM. et al. Identification of a novel transcript disrupted by a novel translocation associated with DiGeorge syndrome. Am J Hum Genet 1996;59:23–31.
42. Levy A, Demczuk S, Aurias A, Depetris D, Mattei MG, Philip N. Interstitial 22q11 deletion excluding the ADU breakpoint in a patient with DGS. Hum Mol Genet 1995;4:2417–8.
43. O'Donnell H, McKeown C, Gould C, Morrow B, Scambler P. Detection of a deletion within 22q11 which has no overlap with the DiGeorge syndrome critical region. Am J Hum Genet 1997;60:1544–8.
44. McQuade L, Christodoulou J, Budarf M, et al. Patient with a 22q11.2 deletion with no overlap of the minimal DiGeorge syndrome critical region (MDGCR). Am J Med Genet 1999;86:27–33.
45. Rauch A, Pfieffer RA, Leipold G, Singer H, Tigges M, Hofbeck M. A novel 22q11.2 microdeletion in DiGeorge syndrome. Am J Hum Genet 1999;64:658–66.
46. Scambler PJ. The 22q11 deletion syndromes. Hum Mol Genet 2000;9:2421–6.
47. Pizzuti A, Novelli G, Ratti A, et al. UFD1L, a developmentally expressed ubiquitination gene, is deleted in CATCH 22 syndrome. Hum Mol Genet 1997;6:259–66.
48. Gottlieb S, Emanuel BS, Driscoll DA, et al. The DiGeorge syndrome minimal critical region contains a Goosecoid-like (GSCL) homeobox gene, which is expressed early in human development. Am J Hum Genet 1997;60:1194–1201.
49. Dunham I, Collins J, Wadey R, Scambler P. Possible role for COMT in psychosis associated with velo-cardio-facial syndrome. Lancet 1992;340:1361–2.
50. Murphy KC, Owen MJ. Evidence for association between polymorphisms of the catechol-*O*-methyltransferase (COMT) and monoamine oxidase (MAO) genes and schizophrenia in adults with velo-cardio-facial syndrome? Am J Med Genet 2000;96:476.
51. Ellenbroek BA, Cools AR. Animal models with construct validity for schizophrenia. Behav Pharmacol 1990;1:469–490.

52. Weinberger DR. From neuropathology to neurodevelopment. Lancet 1995; 346:552–7.
53. Gogos JA, Santha M, Takacs Z, et al. The gene encoding proline dehydroge- nase modulates sensorimotor gating in mice. Nat Genet 1999;21:434–9.
54. Lindsay EA, Botta A, Jurecic V, et al. Congenital heart disease in mice defi- cient for the DiGeorge syndrome region. Nature 1999;401:379–83.
55. Lindsay LA, Vitelli F, Su H, et al. Tbx1 haploinsufficiency in the DiGeorge syndrome region causes aortic arch defects in mice. Nature 2001;410:97–101.
56. Merscher S, Funke B, Epstein JA, et al. TBX1 is responsible for cardiovascular defects in velo-cardio-facial/DiGeorge syndrome. Cell 2001;104:619–29.
57. Jerome LA, Papaioannou VE. DiGeorge syndrome phenotype in mice mutant for the T-box gene, Tbx1. Nat Genet 2001;27:286–91.

9

Williams–Beuren Syndrome

Mònica Bayés and Luis A. Pérez Jurado

1. INTRODUCTION

Williams–Beuren syndrome (WBS) is a genetic neurodevelopmental disorder characterized by distinctive facial features, mental disability with unique cognitive and personality profiles, supravalvular aortic stenosis (SVAS), short stature, occasional transient hypercalcemia in infancy, and connective tissue anomalies *(1,2)*. It was first reported in 1952 under the name "idiopathic infantile hypercalcemia" as a syndrome defined by hypercalcemia, characteristic facial features, and failure to thrive *(3)*. Williams et al. (1961) and Beuren et al. (1962) described the syndrome independently as a disorder involving characteristic facial features, SVAS, and mental retardation *(4,5)*. Subsequent reports clearly demonstrated that the previously described clinical entities were the same, which might include a wider spectrum of abnormalities *(1,6)*.

The estimated incidence of the disease is 1/20,000 newborns with equal frequency in both sexes and all races, and without known predisposing factors *(7)*. Most cases occur sporadically, although there are a few instances of parent-to-child transmission that confirm an autosomal dominant pattern of inheritance *(8,9)*. WBS has also been reported in concordant monozygotic twins and in discordant dizygotic twins *(10,11)*.

In 1993 it was first reported that WBS is caused by a heterozygous deletion at chromosome band 7q11.23 that included the elastin gene (*ELN*) *(12)*. Later, a common deleted interval was found in the great majority of patients that encompasses about 1.5 Mb of DNA and includes *ELN* and several other genes *(13)*.

WBS is of particular interest to neuroscientists because patients exhibit general cognitive deficits with a nonuniform cognitive profile. They show specific difficulties in higher cognitive functions, for example, severe defi-

From: *Contemporary Clinical Neuroscience:*
Genetics and Genomics of Neurobehavioral Disorders
Edited by: G. S. Fisch © Humana Press Inc., Totowa, NJ

cits in visual–spatial processing, but exhibit adequate skills in face processing and some speech and language abilities. The study of the pathophysiology of this disorder is likely to make important contributions toward the understanding of the genetic bases of human cognition.

2. CLINICAL FEATURES AND NATURAL HISTORY

Individuals with WBS are usually born following uncomplicated pregnancies. At birth, they are on average slightly small for gestational age. In early infancy, feeding problems, frequent crying, colics, and constipation are common occurrences, and failure to thrive is often manifested.

WBS subjects have recognizable craniofacial features, characterized by bitemporal narrowing, periorbital fullness, medial eyebrow flare, epicanthic folds, malar flattening, full dropping cheeks, a flat nasal bridge with bulbous nasal tip, a wide mouth with full lips, and a small chin (Fig. 1). Frequently, the iris has a stellate pattern *(14)*. Dental hypoplasia and malocclusion are common. With age, facial features are slightly coarser and hair becomes prematurely gray.

Cardiovascular manifestations are detected in 75% of patients during their lifetimes *(1)*. An obstructive vascular lesion that involves the ascending aorta (SVAS) is the most common and life-threatening problem, with peripheral pulmonic stenosis next in frequency. Involvement of any other muscular arteries may occur, and vascular narrowing may be progressive. Several cases of sudden death have been reported, probably associated with primary or secondary occlusion of the coronary arteries *(15)*. Hypertension is relatively common and may be related to narrowing of the renal artery in some cases *(16)*.

Mild joint laxity is common in infancy but contractures may appear later in life *(17)*. Scoliosis, kyphosis, and lordosis may be present. Individuals with WBS tend to adopt a characteristic posture with kyphotic attitude, sloping shoulders, and mild flexion of hips and knees. Manifestations of connective tissue weakness in other systems may include inguinal hernias, bladder diverticuli, and intestinal diverticulosis. The skin is usually soft and finely wrinkled, particularly on the hands, with decreased subcutaneous fat. The voice is typically hoarse.

There is evidence of hypercalcemia in a minority of patients, which tends to resolve by 2–4 years of age. The hypercalcemia reported in the initial description of the syndrome was probably triggered by the high-dose vitamin D supplements provided to infants for preventing rickets *(6)*. Calcium levels are usually found at the upper end of the normal range. However, the presence of nephrocalcinosis as well as a history of irritability, feeding prob-

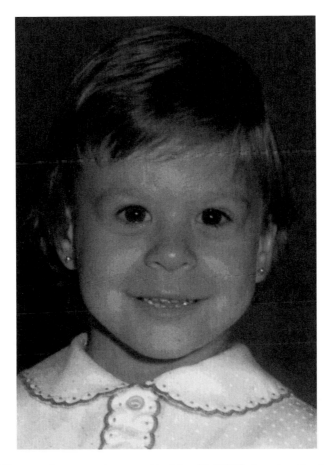

Fig. 1. Picture of a pretty 2-year-old girl with WBS showing the typical facial features.

lems, and constipation might be partly related to undetected hypercalcemia. No consistent abnormality in the regulation of calcium metabolism has been found, except for a delayed renal clearance of calcium following exogenous overload *(18,19)*.

Mild growth retardation is common and the final adult height is usually at the lower end of the normal range, approx 10 cm below average *(20)*. This relatively short stature in WBS is attributable to a combination of factors including prenatal growth delay, failure to thrive in infancy, and premature and short pubertal growth spurt.

Other relatively common clinical manifestations include strabismus, hyperopia and reduced stereoacuity, gastroesophageal reflux, chronic constipation, urinary frequency with bladder dyssynergia, and renal tract abnormalities. Hypothyroidism and celiac disease have been reported to occur more frequently among individuals with WBS than in the general population *(21,22)*.

Regarding psychomotor development, WBS children are globally delayed until about 3–4 years of age, after which they experience some degree of "catch-up" *(23)*. They retain marked deficits, however, in motor coordination and visual–spatial abilities. In contrast, their language skills are relatively preserved *(24,25)*. Mild muscle hypotonia is common and may be due to an actual myopathy *(26)*. However, hyperreflexia and hypertonia may also develop in late childhood; in these cases, symptomatic Chiari type I malformation should be ruled out *(27)*. Hyperacusis is manifested in approx 85% of patients with WBS. The characteristic neurobehavioral phenotype is later described in further detail.

Despite the wide spectrum of possible medical problems, individuals with WBS can have a relatively healthy life in the absence of severe cardiovascular manifestations. They may acquire relative independence in daily tasks such as toileting, washing and dressing, and even moving around using public transportation. However, the majority continues to live at home as adults and remain heavily dependent on their families for their self-care.

3. DIAGNOSIS, COUNSELING, AND FOLLOW-UP

The diagnosis of WBS can usually be made on clinical grounds by expert physicians, and with a high degree of specificity. It can and should be confirmed by molecular methods. The deletion can be detected by fluorescence *in situ* hybridization (FISH) with a probe for the *ELN* locus *(28)*, or using alternative methods such as typing polymorphic markers to detect failure of parental inheritance. Recurrence risk for parents and other relatives of patients with WBS with a deletion is very low, <1%, and probably close to that of the general population. However, individuals with WBS transmit the deletion, and therefore the disorder, to 50% of their offspring in an autosomal dominant fashion.

Medical care by the appropriate specialists should be individualized for every child, adolescent, or adult with WBS *(29)*. Medical surveillance should specially include monitoring of blood pressure and renal function. There is no specific treatment except for the associated medical complications if they occur. In general, vitamin D or multivitamin supplementations should probably be avoided and a dietary regimen to prevent constipation is recommended. An early psychological evaluation and subsequent follow-up are very important to provide adequate educational needs. In cases of attention deficit–hyperactivity disorder, environmental modifications should be implemented and psychostimulant medication may be beneficial. There are excellent guidelines for medical monitoring of patients with WBS written by a panel of experts on WBS and published recently *(30)*.

4. NEUROBEHAVIORAL FEATURES

Patients with WBS show mild to moderate mental retardation, with a mean full scale IQ score around 60, ranging from 40 to 90 *(24,31,32)*. However, the hallmark of this syndrome is an uneven cognitive profile that includes apparent relative strength in language abilities and face processing, but extreme difficulty with visual–spatial construction *(24,25)*. Developmental motor disabilities are also significant including poor balance, coordination, and motor planning. Adaptive behaviors in individuals with WBS show relative strengths in socialization and communication skills, and relative weakness in daily living and motor skills. Although there is some controversy regarding the specific characteristics of the features, their uniqueness to WBS, and their change with chronological age, there is a major agreement that WBS subjects show common neurobehavioral characteristics that constitute a common profile. This profile has been termed the Williams syndrome cognitive profile (WSCP), and a quantitative method for evaluation of several features of this profile has been proposed *(32)*.

4.1. Visual–Spatial Construction

The visual–spatial profile is very unusual *(33)*. Individuals with WBS have a stereotypical pattern of visual processing in which objects are reproduced as a disorganized collection of parts with no sense of coherence of the whole. They perform especially poorly on tasks involving pattern construction, drawing, or assembling pieces in three dimensions (Fig. 2). This visual–spatial processing dysfunction with lack of global organization translates into markedly impaired visual learning abilities, causing troubles for common tasks of everyday life. It may also contribute to their poor motor skills and gait instability. In contrast, while their overall performance on specific tests is below that of normal individuals of the same age, a clear strength in face recognition and processing is evident *(34)*. This ability appears to be related to their tendency to focus on specific features instead of using holistic processes.

4.2. Language

Children with WBS show delayed acquisition of expressive and receptive language milestones, although they finally develop a relatively appropriated

WBS girl, 10 years old
global IQ of 60

WBS boy, 11 years old
global IQ of 58

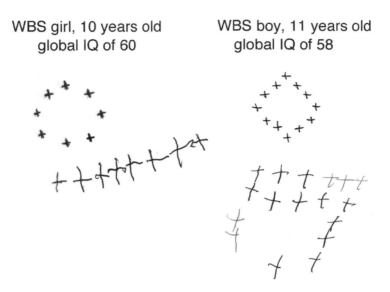

Fig. 2. Impaired visual–spatial construction in individuals with WBS. The figure shows the drawings made by two children with WBS that were asked to copy a global figure composed of small crosses. In both cases, the patients tend to reproduce the crosses but failed in producing the global form.

overall level of language skills. After 3–5 years of age, measures of differences between the greater verbal and the poorer nonverbal abilities are always significant and can exceed 2 standard deviations. Their speech has been described as fluent and loquacious, rich in clichés, emphatic intonations, and unusual aphorisms. However, their command of grammar and comprehension is not as good as it appears *(35)*. Formal assessment of language abilities shows strengths in phonological processing, verbal fluency, vocabulary, and some aspects of morphosyntax, but an overall delay of language abilities *(36,37)*. Their sensitivity to sound patterns is much stronger than their sensitivity to meaning. For these reasons, it has been suggested that the apparent language proficiency in WBS individuals may be linked to their excellent capacity for auditory short-term memory *(38)*.

4.3. Personality

The personality of individuals with WBS is overfriendly and empathetic, with a strong impulse toward social contact and affective expression. Their degree of fearlessness and lack of judgment skills with regard to social interaction with strangers clearly exceed that of normal subjects or other clinical populations *(39)*. Their hypersociability is apparent at an early age and may be a major concern for parents. Persons with WBS show abnormally positive social judgments of strangers, similar to that which has been described for individuals with bilateral damage to the amygdala *(40)*. An undercurrent of anxiety related to common situations, some features of obsessive–compulsive disorder, and a high incidence of simple phobias are also characteristic. In adolescence and adulthood, excessive preoccupations, anxiousness about new situations, and inappropriate interpersonal relating may lead to emotional and behavioral problems *(41)*. Hyperactive behavior and short attention span may be present, compounding the existing learning problems.

4.4. Musicality

Musical ability is usually described in WBS and there are anecdotal reports of individuals with WBS with exceptional musical talent or even "perfect pitch" *(42)*. A possible relation of musical ability to hyperacusis has been suggested. In a formal evaluation of 14 children and adolescents with WBS, they showed similar levels of musical expressiveness compared to age peers, but were less able to discriminate pitch and rhythm, or to attach a semantic interpretation to emotion in music *(43)*. The musical strength in individuals with WBS has been proposed to involve rather a strong engagement with music as a means of expression and play than formal analytic skill in pitch and rhythm discrimination. However, additional contrasted and objective data are needed in this regard.

4.5. Brain Morphology

Using magnetic resonance imaging (MRI), some neuroanatomical abnormalities have been found *(44)*. Brain and brain stem sizes are globally decreased relative to age-matched controls, with relative preservation of the cerebellum and temporal gyrus. There is also some gross discrepancy in size between the larger frontal and temporal limbic cerebral regions, and the smaller parietal and occipital areas. This frontal/temporal sparing correlates with the preservation of language and social skills relative to motor and visual abilities. The overall volume of the cerebellum is normal with preservation of the neocerebellum and the paleocerebellar vermis and a relative increase of the neocerebellar tonsils. The corpus callosum midline length is decreased, likely due to a decreased size of the splenium. There is a relative preservation of cerebral gray matter volume and a disproportionate reduction in cerebral white matter volume. Asymmetries have been noted in the occipital lobes and the planum temporale, with a relative decrease of the gray matter volume on the right side. A consistent finding is a short central sulcus that does not become opercularized in the interhemispheric fissure, suggesting a possible developmental anomaly affecting the dorsal half of the hemispheres *(45)*. Chiari type I malformation can also be found by MRI in subjects with WBS even in the absence of neurological signs *(27)*. Histopathological studies in a few cases have shown that the cortical cytoarchitecture is relatively normal in most brain areas, except for some regions that show increased cell size and decreased cell-packing density. Acquired pathology of microvascular origin has been reported and is likely related to underlying hypertension *(45)*.

4.6. Brain Electrophysiology

Event related potentials during two relatively spared cognitive functions, face processing and language processing, have shown consistent differences between patients with WBS and controls *(46)*. These data, along with other empirical findings, are suggestive of an abnormal cerebral specialization in WBS patients, who might be using different pathways to achieve the proficiency for those functions.

5. MOLECULAR BASIS

WBS is a contiguous gene disorder caused by a heterozygous submicroscopic deletion at chromosome band 7q11.23. The great majority of patients show a common deleted interval that was first defined by deletion mapping with polymorphic markers, and confirmed by the detection of common junction fragments *(47,48)*. The commonly deleted interval has been estimated to encompass approx 1.5 Mb containing 25–30 genes *(13,49–52)*.

5.1. Mutational Mechanism

The fact that the great majority of WBS cases are sporadic indicates a high rate of *de novo* deletions, approx 0.5×10^{-4} per gamete per generation. The deletions occur with similar frequency in the maternally or paternally inherited chromosome. Evidence of recombination between polymorphic markers proximal and distal to the deletion has shown that most deletions arise from crossover events between both chromosome 7 homologues during meiosis. However, absence of recombination in other cases suggests that intrachromosomal rearrangements may also occur *(53,54)*. Physical mapping of the genomic region has been difficult owing to the presence of several segmental repeats recently characterized *(49,50)*. A complex arrangement of large blocks (approx 100 kb) of chromosome 7-specific segmental duplications or low-copy repeat elements (LCRs) flanks the WBS deletion interval (Fig. 3). Fine mapping of deletion ends in patients has revealed that most chromosomal deletion breakpoints are located in two spe-

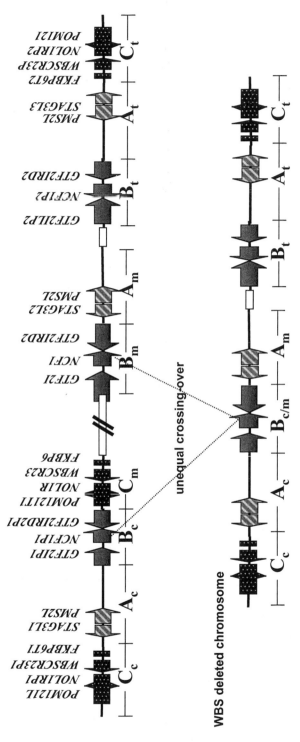

Fig. 3. Schematic diagram of the 7q11.23 genomic region around the WBS deletion. The whole region on a normal chromosome is shown at the **top**, while the most common WBS chromosome resulting from unequal crossing-over between centromeric and middle blocks B is displayed at the **bottom**. The single copy region that is commonly deleted in WBS patients (interrupted square from *FKBP6* to *GTF2I* in the **upper panel**) contains 25–30 genes and is flanked by a complex arrangement of blocks of chromosome 7-specific segmental duplications (called A, B, and C) (*47*). **Middle block A** (A_m) contains sequences related to the *PMS2* mismatch repair gene (*PMS2L*) and the stromal antigen 3 gene (*STAG3L*) that are also present in other chromosome 7 locations. **Middle block B** (B_m) contains the *GTF2I* and *NCF1* genes, and another gene related to *GTF2I* (*GTF2IRD2*). **Middle block C** (C_m) comprises a truncated *POM121* gene, the novel *NOL1R* and *WBSCR23* genes, and the four first exons of *FKBP6*. The centromeric (A_c, B_c, C_c) and telomeric (A_t, B_t, C_t) blocks are paralogs containing additional copies of the same genes or pseudogenes.

217

cific blocks of LCRs (centromeric and middle blocks B) *(50,55)*. These blocks are in tandem, share >99.5% sequence identity along approx 100 kb and have a high density of short interspersed elements. Middle block B contains three genes (*GTF2I*, *NCF1*, and *GTF2IRD2*), while the centromeric block harbors the corresponding pseudogenes *(50)*. Therefore, it appears that a common mutational mechanism accounts for the majority of 7q11.23 deletions causing WBS that somehow explains the high mutation rate. That is, WBS deletions arise as a consequence of misalignment during chromosome pairing and unequal crossing over between highly homologous sequences. A minority (5%) of cases displays slightly larger deletion sizes (approx 1.65 Mb), with breakpoints located in the blocks A (Fig. 4).

Recent data demonstrate the existence of at least two types of genomic rearrangements at 7q11.23 in some of the progenitors transmitting the WBS chromosome: (1) approx one third carry a chromosome with an inversion of the whole interval between the centromeric and telomeric LCRs *(56)*; (2) approx 5% carry a chromosome with either two or four flanking LCRs, instead of the normal number of three (Bayés et al., *unpublished data*). Heterozygosity for such alleles would predispose to unequal chromosome pairing in meiotic prophase. A crossing over event within the misaligned blocks during cell division would lead to the WBS deletion. Since a recombination rate of 1% corresponds approx to 1 Mb, the frequency of recombination in the small misaligned genomic region (approx 100 kb) can be estimated to be about 1/1000. This recombination rate may explain why the recurrence risk for WBS appears not to be significantly increased in families despite the finding of these "predisposing" alleles.

There is evidence for the existence of orthologous LCRs in other primates but not in mouse or other mammals *(50,57)*. In the mouse, the order of the genes within the WBS deletion is fully conserved but the entire region is inverted with respect to the flanking genes in the human map *(50)*. Additional comparative mapping has suggested that the human 7q11.23 chromosomal region evolved through serial, evolutionarily recent, complex inversions and additional rearrangements leading to segmental genomic duplications.

5.2. Genes Within the WBS Deletion

The Human Genome Project has greatly accelerated the gene identification process in the WBS deleted region *(58,59)*. To date, 20 genes located within this hemizygously deleted interval have been reported *(13,60)*. They include genes that code for structural proteins, transcription factors, transmembrane receptors, and other proteins involved in signal transduction and neuronal tasks (Table 1), although functional information is still lacking for

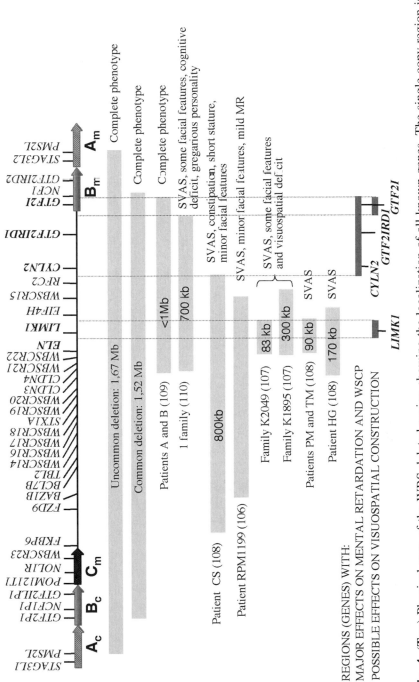

Fig. 4. (**Top**) Physical map of the WBS deleted region showing the localization of all known genes. The single copy region is shown as a black line and the flanking blocks of segmental duplications are depicted as arrows. (**Middle panel**) Horizontal bars represent the sizes of the common and atypical deletions described to date. A summary of the clinical phenotype of each patient with the reference is shown by the corresponding deletion. The candidate regions and genes contributing to the mental retardation, cognitive profile (WSCP) and visuospatial construction by deletion mapping and clinical-molecular correlations are shown at the bottom.

219

Table 1
Genes Commonly Deleted in WBS Ordered from Centromere to Telomere

Gene	Protein products	Putative function/functional clues
NOL1R	NOL1Related	Homology to the proliferating nucleolar protein P120
WBSCR23	Predicted protein	Putative zinc-finger nuclear phosphoprotein
FKBP6	FK-506 binding protein 6	Immunophilin family member
FZD9	Frizzled 9	Transmembrane receptor for wingless-related proteins
BAZ1B/WBSCR9/WSTF	*Drosophila Acf1* homolog	Transcription factor? Chromatin assembly
BCL7B	B-cell lymphoma 7B	Atopy-related IgE autoantigen in atopic dermatitis
TBL2/WS-βTRP	Transducin β-like 2	β-Transducin family member of unknown function
WBSCR14/WS-bHLH	Basic helix–loop–helix protein	Transcription repressor, interacts with Mlx, involved in cell proliferation/differentiation
STX1A	Syntaxin 1A	Presynaptic membrane protein, involved in exocytosis of neurotransmitter-containing vesicles
CLDN3 and *CLDN4*	Claudin family members *Clostridium perfringens* enterotoxin receptors	Part of tight junction structures/paracellular barrier in epithelial tissues

Gene	Protein	Function
ELN	Elastin	Main component of the elastic fibers in the extracellular matrix
LIMK1	LIM-kinase 1	Signal transduction in neuronal synapses involved in actin cytoskeleton depolymerization
EIF4H/WBSCR1	Eukaryotic initiation factor eIF4H	Positive regulator of translation initiation
WBSCR15	Protein without known motifs	Unknown
RFC2	Subunit 2 of the pentameric replication factor C	DNA elongation during replication
CYLN2	Neuronal cytoplasmatic linker protein CLIP-115	Links organelles to cytoskeleton via microtubules
GTF2IRD1/WBSCR11/ GT3	GTF2I-related domain	Enhancer-binding protein and transcriptional regulator
GTF2I	TFII-I/BAP135/SPIN	Transcription initiator factor involved in both basal and activated transcription
NCF1	Neutrophilic cytosolic factor 1, p47-phox	Phagocyte NADPH oxidase subunit. Antimicrobial activity

221

many of them. However, only those genes that are dosage sensitive are likely to be relevant and contribute to the WBS phenotype.

POM121, *NOL1R*, and *WBSCR23* are multiple copy genes present in the blocks C of the 7q11.23 LCRs (Fig. 3) *(50)*. The middle block C is included in the common deletion, while the other two copies are not. This middle block contains a truncated *POM121* and the complete other two genes. The nondeleted copies of these three genes (centromeric and telomeric LCRs) are also expressed and might encode functional proteins as well. *POM121* encodes a pore membrane protein present in the nuclear envelope but also in stacked membrane arrays (annulate lamella) in the cytoplasm *(61)*. *NOL1R* and *WBSCR23* have been identified downstream to *POM121* but in the opposite transcriptional direction. They encode a protein related to the human proliferating cell nucleolar protein P120 (*NOL1R*) and a protein with several domains conserved in zinc-finger nuclear phosphoproteins (*WBSCR23*) (Magano et al., *unpublished*).

FKBP6 belongs to the family of immunophilins, which are cellular receptors for the immunosuppressive drugs FK506 and rapamycin. The expression of *FKBP6* transcripts is detected in all human tissues examined, with exceptionally high levels in testis and lower levels in brain *(62)*. Its function is unknown although other immunophilin family members are involved in modulation of intracellular calcium release.

FZD9 (previously called FZD3) belongs to the frizzled family of WNT receptors that share a cysteine-rich extracellular domain and seven-transmembrane domains *(63)*. The *FZD9* transcript is abundantly found in all areas of the brain, and also in testis and skeletal muscle. *In situ* hybridization studies in mouse embryos show that it is expressed in a variety of tissues throughout development, and particularly in the developing nervous system *(64)*. In transfected cells, FZD9 localizes to the plasma membrane where it can interact with the *Drosophila wingless* protein (*wg*) *(63)*. In mouse, the *wg*-homologous *Wnt1* gene is involved in the early development of the central nervous system. It has been proposed that haploinsufficiency for human *FZD9* could contribute to the neurobehavioral traits of WBS by subtle effects on embryonic brain differentiation.

BAZ1B (also called *WBSCR9* and *WSTF*) encodes a protein with a C-terminal bromodomain, as well as several other conserved motifs *(65,66)*. The bromodomain is a structural motif characteristic of proteins involved in chromatin-dependent regulation of transcription. Northern blot analysis detected ubiquitous expression of *BAZ1B* in adult issues. Proteins of this family have been identified as integral components of chromatin remodeling complexes and frequently possess histone acetyltransferase activity.

BCL7B shows high homology to *BCL7A*, a gene disrupted by a complex translocation in a Burkitt lymphoma cell line. It is highly expressed in most embryonic and adult tissues with the exception of brain *(67)*. BCL7B has been identified as an atopy-related IgE autoantigen *(68)*. The functions of the BCL7 family of proteins are unknown.

TBL2 (also called *WBSCR13* and *WS-βTRP*) encodes a protein of unknown function with four WD40 repeats that belongs to the β-transducin family of proteins *(69,70)*. *TBL2* is expressed predominantly in testis, skeletal muscle, heart, and some endocrine tissues. Because haploinsufficiency causing disease has been shown for other WD40 protein genes, the loss of one copy of *TBL2* in WBS might have a phenotypic effect.

WBSCR14 (also called *WS-bHLH*) encodes a basic helix–loop–helix leucine zipper (bHLHZip) transcription factor of the Myc/Max/Mad superfamily *(71)*. *WBSCR14* is expressed in multiple tissues, including regions of the brain, the liver, and the intestinal tract *(72)*. WBSCR14 forms functional heterodimers with another bHLHZip protein, MLX, and represses E-box-dependent transcription. The actual gene targets of WBSCR14 are unknown, but preliminary results suggest a possible role of WBSCR14 in growth control. Haploinsufficiency for *MITF*, another bHLHZip protein, has been involved in a dominant developmental disorder, the Waardenburg syndrome type II.

STX1A is a plasma membrane component of the SNARE complex, which is involved in vesicle membrane fusion *(73)*. Synaptic vesicles store neurotransmitters that are released at the presynaptic active zones with the intervention of calcium channels. STX1A is involved in the intracellular membrane transport and may play a key role in the exocytosis process of neurotransmitters. In addition, recent data suggest that STX1A up-regulates GABA transporter levels by subcellular redistribution *(74)*. *STX1A* expression is restricted to the central nervous system. It is highly expressed in embryonic spinal cord and ganglia, and in adult cerebellum and cerebral cortex *(75)*.

CLDN3 and *CLDN4* (also called *CPETR2* and *1*, respectively) *(76)* encode members of the claudin family of integral membrane proteins that are major components of tight junction strands. In epithelial and endothelial cells, tight junctions constitute physical barriers that prevent the diffusion of solutes through the paracellular space. *CLDN3* is mainly expressed in lung and liver, while *CLDN4* is found in lung and kidney *(77)*. Both proteins were initially identified as high-affinity receptors for *Clostridium perfringens* enterotoxin *(78)*.

ELN codes for elastin, one of the main components of the elastic fibers found in the extracellular matrix of many tissues *(79)*. It was the first gene identified in the WBS critical region *(12)* and it is the only one that has been unequivocally linked to any aspect of the WBS phenotype. Studies of patients with familial or sporadic isolated SVAS have found deletions or point mutations confined to this gene. Therefore, it can be inferred that *ELN* haploinsufficiency is responsible for the cardiovascular phenotype but not for the other features or cognitive anomalies of WBS *(80,81)*. Pathological specimens from the aorta, skin, and pulmonary arteries of WBS patients have demonstrated disorganized elastin deposition *(82,83)*. Elastin is synthesized by the arterial smooth muscle during late pregnancy and early postnatal life. Hemizygosity at *ELN* leads to a reduced amount of elastin protein that affects arterial compliance. Compensatory increases in elastin lamellae and smooth muscle during development also contribute to increased arterial wall thickness. Further confirmation that *ELN* haploinsufficiency causes the cardiovascular phenotype of WBS comes from mouse models that are deficient for elastin. As in humans, hemizygous animals show an increase of 35% in the number of elastin lamellae and smooth muscle rings in the arteries, and the homozygotes die of an obstructive arterial disease early after birth *(84,85)*. No other phenotypic abnormality has been described in *Eln* knockouts. Likely, *ELN* gene haploinsuffiency may also be responsible for other connective tissue manifestations of the WBS phenotype, including some but not all the facial features (mostly the periorbital fullness and thick lips), the inguinal hernias, the skin and joint changes, and the diverticuli of bladder and intestine.

LIMK1 encodes a serine-only protein kinase that is highly expressed in both adult and fetal central nervous system, with the highest levels in the cerebral cortex *(86)*. LIMK1 phosphorylates cofilin, an actin depolymerization factor, which is then unable to bind and depolymerize F-actin. LIMK1 is activated by Rac-GTP and Rho and therefore is involved in signal transduction of stimulus-induced actin organization. In addition, the LIM domain (a highly conserved cysteine-rich structure containing two zinc fingers) interacts with the cytoplasmic domain of pro-neuregulin-1 and may play a role in synapse formation and maintenance *(87)*. A decrease in *LIMK1* expression in WBS might affect the neuron actin cytoskeleton and the axonal guidance during brain development. Therefore, it has been suggested that hemizygosity at *LIMK1* could account for the abnormally clustered and aligned neurons seen in WBS patients' brains. However, normal LIMK1 immunostaining has been found in the brain of a WBS patient *(45)*.

RFC2 codes for an auxiliary factor for the DNA polymerases δ and ε. It is one of the five subunits of the human replication factor (RFC) that, in the presence of ATP, assembles proliferating-cell nuclear antigen (PCNA) and DNA polymerase on primed DNA templates. The RFC2 protein binds to

ATP and is required not only for chromosomal DNA replication but also for a cell cycle checkpoint in *Saccharomyces cerevisiae (88)*. Haploinsufficiency for *RFC2* could affect DNA replication efficiency and therefore may contribute to growth and developmental deficits in WBS *(89)*.

WBSCR15 (also called *WBSCR5*) encodes a 243-amino-acid sequence with no significant similarity to any characterized protein. Interestingly, unlike other genes in the region that are closely related in human and mouse, human *WBSCR15* is only 48% identical to the mouse orthologue. Northern blot analysis detected strong expression of WBSCR15 in peripheral blood leukocytes, placenta, and lung, with lower expression in spleen, heart, brain, liver, and pancreas *(90)*.

EIF4H (also called *WBSCR1*) encodes a eukaryotic translation initiation factor with an RNA recognition motif. Because its affinity for RNA is weak, it has been suggested that eIF4H functions in translation initiation through protein–protein interactions with other eIF4 initiation factors. Recent studies confirm that it stimulates translational, RNA-dependent ATPase and helicase activities of eIF4A *(91,92)*. Northern blot analysis shows that *EIF4H* is expressed ubiquitously in human tissues *(86)*.

CYLN2 (also named CLIP-115) belongs to the family of cytoplasmic linker proteins that mediate interactions between specific membranous organelles and microtubules *(93,94)*. The association of membrane-bound cell organelles to microtubules is crucial for determination of their shape, intracellular localization, and translocation. The CYLN2 protein is most abundantly expressed in brain, and it is almost exclusively found in neurons. Electron microscopy showed that CYLN2 is highly enriched in the dendritic lamellar body (DLB), an organelle present in bulbous dendritic appendages of neurons linked by dendrodendritic gap junctions. In addition, *CLYN2* is ubiquitously expressed in the Bergmann glia cells of the cerebellum, which are also connected by extensive gap junction plaques. These observations lead to the suggestion of a role for CLYN2 in the turnover of gap junctions. In this sense, it has been speculated that haploinsufficiency at the *CLYN2* gene would affect neuron coupling and disturb brain function in specific regions in WBS.

GTF2IRD1 (also called *WBSCR11*, *CREAM1*, *MusTRD1*, *BEN*) encodes a ubiquitous transcription factor containing five internal repeats of a characteristic helix–loop–helix motif and related to the general transcription factor TFII-I *(95,96)*. It has been shown recently that GTF2IRD1 regulates transcriptional functions of TFII-I by controlling its nuclear residency. GTF2IRD1 promotes TFII-I nuclear exclusion and thus represses TFII-I transcriptional activity *(97)*. A transgenic mouse has been generated in

which the integration of the c-*myc* transgene resulted in disruption of the 5'
end of the mouse *Gtf2ird1* and greatly reduces its expression *(98)*. The
absence of phenotype in these mice suggests that the deletion of *GTF2IRD1*
alone is not likely to contribute to WBS developmental features.

GTF2I, NCF1, and another gene related to GTF2I (GTF2IRD2) are
located in the middle block B (Fig. 3) *(50)*. Corresponding genes or pseudogenes are found at the centromeric (*GTF2IP1, NCF1P1, GTF2IRD2P1*) and
telomeric (*GTF2IP2, NCF1P2, GTF2IRD2*) blocks B. *GTF2I* is always
included in the deleted interval while *NCF1* and *GTF2IRD2* may or may not
be deleted depending on the location of the chromosomal breakpoints (Fig. 4).

GTF2I encodes TFII-I (also called BAP-135 and SPIN), a transcription
factor that shuttles between the cytoplasm and nucleus and is regulated by
serine and tyrosine phosphorylation *(99)*. It is characterized by the presence
of six internal repeats, each containing a potential helix–loop–helix motif
implicated in protein–protein interactions. TFII-I can bind specifically to
several DNA sequence elements in TATA-less promoters and is implicated
in both basal and activated transcription *(100)*. It is strongly expressed at
all developmental stages in most tissues, including several regions of the
brain *(101)*.

NCF1 encodes the p47 cytosolic component of the phagocyte NADPH
oxidase complex, critical for superoxide production for host defense against
microbial infection *(102)*. Impaired NCF1 function leads to the autosomal
recessive form of chronic granulomatous disease (CGD), with recurrent
microbial infections *(103)*. The most common mutation is most probably
caused by either recombination or gene conversion events between the gene
and its highly homologous pseudogenes (*NCF1P1* and *NCF1P2*) *(104)*.
Hemizygosity at this locus is not expected to contribute to the WBS phenotype, as carriers of CGD are completely asymptomatic.

GTF2IRD2 encodes a novel protein of unknown function with two internal repeats related to GTF2I and GTF2IRD1. In at least half of the patients,
the middle gene copy is not affected by the deletion, suggesting that it does
not play a major role in WBS *(55)*.

Seven novel genes (provisionally named *WBSCR16-22*) located between
WBSCR14 and *ELN* have been identified and are still under characterization. Homology searches and prediction of putative protein domains suggest
that these new genes code for: (1) a DNAJ family member, (2) an α/β
hydrolase, (3) a new claudin family member, (4) two different methyltransferases, and (5) two novel proteins with no predicted domains *(52,105)*.

Possibly there are more genes to be found within the deleted region, but
the number will likely be small. In addition, the expression of some addi-

tional genes located nearby but outside the critical interval could be affected owing to altered chromatin conformation or elimination of regulatory elements in WBS chromosomes with a deletion.

5.3. Genes Involved in the WBS Phenotype. Genes Involved in Cognition

Haploinsufficiency for genes affected by the deletion must be the pathogenic mechanism for the entire WBS phenotype, including the neurobehavioral impairment. Despite the number of known genes commonly deleted, however, except for the cardiovascular problems related to *ELN* hemizygosity, the other features of WBS have not yet been clearly attributed to specific genes. Several candidate genes for the neurocognitive deficits have been proposed based on their predicted or demonstrated functions and expression profiles. *STX1A* and/or *CYLN2* are excellent functional candidates because both genes show brain-specific expression and are involved in putatively important functions, neurotransmitter release (STX1A) and intracellular neuronal organization and shape (CYLN2). In addition, LIMK1 has high neuronal expression and a putative action over axonal guidance during development, and several HLH transcription factors (BAZ1B, WBSCR14, GTF2IRD1, GTF2I) could also be master regulators of important genes for brain development and function.

5.3.1. Deletion Mapping

A few atypical patients with smaller deletions and either a full phenotype or partial phenotype have been reported *(36,60,106–110)* (Fig. 4). Clinical–molecular relationships in those patients have led to the proposal of a map for the WBS phenotype and the cognitive features. Based on two families with small deletions involving only *ELN* and *LIMK1*, hemizygosity of *LIMK1* was proposed as a contributing factor to impaired visual–spatial constructive cognition in WBS *(107)*. However, this claim was not confirmed in two different patients with similar heterozygous *LIMK1* deletions who showed no cognitive deficits on repeated testing *(37,108)*. In addition, two patients have been reported with deletions encompassing the region between *BAZ1B* and *EIF4H* who show only SVAS and, possibly, a subtle cognitive deficit *(106,108)*. This implies that other genes close to *ELN* (including *RFC2, EIFH4, STX1A*) appear to be excluded from contributing significantly to the phenotype. A recent description of two patients with the full WBS phenotype and harboring a deletion from *ELN* to *GTF2I* suggests that the genes mainly responsible for abnormal cognition map to the telomeric interval of the deletion, *CYLN2, GTF2IRD1*, and *GTF2I (109)*. A similar deletion that does not include *GTF2I* has been recently reported in all affected members of a three-generation family with SVAS, absence of WBS craniofacial features, milder general cognitive deficits, gregarious and enthusiastic personality, but normal visual–spatial construction *(110)*. Comparing the full phenotype cases reported by Botta et al. *(109)* with this last family, it has been proposed that *GTF2I* could contribute to some craniofacial features, the IQ deficit, and some aspects of the cognitive profile, including visual–spatial constructive cognition. Genes from *POM121* to *WBSCR14*, at the centromeric edge of the deletion, might contribute to other phenotypic aspects including mental retardation. However, these conclusions still lack strong supportive evidence and additional clinical and molecular studies are required.

5.4. Phenotypic Variability

There is a wide range of clinical variability among patients with WBS. In addition, a striking intrafamilial variation in the clinical presentation has been also reported in two WBS families *(111)*. The observed phenotypic variability of the cardiovascular features in WBS (25% nonpenetrance and diverse degrees of severity) is similar to that observed in isolated SVAS, where the variability within families is as great as that seen between families *(81)*. The only correlation found is that the severity of both supravalvular aortic stenosis and total cardiovascular disease is significantly greater in male than in female patients *(112)*. These differences by sex in the penetrance and severity of arterial stenoses might be related to prenatal hormonal effects.

As might be expected, the range of phenotypic variability of the neurobehavioral phenotype is even greater among WBS individuals, despite the presence of identical molecular deletions. Divergences in full-scale IQ scores and a wide range of recorded values for many tests are a common finding. The molecular basis of this phenotypic variability, if any, remains unknown, but it is considered typical of phenotypes produced by haploinsufficiency. Environmental factors, genetic variants in the nondeleted allele, subtle imprinting effects, and the genetic background may all contribute to the variable expression of the phenotype.

6. CONCLUDING REMARKS

Identification of the genes whose haploinsufficiency underlies the characteristic cognitive and personality profiles of WBS should provide new insight into the complex processes regulating the development and functioning of the central nervous system. However, the task of determining which of the deleted gene or combination of genes in WBS contributes to the neurobehavioral features of the phenotype is difficult. The identification of mutations in single genes from the WBS region in patients with distinct features of the WBS phenotype would be definitive. However, single gene defects may not be sufficient, and additive effects of haploinsufficiency for two or more genes may be necessary for a neurobehavioral phenotypic effect.

Quantitative and uniformly standardized methods need to be established to define the phenotype precisely, particularly the neurobehavioral features. These should include tests to assess cerebral morphology and electrophysiology. The profile provided by each test, and the range of variation, need to be determined for a large number of patients with WBS with identical molecular deletions. At that point, profiles generated by standardized tests can be used to establish precise phenotype–genotype correlations for those rare cases in which a partial deletion or single gene mutations are extent within the critical 7q11.23 interval.

Future studies should also focus on the functional characterization of the protein products of the deleted genes, including their subcellular localization, the identification of interacting proteins, and their involvement in cellular pathways. Some of the genes deleted in WBS encode transcriptional master regulators of several downstream genes. Therefore, global approaches to determine mRNA and/or protein expression in tissues, and comparative studies in patients with typical and atypical deletions can be used to sort out the pathways affected in WBS. Recent advances in genomic and proteomic technology and the resources generated by the Human Genome Project *(58,59)* provide the tools to approach these goals.

Finally, the answer to many of the remaining open questions about WBS, including the specific contribution of genes to the phenotype and the underlying pathophysiologic mechanisms of the disease, may need to rely on animal experimentation. Mice carrying identical deletion to humans as well as single and multiple gene knockouts should be generated and studied for developmental and neurobehavioral features. The recent success of gene targeting and chromosomal engineering in mice to dissect another complex microdeletion disorder, the DiGeorge/velo–cardio–facial syndrome, is highly encouraging *(113–115)*.

NOTE ADDED IN PROOF

Two recent manuscripts reporting mouse single gene knockouts further suggest that *LIMK1* and *CYLN2* are good candidates for involvement in the neurobehavorial features of WBS *(116,117)*. Homozygous (but not heterozygous) *Limk1* knockout mice exhibited significant abnormalities in dendritic spine morphology and synaptic function, associated with impaired spatial learning and increased locomotor activity *(116)*.

Haploinsufficiency for *Cyln2* in a different knockout mouse produced mild growth deficiency, hippocampal dysfunction, and deficits in motor coordination that may be owing to an aberrant regulation of dynein motor activity in neurons, while homozygous animals showed a slightly more severe phenotype *(117)*.

REFERENCES

1. Morris CA, Demsey SA, Leonard CO, Dilts C, Blackburn BL. Natural history of Williams syndrome: physical characteristics. J Pediatr 1988;113:318–26.
2. Burn J. Williams syndrome. J Med Genet 1986;23:389–95.
3. Fanconi VG, Giardet P, Schlesinger B, Butler N, Black J. Chronische hypercalcamie kambiniert mit osteosklerose, hyperazotamie, minderwuschs und kongenitalen missbildungen. Helv Paediatr Acta 1952;7:314–49.
4. Williams JCP, Barratt-Boyes BG, Lowe JB. Supravalvular aortic stenosis. Circulation 1961;24:1311–8.
5. Beuren AJ, Apitz J, Harmjanz D. Supravalvular aortic stenosis in association with mental retardation and a certain facial appearance. Circulation 1962;26:1235–40.
6. Jones KL. Williams syndrome: an historical perspective of its evolution, natural history, and etiology. Am J Med Genet 1990;6(Suppl):89–96.
7. Greenberg F. Williams syndrome professional symposium. Am J Med Genet 1990;6(Suppl):85–8.
8. Morris CA, Thomas IT, Greenberg F. Williams syndrome: autosomal dominant inheritance. Am J Med Genet 1993;47:478–81.
9. Sadler LS, Robinson LK, Verdaasdonk KR, Gingell R. The Williams syndrome: evidence for possible autosomal dominant inheritance. Am J Med Genet 1993;47:468–70.
10. Murphy MB, Greenberg F, Wilson G, Hughes M, DiLiberti J.Williams syndrome in twins. Am J Med Genet 1990;6(Suppl):97–9.
11. Hokama T, Rogers JG. Williams syndrome in one dizygotic twin. Acta Paediatr Jpn 1991;33:678–80.
12. Ewart AK, Morris CA, Atkinson D, et al. Hemizygosity at the elastin locus in a developmental disorder, Williams syndrome. Nat Genet 1993;5:11–6.
13. Francke U. Williams syndrome: genes and mechanisms. Hum Mol Genet 1999;8:1947–54.
14. Winter M, Pankau R, Amm M, Gosch A, Wessel A. The spectrum of ocular features in the Williams–Beuren syndrome. Clin Genet 1996;49:28–31.
15. Bird LM, Billman GF, Lacro RV, et al. Sudden death in Williams syndrome: report of ten cases. J Pediatr 1996;129:926–31.
16. Broder K, Reinhardt E, Ahern J, et al. Elevated ambulatory blood pressure in 20 subjects with Williams syndrome. Am J Med Genet 1999;83:356–60.

17. Kaplan P, Kirschner M, Watters G, Costa MT. Contractures in patients with Williams syndrome. Pediatrics 1989;84:895–9.
18. Forbes GB, Bryson MF, Manning J, Amirhakimi GH, Reina JC. Impaired calcium homeostasis in the infantile hypercalcemic syndrome. Acta Paediat Scand 1972;61:305–9.
19. Kruse K, Pankau R, Gosch A, Wohlfahrt K. Calcium metabolism in Williams–Beuren syndrome. J. Pediatr 1992;121:902–7.
20. Partsch CJ, Dreyer G, Gosch A, et al. Longitudinal evaluation of growth, puberty, and bone maturation in children with Williams syndrome. J Pediatr 1999;134:82–9.
21. Cammareri V, Vignati G, Nocera G, Beck-Peccoz P, Persani L. Thyroid hemiagenesis and elevated thyrotropin levels in a child with Williams syndrome. Am J Med Genet 1999;85:491–4.
22. Santer R, Pankau R, Schaub J, Burgin-Wolff A. Williams–Beuren syndrome and celiac disease. J Pediatr Gastroenterol Nutr 1996;23:339–40.
23. Jarrold C, Baddeley AD, Hewes AK, Phillips C. A longitudinal assessment of diverging verbal and non-verbal abilities in the Williams syndrome phenotype. Cortex 2001;37:423–31.
24. Bellugi U, Lichtenberger L, Jones W, Lai Z, St George M. The neurocognitive profile of Williams Syndrome: a complex pattern of strengths and weaknesses. J Cogn Neurosci 2000;12(Suppl 1):7–29.
25. Mervis CB, Klein-Tasman BP. Williams syndrome: cognition, personality, and adaptive behavior. Ment Retard Dev Disabil Res Rev 2000;6:148–58.
26. Voit T, Kramer H, Thomas C, et al. Myopathy in Williams–Beuren syndrome. Eur J Pediatr 1991;150:521–6.
27. Mercuri E, Atkinson J, Braddick O, et al. Chiari I malformation in asymptomatic young children with Williams syndrome: clinical and MRI study. Eur J Paediatr Neurol 1997;1:177–81.
28. St Heaps L, Robson L, Smith A. Review of referrals for the FISH detection of Williams syndrome highlights the importance of testing in supravalvular aortic stenosis/pulmonary stenosis. Am J Med Genet 2001;98:109–11.
29. Lashkari A, Smith AK, Graham JM. Williams–Beuren syndrome: an update and review for the primary physician. Clin Pediatr (Phila) 1999;38:189–208.
30. Committee on Genetics American Academy of Pediatrics: Health care supervision for children with Williams syndrome. Pediatrics 2001;107:1192–204.
31. Udwin O, Yule W. A cognitive and behavioural phenotype in Williams syndrome. J Clin Exp Neuropsychol 1991;13:232–44.
32. Mervis CB, Robinson BF, Bertrand J, et al. The Williams syndrome cognitive profile. Brain Cogn 2000;44:604–28.
33. Mervis CB, Robinson BF, Pani JR. Visual–spatial construction. Am J Hum Genet 1999;65:1222–9.
34. Deruelle C, Mancini J, Livet MO, Casse-Perrot C, de Schonen S. Configural and local processing of faces in children with Williams syndrome. Brain Cogn 1999;41:276–98.

35. Stojanovik V, Perkins M, Howard S. Language and conversational abilities in Williams syndrome: how good is good? Int J Lang Commun Disord 2001;36(Suppl):234–9.
36. Bellugi U, Lichtenberger L, Mills D, Galaburda A, Korenberg JR. Bridging cognition, the brain and molecular genetics: evidence from Williams syndrome. Trends Neurosci 1999;22:197–207.
37. Donnai D, Karmiloff-Smith A. Williams syndrome: from genotype through to the cognitive phenotype. Am J Med Genet 2000;97:164–71.
38. Klein BP, Mervis CB. Contrasting patterns of cognitive abilities of 9 and 10-year-olds with Williams syndrome or Down syndrome. Dev Neuropsycol 1999;16:177–196.
39. Bellugi U, Adolphs R, Cassady C, Chiles M. Towards the neural basis for hypersociability in a genetic syndrome. NeuroReport 1999;10:1653–7.
40. Park NW, Conrod B, Rewilak D, et al. Automatic activation of positive but not negative attitudes after traumatic brain injury. Neuropsychologia 2001;39:7–24.
41. Davies M, Howlin P, Udwin O. Independence and adaptive behavior in adults with Williams syndrome. Am J Med Genet 1997;70:188–95.
42. Lenhoff HM, Wang PP, Greenberg F, Bellugi U. Williams syndrome and the brain. Sci Am 1997;277:68–73.
43. Hopyan T, Dennis M, Weksberg R, Cytrynbaum C. Music skills and the expressive interpretation of music in children with Williams–Beuren syndrome: pitch, rhythm, melodic imagery, phrasing, and musical affect. Neuropsychol Dev Cogn C Child Neuropsychol 2001;7:42–53.
44. Schmitt JE, Eliez S, Bellugi U, Reiss AL. Analysis of cerebral shape in Williams syndrome. Arch Neurol 2001;58:283–7.
45. Galaburda AM, Bellugi U. Multi-level analysis of cortical neuroanatomy in Williams syndrome. J Cogn Neurosci 2000;12(Suppl 1):74–88.
46. Mills DL, Alvarez TD, St George M, et al. Electrophysiological studies of face processing in Williams syndrome. J Cogn Neurosci 2000;12(Suppl 1):47–64.
47. Pérez Jurado LA, Peoples R, Wang YK, et al. Molecular definition of the chromosome 7 deletion in Williams syndrome and parent-of-origin effects on growth. Am J Hum Genet 1996;59:618–25.
48. Wu YQ, Sutton VR, Nickerson E, et al. Delineation of the common critical region in Williams syndrome and clinical correlation of growth, heart defects, ethnicity, and parental origin. Am J Med Genet 1998;78:82–9.
49. Peoples R, Franke Y, Wang YK, et al. A physical map, including a BAC/PAC clone contig, of the Williams–Beuren syndrome deletion region at 7q11.23. Am J Hum Genet 2000;66:47–68.
50. Valero MC, de Luis O , Cruces J, Pérez Jurado LA. Fine-scale comparative mapping of the human 7q11.23 region and the orthologous region on mouse chromosome 5G: the low-copy repeats that flank the williams-beuren syndrome deletion arose at breakpoint sites of an evolutionary inversion(s). Genomics 2000;69:1–13.
51. Hockenhull EL, Carette MJ, Metcalfe K, et al. A complete physical contig and partial transcript map of the Williams syndrome critical region. Genomics 1999;58:138–45.

52. DeSilva U, Elnitski L, Idol JR, et al. Generation and comparative analysis of approximately 3.3 Mb of mouse genomic sequence orthologous to the region of human chromosome 7q11.23 implicated in Williams syndrome. Genome Res 2002;12:3–15.

53. Urbán Z, Helms C, Fekete G, et al. 7q11.23 deletions in Williams syndrome arise as a consequence of unequal meiotic crossover. Am J Hum Genet 1996;59:958–62.

54. Dutly F, Schinzel A. Unequal interchromosomal rearrangements may result in elastin gene deletions causing the Williams–Beuren syndrome. Hum Mol Genet 1996;5:1893–8.

55. Bayés M, de Luis O, Magano LF, Pérez Jurado LA. Fine mapping of deletion breakpoints in Williams–Beuren syndrome patients. Eur J Hum Genet 2001;9(Suppl):P1446.

56. Osborne L, Li M, Pober B, et al. A 1.5 million base-pair inversion polymorphism in families with Williams–Beuren syndrome. Nat Genet 2001; 29:321–5.

57. DeSilva U, Massa H, Trask BJ, Green ED. Comparative mapping of the region of human chromosome 7 deleted in Williams syndrome. Genome Res 1999;9:428–36.

58. Venter JC, Adams MD, Myers EW, et al. The Sequence of the Human Genome. Science 2001;291:1304–51.

59. International human genome sequencing consortium. Initial sequencing and analysis of the human genome. Nature 2001;409:860–921.

60. Osborne LR. Williams-Beuren syndrome: unraveling the mysteries of a microdeletion disorder. Mol Genet Metab 1999;67:1–10.

61. Imreh G, Hallberg E. An integral membrane protein from the nuclear pore complex is also present in the annulate lamellae: implications for annulate lamella formation. Exp Cell Res 2000;259:180–90.

62. Meng X, Lu X, Morris CA, Keating MT. A novel human gene FKBP6 is deleted in Williams syndrome. Genomics 1998;52:130–7.

63. Wang Y-K, Harryman-Samos C, Peoples R, et al. A novel human homologue of the *Drosophila* frizzled wnt receptor gene binds wingless protein and is in the Williams syndrome deletion at 7q11.23. Hum Mol Genet 1997;6:465–72.

64. Wang YK, Sporle R, Paperna T, Schughart K, Francke U. Characterization and expression pattern of the frizzled gene Fzd9, the mouse homolog of FZD9 which is deleted in Williams–Beuren syndrome. Genomics 1999;57:235–48.

65. Lu X, Meng X, Morris CA, Keating MT. A novel human gene, WSTF, is deleted in Williams syndrome. Genomics 1998;54:241–9.

66. Peoples RJ, Cisco MJ, Kaplan P, Francke U. Identification of the WBSCR9 gene, encoding a novel transcriptional regulator, in the Williams–Beuren syndrome deletion at 7q11.23. Cytogenet Cell Genet 1998;82:238–46.

67. Jadayel DM, Osborne LR, Coignet LJ, et al. The BCL7 gene family: deletion of BCL7B in Williams syndrome. Gene 1998;224:35–44.

68. Natter S, Seiberler S, Hufnagl P, et al. Isolation of cDNA clones coding for IgE autoantigens with serum IgE from atopic dermatitis patients. FASEB J 1998;12:1559–69.

69. Pérez Jurado LA, Wang YK, Francke U, Cruces J. TBL2, a novel transducin family member in the WBS deletion: characterization of the complete

sequence, genomic structure, transcriptional variants and the mouse ortholog. Cytogenet Cell Genet 1999;86:277–84.

70. Meng X, Lu X, Li Z, et al. Complete physical map of the common deletion region in Williams syndrome and identification and characterization of three novel genes. Hum Genet 1998;103:590–9.

71. Cairo S, Merla G, Urbinati F, Ballabio A, Reymond A. WBSCR14, a gene mapping to the Williams–Beuren syndrome deleted region, is a new member of the Mlx transcription factor network. Hum Mol Genet 2001;10:617–27.

72. de Luis O, Valero MC, Pérez Jurado LA. WBSCR14, a putative transcription factor gene deleted in Williams-Beuren syndrome: complete characterisation of the human gene and the mouse ortholog. Eur J Hum Genet 2000;8:215–22.

73. Schulze KL, Broadie K, Perin MS, Bellen HJ. Genetic and electrophysiological studies of Drosophila syntaxin-1A demonstrate its role in non neuronal secretion and neurotransmission. Cell 1995;80:311–20.

74. Horton N, Quick MW. Syntaxin 1A up-regulates GABA transporter expression by subcellular redistribution. Mol Membr Biol 2001;18:39–44.

75. Botta A, Sangiuolo F, Calza L, et al. Expression analysis and protein localization of the human HPC-1/syntaxin 1A, a gene deleted in Williams syndrome. Genomics 1999;62:525–8.

76. Paperna T, Peoples R, Wang Y-K, Kaplan P, Francke U. Genes for the CPE-receptor (CPETR1) and the human homolog of RVP (CPETR2) are localized within the Williams–Beuren syndrome deletion. Genomics 1998;54:453–9.

77. Morita K, Furuse M, Fujimoto K, Tsukita S. Claudin multigene family encoding four-transmembrane domain protein components of tightjunction strands. Proc Natl Acad Sci USA 1999;96:511–6.

78. Katahira J, Sugiyama H, Inoue N, et al. *Clostridium perfringens* enterotoxin utilizes two structurally related membrane proteins as functional receptors in vivo. J Biol Chem 1997;272:26652–8.

79. Rosenbloom J, Abrams WR, Mecham R. Extracellular matrix 4: the elastic fiber. FASEB J 1993;7:1208–18.

80. Curran ME, Atkinson DL, Ewart AK, et al. The elastin gene is disrupted by a translocation associated with supravalvular aortic stenosis. Cell 1993;73:159–68.

81. Chowdhury T, Reardon W. Elastin mutation and cardiac disease. Pediatr Cardiol 1999;20:103–7.

82. Dridi SM, Ghomrasseni S, Bonnet D, et al. Skin elastic fibers in Williams syndrome. Am J Med Genet 1999;87:134–8.

83. O'Connor WN, Davis JB, Geissler R, et al. Supravalvular aortic stenosis. Clinical and pathologic observations in six patients. Arch Pathol Lab Med 1985;109:179–85.

84. Li DY, Brooke B, Davis EC, et al. Elastin is an essential determinant of arterial morphogenesis. Nature 1998;393:276–80.

85. Li DY, Faury G, Taylor DG, et al. Novel arterial pathology in mice and humans hemizygous for elastin. J Clin Invest 1998;102:1783–7.

86. Osborne L, Martindale D, Scherer SW, et al. Identification of genes from a 500 kb region that is commonly deleted in Williams syndrome. Genomics 1996;36:328–36.

87. Stanyon CA, Bernard O. LIM-kinase1. Int J Biochem Cell Biol 1999; 31:389–94.

88. Noskov VN, Araki H, Sugino A. The RFC2 gene, encoding the third-largest subunit of the replication factor C complex, is required for an S-phase checkpoint in Saccharomyces cerevisiae. Mol Cell Biol 1998;18:4914–23.

89. Peoples RJ, Pérez Jurado LA, Wang Y-K, Kaplan P, Francke U. The gene for the replication factor C subunit 2 (RFC2) is within the 7q11.23 Williams syndrome deletion. Am J Hum Genet 1996;58:1370–3.

90. Doyle JL, DeSilva U, Miller W, Green ED. Divergent human and mouse orthologs of a novel gene (WBSCR15/Wbscr15) reside within the genomic interval commonly deleted in Williams syndrome. Cytogenet Cell Genet 2000;90:285–90.

91. Richter-Cook NJ, Dever TE, Hensold JO, Merrick WC. Purification and characterization of a new eukaryotic protein translation factor. Eukaryotic initiation factor 4H. J Biol Chem 1998;273:7579–87.

92. Richter NJ, Rogers GW Jr, Hensold JO, Merrick WC. Further biochemical and kinetic characterization of human eukaryotic initiation factor 4H. J Biol Chem 1999;274:35,415–24.

93. De Zeeuw CI, Hoogenraad CC, Goedknegt E, et al. CLIP-115, a novel brain-specific cytoplasmic linker protein, mediates the localization of dendritic lamellar bodies. Neuron 1997;19:1187–99.

94. Hoogenraad CC, Eussen BHJ, Langeveld A, et al. The murine CYLN2 gene: genomic organization, chromosome localization, and comparison to the human gene that is located within the 7q11.23 Williams syndrome critical region. Genomics 1998;53:348–58.

95. Osborne LR, Campbell T, Daradich A, Scherer SW, Tsui LC. Identification of a putative transcription factor gene (WBSCR11) that is commonly deleted in Williams–Beuren syndrome. Genomics 1999;57:279–84.

96. Franke Y, Peoples RJ, Francke U. Identification of GTF2IRD1, a putative transcription factor within the Williams-Beuren syndrome deletion at 7q11.23. Cytogenet Cell Genet 1999;86:296–304.

97. Tussie-Luna MI, Bayarsaihan D, Ruddle FH, Roy AL. Repression of TFII-I-dependent transcription by nuclear exclusion. Proc Natl Acad Sci USA 2001;98:7789–94.

98. Durkin ME, Keck-Waggoner CL, Popescu NC, Thorgeirsson SS. Integration of a c-myc transgene results in disruption of the mouse Gtf2ird1 gene, the homologue of the human GTF2IRD1 gene hemizygously deleted in Williams–Beuren Syndrome. Genomics 2001;73:20–7.

99. Pérez Jurado LA, Wang Y-K, Peoples R, et al. A duplicate gene in the breakpoint regions of the Williams–Beuren syndrome deletion encodes the initiator binding protein TFII-I and BAP-135, a phosphorylation target of BTK. Hum Mol Genet 1998;7:325–34.

100. Roy AL, Du H, Gregor PD, et al. Cloning of an inr- and E-box-binding protein, TFII-I, that interacts physically and functionally with USF1. EMBO J 1997;16:7091–104.

101. Wang YK, Pérez Jurado LA, Francke U. A mouse single-copy gene, Gtf2i, the homolog of human GTF2I, that is duplicated in the Williams–Beuren syndrome deletion region. Genomics 1998;48:163–70.

102. Nauseef WM. The NADPH-dependent oxidase of phagocytes. Proc Assoc Am Phys 1999;111:373–82.

103. Casimir CM, Bu-Ghanim HN, Rodaway AR, et al. Autosomal recessive chronic granulomatous disease caused by deletion at a dinucleotide repeat. Proc Natl Acad Sci USA 1991;88:2753–7.

104. Gorlach A, Lee PL, Roesler J, et al. A p47-phox pseudogene carries the most common mutation causing p47-phox- deficient chronic granulomatous disease. J Clin Invest 1997;100:1907–18.

105. Magano LF, Bayés M, Flores R, Pérez Jurado LA. Towards a complete transcription map of the Williams–Beuren syndrome deletion region. Eur J Hum Genet 2001;9(Suppl):P0744.

106. Korenberg JR, Chen XN, Hirota H, et al. Genome structure and cognitive map of Williams syndrome. J Cogn Neurosci 2000;12(Suppl 1):89–107.

107. Frangiskakis JM, Ewart AK, Morris CA, et al. LIM-kinase 1 hemizygosity implicated in impaired visuospacial cognitive cognition. Cell 1996;86:59–69.

108. Tassabehji M, Metcalfe K, Karmiloff-Smith A, et al. Williams syndrome: use of chromosomal microdeletions as a tool to dissect cognitive and physical phenotypes. Am J Hum Genet 1999;64:118–25.

109. Botta A, Novelli G, Mari A, et al. Detection of an atypical 7q11.23 deletion in Williams syndrome patients which does not include the STX1A and FZD3 genes. J Med Genet 1999;36:478–80.

110. Del Campo M, Magano LF, Martínez Iglesias J, Pérez Jurado LA. Partial features of Williams–Beuren syndrome in a family with a novel 700 Kb 7q11.23 deletion. Eur J Hum Genet 2001;9(Suppl):C056.

111. Pankau R, Siebert R, Kautza M, et al. Familial Williams–Beuren syndrome showing varying clinical expression. Am J Med Genet 2001;98:324–9.

112. Sadler LS, Pober BR, Grandinetti A, et al. Differences by sex in cardiovascular disease in Williams syndrome. J Pediatr 2001;139:849–53.

113. Guris DL, Fantes J, Tara D, Druker BJ, Imamoto A. Mice lacking the homologue of the human 22q11.2 gene CRKL phenocopy neurocristopathies of DiGeorge syndrome. Nat Genet 2001;27:293–8.

114. Jerome LA, Papaioannou VE. DiGeorge syndrome phenotype in mice mutant for the T-box gene, Tbx1. Nat Genet 2001;27:286–91.

115. Merscher S, Funke B, Epstein JA, et al. TBX1 is responsible for cardiovascular defects in velo-cardio-facial/DiGeorge syndrome. Cell 2001;104:619–29.

116. Meng Y, Zhang Y, Tregoubov V, et al. Abnormal spine morphology and enhanced LTP in Limk-1 knockout mice. Neuron 2002;35:121–33.

117. Hoogenraad CC, Koekkoek B, Akhmanova A, et al. Targeted mutation of Cyln2 in the Williams syndrome critical region links CLIP-115 haploinsufficiency to neurodevelopmental abnormalities in mice. Nat Genet 2002;32:117–27.

10

Behavioral Phenotype in Myotonic Dystrophy (Steinert's Disease)

Jean Steyaert

1. INTRODUCTION

Myotonic dystrophy is a heritable, slowly progressive muscle disorder with involvement of multiple organ systems. Not only the muscles are affected, but also the eye, heart, gastrointestinal tract, skin, immune system, endocrine system, skull, kidneys *(1)*, and brain *(2)*. Moreover, these systems may be affected differentially, the age at onset is variable, as well as the course of the disease. The severity of the disease tends to increase from one generation to the next, while the age of onset decreases. This phenomenon is called anticipation. The underlying genetic mechanism of myotonic dystrophy is that of dynamic mutations, which it shares with fragile X syndrome, Huntington's disease, and almost 20 other diseases affecting the central nervous system (NS). The molecular mechanisms of myotonic dystrophy have been partly elucidated in the last 10 years. All these characteristics make myotonic dystrophy "perhaps the most variable of human disorders" *(3)*.

Myotonic dystrophy affects the brain, and patients with the disorder have a wide range of behavioral symptoms. Perhaps the most common symptom is daytime sleepiness. Children with myotonic dystrophy have mild to moderate developmental delays, or may have more specific behavior problems. In this chapter, I focus on the effects of myotonic dystrophy in brain and what is known about the consequent cognitive and behavioral problems. First, I give an overview of the clinical and genetic features of the disease. The reader wanting to know more about the clinical, genetic, and molecular aspects of myotonic dystrophy will find the most comprehensive overview in Harper's textbook on the subject *(3)*.

From: *Contemporary Clinical Neuroscience:*
Genetics and Genomics of Neurobehavioral Disorders
Edited by: G. S. Fisch © Humana Press Inc., Totowa, NJ

2. HISTORY

Myotonic disorders are characterized by myotonia, the stiffness of a muscle after contraction. The first description of this rare clinical sign was made in 1876 by Dr. Julius Thomsen, a German neurologist who was affected himself. He described a benign hereditary myotonia beginning in early childhood in his family: Thomsen's disease or myotonia congenita. In the following years, it became clear that a variant of this clinical entity existed. The new variant started later in life, and was accompanied by progressive muscle weakness and muscle wasting. In 1909, Steinert, another German neurologist, delineated this new hereditary myotonia as a separate entity, which was later named after him. Steinert was the first to describe clinical signs in systems other than the muscles. Later, the disease was called dystrophia myotonica, referring to the combination of muscle wasting and myotonia.

Since then, considerable progress has been made on the clinical and genetic aspects of this disease. Research in myotonic dystrophy can be arbitrarily divided in three phases; The first was an early phase, approximately from 1909 to the 1970s, during which most of the symptoms were described by experienced clinicians who reported case studies or small groups of patients. The second phase of research in myotonic dystrophy is from the 1970s to 1992, when the discovery of the gene and the mechanism of the mutation were published (4–6). This phase is characterized by systematic clinical studies on one hand and a hunt for the myotonic dystrophy gene on the other. In this "middle phase" it became clear how variable the phenotype of myotonic dystrophy could be. Unfortunately, knowledge of the different subtypes was not universally shared. Consequently, many high-quality studies contain heterogeneous groups of subjects and are difficult to compare with each other. The present phase of research on myotonic dystrophy began with the discovery of the mutation, after which the diagnosis could easily be made through a DNA test. This phase is characterized by fundamental research on the pathway between the mutation and phenotype, clinical studies on different aspects of the disease, and in specific forms of myotonic dystrophy. Several clinical studies have looked for correlations between clinical characteristics and length of the mutation (*see* Subheading 4.2.). One of the consequences of the easy and definite diagnosis through DNA testing is that subjects with a mild form of the disease, or at a very early stage of the disease, can be included. This has, for instance, led to the finding that in a particular form of the disease, namely the juvenile onset myotonic dystrophy, behavioral symptoms can precede neuromuscular symptoms (7,8).

3. CLINICAL ASPECTS

3.1. Prevalence

Myotonic dystrophy is the most common of myotonic diseases. Its prevalence is estimated at around one in 8000 persons *(9)*. However, this may be an underestimation as it is based on the prevalence of the congenital and classical or adult type of the disease, and probably does not include patients who were not diagnosed because they had not yet manifested significant symptoms.

3.2. The Classical Type of Myotonic Dystrophy

The classical form of myotonic dystrophy begins in late adolescence or adulthood, generally in the third or fourth decade of life (*see* Table 1 for overview of symptoms). Retrospectively, it is often difficult to pinpoint the time when symptoms first occur. Patients may have had vague cognitive or gastrointestinal complaints well before any neuromuscular sign appeared. Clinicians who are not very familiar with the disease may not interpret this as possible early symptoms of myotonic dystrophy. Before the first complaints of muscle weakness, the disease often begins with myotonia: muscles that relax only gradually after an effort. This phenomenon can impair smooth and precise manual activities. It becomes more severe in cold weather, and is most pronounced after forceful movements have been made, hand movements in particular. Most patients experience this only as a minor discomfort and rarely seek medical attention for the problem. Tongue fasciculations, fine and rapid uncontrolled movements of the tongue muscles, are another sign of myotonia.

Muscle weakness generally begins in the face, jaw, neck and forearms. Patients typically exhibit little facial expression, and have progressive ptosis of the eyelids, wasting of the temporal and jaw muscles, and articulation and swallowing problems. Gradually, the muscle wasting and weakness worsens and patients may eventually become wheel chair bound with severe respiratory problems, partly owing to weakness of the diaphragm and other respiratory muscles.

One of the most common complaints in adult myotonic dystrophy patients is somnolence during the day. Patients can fall asleep anywhere and at any time. Besides these prominent and progressive muscle problems and typical daytime sleepiness, other organ systems are involved to a varying degree.

A frequent nonmuscular symptom of myotonic dystrophy is progressive cataract: the eye lens becomes gradually more opaque and sight is impaired. In some patients with myotonic dystrophy, cataract may be the only symp-

Table 1
Principal Clinical Manifestations in Myotonic Dystrophy

System affected	Symptoms
Skeletal muscles	Myotonia, in particular in adult and mild forms, absent in congenital form Progressive wasting and weakness, beginning in face, head, and neck, distal limb muscles, respiratory muscles Speech problems In adult and mild form: myotonia In congenital form: severe muscle hypotonia, clubfoot
Gastrointestinal	Swallowing problems, esophageal dysfunction, obstipation, megacolon, laxity of anal sphincter, diarrhea, vague complaints due to motility problems
Heart	Conduction problems leading to arrhythmia, cardiomyopathy
Respiratory system	Weakness of respiratory muscles and poor regulation of respiratory rhythm due to CNS problems (?); ensuing poor ventilation and lung infections
Endocrine	Testicular atrophy and infertility; insulin resistance with diabetes mellitus
Eye	Ptosis of the eyelids, cataract, slow reactions of the pupil muscles, slow eye movements
Skin	Early balding, hair follicle tumors
Immune system	Reduced levels of immunoglobulins
Peripheral nerve	Polyneuropathy
CNS	Excessive daytime sleepiness, excessive nighttime sleep, apathy, specific memory problems, possible personality changes Mental retardation in congenital myotonic dystrophy Learning problems in childhood onset myotonic dystrophy Other behavior problems in children: social functioning, ADHD

It should be noted that the presence and degree of these symptoms vary widely.
Adapted from Thornton *(1)*.

tom. These will often occur in members of the older generations in families with myotonic dystrophy, while members of younger generations are more severely affected, evincing symptoms in several organ systems. This phenomenon puzzled early researchers on myotonic dystrophy (Fleisher, [1918] cited by Harper [3]) and could be explained once the molecular mechanism of a dynamic mutation (*see* Subheading 4.1.) was found to cause myotonic dystrophy.

Myotonic dystrophy affects not only skeletal muscles, but smooth muscle tissue also. Smooth muscles are responsible for the motility of the gastrointestinal tract from the pharynx and the esophagus to the anal sphincter. Smooth muscles control the functions of the urinary bladder, as well as the working of the iris and the lens in the eye. In myotonic dystrophy, the smooth muscles of the gastrointestinal tract are generally the most affected and this leads to a wide range of complaints and symptoms. Involvement of the pharynx and esophagus can lead to swallowing problems and frequent tracheal aspiration. Problems of the colon range from vague complaints due to motility problems to more impairing dysfunctions. Some patients have chronic diarrhea, while others have constipation, spastic colon, laxity of the anal sphincter, and fecal soiling. Among patients who have only minimal impairment of skeletal muscle function, gastrointestinal problems can be the first real impairment and reason to seek medical attention.

Cardiac rhythm problems are another complication of myotonic dystrophy. Owing to an abnormality in the conduction fibers of the heart, its electrical activity can be disrupted, leading to slow and/or irregular heart rhythm. Abnormalities of the electrocardiogram are frequent in myotonic dystrophy patients, but only a limited number of them have clinically significant cardiac problems. In the worst case, sudden death occurs. It is unclear how many premature deaths in myotonic dystrophy are due to cardiac arrhythmias.

Another frequent symptom of myotonic dystrophy is early balding, which is more pronounced in males than in females. The combination of muscle wasting of the jaw and temporal muscles, lack of facial expression and ptosis of the eyelids, and early balding give the typical facial appearance of the adult patient with myotonic dystrophy. Patients with myotonic dystrophy frequently have an otherwise seldom benign tumor of the hair follicles.

These abnormalities are the most prominent and well known. Other problems of myotonic dystrophy include endocrine dysfunctions and disorders of the immune system, the liver, gallbladder, kidney, and of the peripheral nerves. The endocrine dysfunctions consist of insulin resistance that may influence brain metabolism (10), abnormal secretion of growth hormone, testicular atrophy, and others. Infertility is frequent in patients with myotonic dystrophy, particularly in males.

Behavioral changes in adult patients, due to involvement of the CNS, have been known since early research in myotonic dystrophy. In addition to daytime sleepiness, other cognitive and personality changes have been described (3). These are reviewed in Subheading 5. Myotonic dystrophy is a progressive degenerative disorder and, as such, problems become worse with age. Although the variability in symptoms and degree of impairment varies widely in myotonic dystrophy, the disease can be a cause of early death. The mean age at death in patients with the classic form of myotonic dystrophy is approx 54 years *(11)*, the main causes of which are respiratory and cardiac problems.

3.3. The Congenital Type of Myotonic Dystrophy

In 1960 Vanier *(12)* gave the first description of myotonic dystrophy in infants. This was much later than the descriptions of the classical type of myotonic dystrophy in adults. Frequent neonatal deaths in families with myotonic dystrophy had previously probably not been recognized as children with a severe form of the disease. Alternatively, they may have been attributed to maternal problems due to myotonic dystrophy. Indeed, children with congenital myotonic dystrophy generally inherit the disorder from their mother (*see* Subheading 4.1.), while patients with the classical adult form may inherit it from either parent. Only when children with congenital myotonic dystrophy could be kept alive by means of improved neonatal resuscitation techniques did it become clear that a congenital form of myotonic dystrophy existed. Symptoms are already present before birth, as these children show reduced fetal movements. Neonates have severe muscle weakness, with potentially fatal feeding and respiratory problems. If they survive this initial phase of extreme hypotonia, muscle strength improves and the child will develop slowly. Muscle weakness is pronounced, but improves with age. Unlike patients with adult onset myotonic dystrophy, these children have no marked muscle wasting. Muscle weakness is particularly evident in the face, with an open mouth and tented upper lip as clinical hallmarks of congenital myotonic dystrophy. Motor development of these children is delayed, and many will need physiotherapy to learn to walk. A number of infants are born with clubfeet (talipes). Myotonia is markedly absent in the congenital form.

Cognitive development in children with congenital myotonic dystrophy is delayed. They have an average mental age in the mildly retarded range (*see* Subheading 5.1.). As a result of peripheral muscle hypotonia and to developmental problems in the CNS, speech and language development are delayed *(3)*.

As in the classic form of myotonic dystrophy, gastrointestinal symptoms occur in early life. Other systemic features of the classical type of myotonic dystrophy may be present in patients with the congenital form. Longitudinal research looking at the various systemic problems in this form of myotonic

Table 2
The Four Subtypes or Forms of Myotonic Dystony

Subtype	Age at onset	Initial symptoms	Range of number of CTG repeats
Congenital	Prenatal/birth	Reduced fetal movements; swallowing and respiratory problems at birth, hypotonia	1000–5000
Childhood (juvenile)	1–12 years	Learning and/or behavior difficulties; speech problems	500–2000
Adult (classical)	12–50 years	Myotonia, muscle weakness	100–1000
Mild	> 50 years	Cataract	40–80

Adapted from de Die-Smulders *(7)*.

dystrophy is scarce, and it is still unclear whether these symptoms are already present in early life, or whether they appear gradually in the course of development. Most children with congenital myotonic dystrophy generally live into adulthood. In adolescence and early adulthood they have increasing muscle weakness and other characteristics of the classical adult type. Only half of them survive into their 30s and 40s *(13)*.

Although it is now evident that the classical adult form and the congenital form of myotonic dystrophy have the same genetic cause, they seem to belong to two different categories of disorders *(3)*. Adult myotonic dystrophy is a typical progressive degenerative disorder, in which a formerly healthy individual becomes gradually more impaired. Congenital myotonic dystrophy, however, has more characteristics of a developmental disorder, in which an individual with severe problems in early childhood improves progressively although he or she maintains a number of features of the disorder. Only in later life do individuals with congenital myotonic dystrophy show signs of degeneration. Despite the same genetic cause, it is still unclear whether different pathophysiological mechanisms account for the different characteristics in these two forms of myotonic dystrophy.

3.4. Other Phenotypes in Myotonic Dystrophy

Although the classical adult type and the congenital type of myotonic dystrophy are best known and generally well recognized by physicians, two other forms exist: the *mild form* and the *childhood form* (*see* Table 2). In the mild or minimal form of myotonic dystrophy, subjects have no or only minimal muscle weakness and myotonia. Symptoms begin after the age of 50 and are not easy to differentiate from normal senescence *(1)*. Cataract of the eye lens at an earlier age may be considerable and sometimes this is the only reason why affected individuals seek medical attention. In these patients, the diagnosis of myotonic dystrophy is often made only after the diagnosis has been made in more affected relatives.

In the childhood or juvenile type of myotonic dystrophy, children are unaffected at birth and show symptoms before the age of 12. Mild muscle signs develop in late childhood or adolescence, and are seldom impairing *(7)*. These children may have significant cognitive and/or behavioral problems that precede the muscle symptoms *(8,14)*. Medical attention is sought first for behavior or learning difficulties, rather than for physical complaints. If the clinician is unaware that myotonic dystrophy occurs in the family, he or she may miss the fact that the presenting behavior problems may be early symptoms of this disease. In adulthood, children with the juvenile form have progressive muscle weakness and the other system manifestations of myotonic dystrophy. Although these individuals have earlier signs of the disease and manifest earlier impairment, current research does not clarify whether these patients have an average shorter life expectancy than patients with the classical adult type *(13)*.

3.5. Other Myotonies

When the gene and the mutation for myotonic dystrophy were discovered on chromosome 19, the mutation could not be demonstrated in all affected families. Based on clinical differences, the phenotype in these families was called proximal myotonic myopathy (PROMM) *(15,16)*. More recently, the ZNF9 gene with a related kind of mutation was discovered on chromosome 3 in individuals with PROMM/DM2 *(17)*. Based mainly on the different causal genes, a differentiation is made between myotonic dystrophy type 1—with a mutation on chromosome 19 and the most frequent mutation (95% of cases)—and myotonic dystrophy type 2 (about 5% of cases), which is caused by a CCTG tetranucleotide repeat mutation in the ZNF9 gene on chromosome 3. It is unclear whether all cases of PROMM have in fact myotonic dystrophy type 2, or whether there is still another genetic cause. We will not consider PROMM and DM type 2 further in this text, as little is known about CNS involvement in this phenotype.

4. THE GENETICS OF MYOTONIC DYSTROPHY

Myotonic dystrophy is an autosomal dominant inherited disorder: if one carries the mutation causing the disorder, that individual has a 50% risk of transmitting the mutant gene and the disease associated with it to each of his or her children. A striking characteristic of families with myotonic dystrophy is that older generations are only mildly affected and exhibit symptoms at an older age, whereas individuals in younger generations are more severely affected and present symptoms at an earlier age *(18)*. As in some other inherited neuropsychiatric disorders, such as Huntington's disease, the symptoms of myotonic dystrophy may worsen and manifest themselves at an earlier age in each consecutive generation. This phenomenon is called anticipation. The underlying mechanism is that of expanding polynucleotide repeats, or dynamic mutation *(19)*. To understand this mechanism we have to look at the molecular genetics of myotonic dystrophy.

4.1. Molecular Genetics

The mutation causing the disease was discovered in 1991 *(4–6)*. The mutation is within a gene on chromosome 19 (19q13.3) that codes for an enzyme, the myotonic dystrophy protein kinase (DMPK). The precise function of this protein is not yet clear. An untranslated[1] region of the gene contains an unstable repeat sequence of three base pairs: CTG. This locus is called the *DM1* locus. In the general population the number of $(CTG)_n$ repeats varies between 5 and 37 repeats, and the same number of CTG repeats is inherited from generation to generation. In some families however, the number of CTG-repeats increases from one generation to the next. When a threshold of 50 repeats is reached, subjects may be mildly affected. The longer the expansion, the more unstable it becomes and may expand from one generation to the next. The increase in repeat number from one generation to the next and the moderate correlation between repeat number and the severity of the phenotype demonstrates the phenomenon of anticipation *(20)*. There is some evidence that the repeat length increases more during maternal rather than paternal transmission *(7,21)*. Men with moderately long expansions are generally infertile, whereas women are often still fertile. Consequently, an increase from a moderate to a long expansion will almost exclusively occur after maternal inheritance. As longer expansions are often associated with the congenital phenotype, this phenotype will almost always occur after maternal inheritance *(22)*.

Another characteristic of the mutation is that it is not only unstable from one generation to the next, but also within one individual. There is marked somatic mosaicism of the expansion length *(21)* and, at least in peripheral

---

[1]Transcription is the process occurring in the cell nucleus in which the DNA is copies into messenger RNA (mRNA) carries the genetic information from the cell nucleus to the cytoplasm of the cell. In the translation process, the mRNA is used as information in the building of proteins, the final product of genes. In the translation process, only parts of the mRNA are actually used. Some parts have no direct coding function, and though these are transcribed from DNA to mRNA, they will not be translated.

blood cells, the expansion length progresses with age *(23)*. Consequently, the expansion length found in peripheral lymphocytes of an individual of a certain age, is not the same and most likely longer than that in brain cells.

More complicated than the genetics of myotonic dystrophy is the fact that the mutation occurs in an untranslated region of the gene, and that cells containing the mutation in the *DMPK* gene produce the intact protein, although probably in lower quantities. Several theories have been proposed, and are described elsewhere *(24)*. What is important to know from the present findings is that different mechanisms may underlie different groups of symptoms. Some symptoms, such as the cardiac rhythm problems, are likely caused by a limited availability of the gene product of the myotonic dystrophy gene, the DMPK protein. There is evidence that other symptoms may be caused by the messenger RNA (mRNA) transcribed from the mutant gene. This mRNA also contains a long expansion and cannot be processed as effectively as normal mRNA. It accumulates in the cell nucleus and may disrupt normal cell functions by perturbing the processing of other mRNAs such as those for ion channels *(25)*, insulin receptor *(26)*, and cardiac isoform of troponin *(27)*. This is thought to cause the muscle weakness and wasting. Still other mechanisms may be responsible for the cataract of the eye, mediated through haploinsufficiency for the *SIX5* gene *(28–30)*. It is currently not known which mechanism causes the dysfunctions of the central nervous system in myotonic dystrophy.

4.2. Correlation Between Expansion Length and Clinical Form of Myotonic Dystrophy

As we have seen, four clinical forms of myotonic dystrophy can be differentiated from each other: congenital, childhood onset, adult onset, and mild form. As we can see in Table 2 in the forms with an older age at onset, subjects have in average a shorter expansion length. This is a group effect, and there is significant overlap between the groups. At both ends of the range, there seems to be threshold effects: subjects with congenital myotonic dystrophy always have more than 1000 CTG repeats at the mutation site, while patients with the mild form have fewer than 80 CTG repeats *(1)*. For CTG repeats between 80 and 1000, the correlation between phenotype severity and number of repeats is lower. Severity, defined in terms of cognitive and neuromuscular impairment, correlates more with the age of onset than with the expansion length of the CTG repeat. The same is true for life expectancy. Subjects with the congenital form have, on average, a shorter life expectancy than those with childhood or adult onset *(13)*. Here, too, there is significant overlap between the groups. Subjects with the mild form probably have a normal life expectancy.

5. BEHAVIORAL AND COGNITIVE ASPECTS OF MYOTONIC DYSTROPHY

Early studies described behavioral anomalies in adult myotonic dystrophy patients *(3)*. Early researchers noted apathy and neglect as signs of myotonic dystrophy and stated that the myotonic patient's home could be identified through its neglected aspect (Caughey and Myrianthopoulos [1963], cited in *[3]*). Lower intelligence, lack of initiative, and apathy were considered as part of the disease, in studies matching myotonic dystrophy with other muscular dystrophies with comparable muscle impairment. Excessive daytime sleepiness has been frequently described in adult type myotonic dystrophy, and some studies suggest a higher incidence of depression and/or personality disorders in adult patients with myotonic dystrophy. Children with congenital myotonic dystrophy often present with a developmental delay.

These findings raise several questions. (1) Which behavior characteristics are typical for the myotonic dystrophy phenotype, and which are rather anecdotal or coincidental? (2) Are the different subtypes of myotonic dystrophy associated with different behavior problems? (3) Are the behavioral findings a consequence of brain involvement in myotonic dystrophy, or are they secondary to the muscle weakness and chronic disability that patients with myotonic dystrophy experience?

5.1. Cognitive Characteristics

Early research on myotonic dystrophy suggested that the disease may be a cause of mental retardation *(31)*. Larger studies in the 1980s and early 1990s confirmed the fact that, as a group, patients with myotonic dystrophy are cognitively impaired *(32)*. The degree of cognitive delay varied from study to study. Bird and colleagues found that 6 out of 29 patients had IQs <70 *(33)*. Portwood et al. *(34)* studied 43 patients and found significant intellectual impairment in the subgroup of patients with maternal inheritance, but not in the patients with paternal inheritance. Sinforiani et al. *(35)* confirmed this later. Bird et al. *(33)* and Franzese et al. *(36)* found females were intellectually more impaired than males, although these results have not been confirmed. Degree of intellectual impairment was found to correlate with age at onset *(37)*. All these studies were carried out before the genetic mechanism of myotonic dystrophy had been revealed, which made the findings that intellectual impairment correlated with age at onset and with maternal inheritance difficult to understand.

After the discovery of the dynamic mutation in myotonic dystrophy, studies on intellectual impairment could be correlated with the length of the CTG expansion. Turnpenny et al. *(38)* and later Perini et al. *(39)* found that longer expansion lengths at the myotonic dystrophy mutation locus correlate moderately with the degree of intellectual impairment. This is different from what is seen in fragile X syndrome, another disease caused by a dynamic mutation (in this case a CGG_n repeat) and associated with intellectual impairment. In fragile X syndrome there is a sharp threshold phenomenon: subjects with an unmethylated expansion of fewer than 200 repeats have a normal intelligence, while subjects with a larger hypermethylated expansion demonstrate marked cognitive impairment. In myotonic dystrophy the variance is large, and the expansion length does not predict individual functioning accurately. In Turnpenny's study, a younger age at onset correlated more strongly with lower intelligence than expansion length did. However, as mentioned earlier, there are important problems in correlating the expansion length in peripheral blood cells and in brain cells in a group of individuals with a wide age range: there is a continuous growth of the repeat with increasing age, and there is a significant somatic mosaicism *(23)*.

The level of cognitive impairment seems to be directly related to age of onset and repeat length, but not to muscular impairment. There is broad consensus that children with congenital myotonic dystrophy have the lowest IQs *(14,37,40–44)*. At least 75% of them have IQs <70. Most are in the mildly retarded range, but some children are moderately retarded. Theoretically, their cognitive impairment might be caused by a direct effect of the mutation on the brain, or the effect of muscular impairment in infancy on psychomotor development. Subjects with juvenile-onset myotonic dystrophy already have cognitive impairment before they have significant muscular complaints *(14,45)*. Cognitive impairment in adult-onset myotonic dystrophy is generally very mild *(36)* or even absent *(42)*, although these patients may have significant muscle impairment at the time of assessment.

Data on possible cognitive deterioration during the course of the disease are limited and equivocal. Tuikka et al. *(42)* found no cognitive decline in 16 myotonic dystrophy patients after an average follow-up time of 12 years. In our own study of 16 children and adolescents with congenital or juvenile onset myotonic dystrophy, reliable 2-year follow-up data were available for two subjects, both of whom showed a significant decline on the same IQ test, the Wechsler Intelligence Scale for Children Revised *(14)*. Possible cognitive deterioration in myotonic dystrophy is certainly a subject of further research, particularly in children with the congenital and juvenile form of the disease.

Another area in which further research is necessary is whether there is only a global cognitive impairment in some forms of myotonic dystrophy, or if more specific cognitive problems can be observed. Most studies have not found significant differences between verbal and performance intelligence. Palmer et al. *(46)* noted lower intelligence, visual–constructive and executive function problems in patients with maternal inheritance but not in those with paternal inheritance. Memory and visual–perception skills were normal in both groups. It should be noted that individuals with maternal inheritance will more often present with congenital myotonic dystrophy, and thus be more affected as a group. A more recent study with a homogeneous group of noncongenital onset patients, all with normal intelligence, showed that these persons do have specific memory impairment *(47)*. In this group, there was a trend toward impairment of executive function as measured by the Wisconsin Card Sorting Test. Earlier, Woodward and colleagues found more severe impairment of executive function in a group of 17 myotonic dystrophy patients *(32)*. In their study, subjects with myotonic dystrophy scored worse than controls on almost every neuropsychological measure, and the finding of executive function impairment was not specific. In our own research, we found 4 of 16 children with congenital and juvenile myotonic dystrophy to have attention deficit hyperactivity disorder (ADHD) *(14)*, which is significantly higher than the frequency of 3–5% ADHD occurring in the school-age children's population *(48)*. These data were confirmed in a second study limited to children with juvenile onset myotonic dystrophy, where 8 of 24 children were given this diagnosis *(45)*. As the pattern of neuropsychological findings in children with ADHD implicates deficits in executive function *(49,50)*, the finding of ADHD in children with myotonic dystrophy probably reflects deficits in executive function in these children.

5.2. Somnolence, Hypersomnia, and Sleep Apnea

In early observations, the somnolence or excessive daytime sleepiness of individuals with myotonic dystrophy may have been seen as a form of fatigue or as a consequence of respiratory depression due to muscle weakness *(3)*. The symptom is perhaps one of the most common features of myotonic dystrophy, and occurs typically when attention is not focused. Somnolence in myotonic dystrophy is independent of irregular breathing during night sleep and sleep apnea, which may also occur in myotonic dystrophy *(51–53)*. The symptom is significantly more frequent in subjects with myotonic dystrophy than in controls with other neuromuscular disorders *(54,55)*. Rubinsztein et al. *(54)* showed that somnolence is independent of apathy and of depression in patients with myotonic dystrophy. They conclude that it likely reflects CNS involvement and is not secondary to other symptoms. Phillips et al. showed that daytime somnolence in myotonic dystrophy is partially correlated with the degree of muscular disability.

Several authors report that adult patients with myotonic dystrophy also have excessive nighttime sleep *(54,56,57)*. The same observation was made in children with juvenile myotonic dystrophy *(7,14)*.

5.3. Apathy

Apathy, lack of initiative, sitting idly, and indifference have been reported since the early observations on myotonic dystrophy *(3)*. Systematic observations on apathy in myotonic dystrophy have been performed by Ambrosini and Nurnberg *(58)*, and more recently by Rubinsztein et al. *(54)*. The latter study could elegantly demonstrate that apathy is a common and independent feature of myotonic dystrophy, and cannot be accounted for by depression or muscle weakness. It is therefore likely to reflect CNS involvement. One possible consequence of apathy in myotonic dystrophy may be the high level of unemployment found among patients with mild physical disability *(59)*.

5.4. Personality Changes

A more controversial subject is whether individuals with myotonic dystrophy have a particular personality profile, or a higher frequency of personality disorders. Based on personal impressions of their patients, several early researchers on myotonic dystrophy found unusual personality characteristics *(3)*. However, their impressions were not all the same. Some authors found myotonic dystrophy patients to be cheerful and careless, others saw them as hostile and unreliable. Research on personality problems has become more objective, but even then the subject remains unclear in myotonic dystrophy. Using the Minnesota Multiphasic Personality Inventory, Bird et al. *(33)* found significant personality changes in 8 of 25 (32%) subjects with myotonic dystrophy. On the other hand, Franzese et al. *(36)* did not find significant personality traits in a group of 28 patients with juvenile- or adult-onset myotonic dystrophy. Palmer et al. *(46)* found a high incidence of "dependent tendencies" in the personality of myotonic dystrophy subjects, and attributed this to their adjustment to a disabling disorder. In another study, Delaporte *(60)* found a homogeneous personality profile in the group of myotonic dystrophy subjects studied. They used the International Personality Disorder Examination in adults with minimal muscle weakness, a group of healthy controls, and a group of controls, with facioscapulohumeral dystrophy. Most of the 15 subjects with myotonic dystrophy displayed traits of avoidant personality, four of whom exhibited avoidant personality disorder. They concluded that a profile consisting of avoidant, obsessive–compulsive, passive–aggressive, and schizotypic traits, could not be attributed to adjustment to the disease, but reflected CNS involvement in myotonic dystrophy.

In these different studies, age at onset, degree of physical disability, research instruments, and definition of personality changes vary widely. It is thus impossible to compare them accurately. However, most researchers and clinicians agree that many persons with myotonic dystrophy have "something" in the area of emotional functioning and interpersonal relationships that is not observed in patients with comparable degree of muscle weakness due to other progressive neuromuscular diseases. It remains a challenge to identify this something, perhaps because classical personality inventories that were used in these studies are not suitable to detect personality traits that mainly occur in organic personality changes.

5.5. Depression

Several studies have suggested that signs of depression are found more frequently in patients with myotonic dystrophy. Duveneck et al. *(61)* described significantly more depressive tendencies in patients with myotonic dystrophy than in patients with other nonprogressive or progressive neuromuscular disorders. However, the degree of depressive traits was mild and the authors could not conclude that depressive disorder occurs more frequently in myotonic dystrophy. Another study found depressive disorder in 17% of myotonic dystrophy patients with severe muscle impairment *(62)*. Less severely affected individuals were not found to be more severely or more frequently depressed than normal controls *(54,63)*. To the contrary, Bungener et al. *(63)*, found flat affect among persons with myotonic dystrophy. It is possible that some symptoms like flat affect, apathy, somnolence (*see* Subheadings 5.2. and 5.3.), and other characteristics of myotonic dystrophy may give the wrong impression that mildly affected myotonic dystrophy patients appear to be depressed. On the other hand, one can imagine that the threat of further physical decline or even sudden death due to cardiac arrhythmia can cause depressive disorder in already severely affected patients. The risk of transmitting the disease to their children is another severe stressor for parents with myotonic dystrophy *(64)*, and this might also affect these individuals' mood. The question as to whether patients with myotonic dystrophy have a higher incidence of depressive disorder; and, if so, whether this reflects CNS involvement or adjustment problems in having or transmitting the disorder, remains to be answered.

5.6. Child Psychiatric Findings in Myotonic Dystrophy

The congenital and juvenile forms of myotonic dystrophy have been described more recently than the classical adult-onset form. To our knowledge, research on the behavior phenotype in these forms of myotonic dystrophy is limited, apart from the consistent finding that children with congenital myotonic dystrophy have cognitive developmental delays, with an average in the mildly retarded range (*see* Subheading 5.1.). Although children with congenital myotonic dystrophy initially present with neuromuscular problems and developmental delay, we observed that the first complaints in children with juvenile onset myotonic dystrophy—symptoms occur before age 18, but were absent at birth—were often learning and attention problems, even in children with IQs in the low-normal range (*14,45*). Using the Child Behavior Checklist, we found a marked increase of attention deficits and social problems in children with juvenile myotonic dystrophy, all of whom had no or minimal muscle weakness. A standardized child psychiatric interview showed a higher than expected frequency of Attention Deficit Hyperactivity Disorder: 4 of 16 in the first study (*14*), 8 of 24 in the second study (*45*). Symptoms of lack of impulse inhibition and of attention deficit were more pronounced in these children than symptoms of hyperactivity. Both studies also showed an increase of anxiety disorders in children with juvenile myotonic dystrophy.

These studies do not demonstrate convincingly whether the behavior problems and child psychiatric disorders were a direct consequence of CNS involvement, or of adjustment problems to the disease. The latter hypothesis seems unlikely for several reasons. In most subjects, the behavior problems existed before any neuromuscular sign of the disease, and the very significant increase of one particular child psychiatric disorder, ADHD, rather suggests a brain involvement. Indeed, adjustment problems would most likely be transient, more diverse, and in line with the personality development of the individual subjects.

6. BRAIN INVOLVEMENT IN MYOTONIC DYSTROPHY

Individuals with neuromuscular disorders with a genetic origin may show behavioral problems. These problems, however, should not automatically be attributed to a direct effect of the mutant gene on the brain. Having a chronic disability may cause emotional and mood problems in affected individuals, for example, individuals with diabetes mellitus have higher levels of anxiety and mood problems than controls *(65)*. The idea of having transmitted the mutated gene to one's children may add to the stress, as observed in otherwise healthy mothers of children with fragile X syndrome *(66,67)*. In children with congenital myotonic dystrophy, the severe breathing problems at birth might lead to brain damage, and the muscle weakness in early childhood might impede the child's normal development. These would be indirect mechanisms influencing the behavior phenotype. In myotonic dystrophy research, many resources have been used to demonstrate direct effects of the mutated gene on the brain. However, questions remain open concerning the importance of indirect effects of this disabling disorder on development and behavior. Insulin resistance is prominent in myotonic dystrophy patients, and impairs cerebral glucose metabolism *(10)*.

Various approaches have been used to demonstrate direct effects. One has been to take subjects with other forms of neuromuscular impairment as control subjects in behavior studies with myotonic dystrophy patients. Facioscapulohumeral dystrophy and Charcot–Marie–Tooth disease are other hereditary neuromuscular disorders that begin in late childhood or adulthood, with slowly progressive disability. The degree of disability is very similar to that in myotonic dystrophy. This approach demonstrates that personality problems *(60)*, relative underemployment *(59)*, apathy, and hypersomnia *(54)* are specifically associated with myotonic dystrophy, and not with having a neuromuscular disorder. These findings support the idea that myotonic dystrophy is not only a neuromuscular disorder, but that the brain is also directly involved.

A second and more fundamental approach has been to examine the brains of patients with myotonic dystrophy. This approach has provided convincing evidence that myotonic dystrophy is a brain disorder, as much as a neuromuscular disorder *(2)*. Neuropathological studies in adult-onset myotonic dystrophy have shown several neurodegenerative changes in the brain: cell loss, neuronal inclusion bodies, neurofibrillary tangles, and others *(3)*. These changes are somewhat different from those found in Alzheimer's disease, and thus can be directly related to myotonic dystrophy. Neuropathological findings in congenital myotonic dystrophy are less conclusive, although neuronal migration problems have been found in a few cases.

Many brain imaging studies have been performed in myotonic dystrophy. The earliest ones, using air encephalograms, showed enlarged cerebral ventricles *(68)*. This finding was reproduced in later studies with magnetic resonance imaging (MRI) *(37,69)*. In some patients cortical atrophy was also demonstrated *(70)*. Although some studies showed that cognitive impairment correlated with degree of cerebral atrophy *(37)*, others did not confirm this finding *(70)*. An important problem in these equivocal results is that the different forms of myotonic dystrophy had not been clearly delineated in these studies. Hashimoto et al. compared MRI findings in congenital vs adult-onset myotonic dystrophy and demonstrated that the cerebral atrophy is more marked in the congenital form *(71)*. Giubilei et al. found that atrophy of the anterior part of the corpus callosum correlates with sleep breathing irregularities *(72)*.

Another common MRI finding in myotonic dystrophy is the presence of white matter hyperintense lesions *(35,71,73,74)*. Damian et al. found that these white matter lesions correlate with cognitive impairment when they lie in the white matter immediately adjacent to cortex, but had no clear clinical significance when they have a periventricular localization *(73)*. Neurocognitive dysfunctions correlate more strongly with white matter anomalies than with ventricular enlargement *(75)*. Chang et al. *(76)* found evidence of diminished cerebral blood flow, most severe in the frontal and temporoparietal association cortex. Functional magnetic resonance imaging (fMRI) is a noninvasive imaging technique that makes it possible to study the concentration of specific chemical compounds in the brain of living patients. Using fMRI, Chang et al. *(77)* demonstrated changed concentrations of several chemical compounds in the brain of patients with myotonic dystrophy. The degree of changes correlated well with the length of the CTG expansion in the myotonic dystrophy gene.

Brain imaging studies are subject to the same limitation as psychological investigations, which is that different researchers have included different subgroups of the broad spectrum of myotonic dystrophy phenotypes, thus making comparisons across investigations difficult. Nonetheless, the neuropathological studies, and the more recent brain imaging studies, give convincing evidence that the brain is involved in myotonic dystrophy and support the view that at least a substantial part of the behavior phenotype is the direct consequence of a brain disorder. However, elucidating the pathophysiological mechanisms between the molecular changes in myotonic dystrophy, the anatomical and functional signs of brain involvement, and the behavioral phenotype, still requires a lot of work.

7. DIAGNOSIS OF MYOTONIC DYSTROPHY

Until the discovery of the gene and the molecular causes of myotonic dystrophy, the diagnosis was based on clinical observations and family history, and demonstrating electromyographical and pathological changes in the muscles *(3)*. Now that direct detection of the mutated gene through a DNA test has become possible, making the diagnosis has become easier.

This will probably lead to making the diagnosis in unaffected, or only minimally affected, family members of patients with myotonic dystrophy. This raises ethical questions, in particular if parents request asymptomatic children to be tested. The ethical consideration in this group is that if children who are potential carriers of a disease of which they have no signs (yet), and if uncertainty about their carriership has no effect on later prognosis, these children should not be tested for the disease until they are mature enough to decide themselves whether they want to be tested. On the other hand, one should consider that in children, myotonic dystrophy may begin with behavioral rather than neuromuscular symptoms, and that lack of the latter symptoms should not impede making an early diagnosis.

Another possible side effect of the easy and very reliable DNA test is the fact that parts of the clinical assessment may be neglected in these patients with a complex multisystem disease.

8. CONCLUSIONS

Myotonic dystrophy is a multisystem disease with a wide spectrum of clinical manifestations. Depending on the widely varying age at onset and degree of impairment, four forms of myotonic dystrophy can be distinguished. The congenital form may present (initially) as a developmental disorder, with severe symptoms in infancy and consequent improvement. The other three forms present as a slowly progressive degenerative disorder, which is also the fate in adulthood of patients with congenital myotonic dystrophy. There is convincing evidence that the brain is directly affected, contrarily to many other neuromuscular disorders. The path from mutant gene to brain pathology, neurophysiological changes, and finally to behavior is still unclear.

The behavioral phenotype is quite characteristic, but its degree of expression is variable. As a rule, an early age at onset of the disorder correlates with a more severe behavioral phenotype. There is a weaker correlation between age of onset and length of the CTG expansion at the mutation site in the gene.

Mild mental retardation is common in congenital myotonic dystrophy, and milder learning problems are frequent in juvenile myotonic dystrophy. Often, they even precede neuromuscular symptoms in these children, and should thus warrant the possibility of myotonic dystrophy in children with learning problems in myotonic dystrophy families. It is equivocal whether adult-onset patients as a group have a lower intelligence, and there is a marked lack of follow-up data on the evolution of intelligence in all forms of myotonic dystrophy.

Besides these global impairments in cognitive ability, impairment of executive functions is present in all forms of myotonic dystrophy, but not in all individuals with the disease. In children with juvenile onset, deficits of attention and impulse control may be signs of poor executive functioning. Apathy is a very common symptom in myotonic dystrophy and is independent of sleep anomalies and depression *(54)*. In neuropsychological literature, apathy is mentioned as a sign of frontal lobe dysfuntion and as such may correlate with poor executive function *(78)*. Specific memory dysfunctions have been found in adult-onset myotonic dystrophy. Somnolence (excessive daytime sleepiness) and hypersomnia are frequent symptoms in myotonic dystrophy, and reflect brain involvement rather than fatigue due to muscle weakness.

It is equivocal whether myotonic dystrophy patients have a higher incidence of depressive disorders, and if so, what the pathological mechanism is. Some researchers have found a higher prevalence of particular personality traits, and/or personality disorders in myotonic dystrophy, whereas others have not. It is not clear whether these possible personality problems are independent of the apathy, poor executive functions, and other neurocognitive signs that we discussed previously.

Finally, to our knowledge, nothing is known about the behavioral phenotype in patients with the mild, late-onset form of myotonic dystrophy. Considering the reflections on age at onset and degree of behavioral impairment, it is most likely that these patients have no or only minimal behavioral characteristics.

REFERENCES

1. Thornton C. The myotonic dystrophies. Semin Neurol 1999;19:25–33.
2. Ashizawa T. Myotonic dystrophy as a brain disorder. Arch Neurol 1998;55:291–3.
3. Harper PS. Myotonic dystrohpy. In: Warlow CP, ed. Major problems in neurology. vol. 37. London: WB Saunders, 2001.
4. Harley HG, Brook JD, Rundle SA, et al. Expansion of an unstable DNA region and phenotypic variation in myotonic dystrophy. Nature 1992;355:545–6.
5. Aslanidis C, Jansen G, Amemiya C, et al. Cloning of the essential myotonic dystrophy region and mapping of the putative defect. Nature 1992;355:548–51.
6. Buxton J, Shelbourne P, Davies J, et al. Detection of an unstable fragment of DNA specific to individuals with myotonic dystrophy. Nature 1992; 355:547–8.
7. de Die-Smulders C. Long-term clinical and genetic studies in myotonic dystrophy. Faculty of Medicine. Maastricht: Universiteit Maastricht, 2000;191.
8. Steyaert J, de Die-Smulders C, Fryns JP, Goossens E, Willekens D. Behavioral phenotype in childhood type of dystrophia myotonica. Am J Med Genet 2000;96:888–9.

9. Wieringa B. Myotonic dystrophy reviewed: back to the future? Hum Mol Genet 1994;3:1–7.
10. Annane D, Fiorelli M, Mazoyer B, et al. Impaired cerebral glucose metabolism in myotonic dystrophy: a triplet- size dependent phenomenon. Neuromuscul Disord 1998;8:39–45.
11. de Die-Smulders CE, Howeler CJ, Thijs C, et al. Age and causes of death in adult-onset myotonic dystrophy. Brain 1998;121:1557–63.
12. Vanier TM. Dystrophia myotonica in childhood. Br Med J 1960;2:1284–8.
13. Mathieu J, Allard P, Potvin L, Prevost C, Begin P. A 10-year study of mortality in a cohort of patients with myotonic dystrophy. Neurology 1999; 52:1658–62.
14. Steyaert J, Umans S, Willekens D, et al. A study of the cognitive and psychological profile in 16 children with congenital or juvenile myotonic dystrophy. Clin Genet 1997;52:135–41.
15. Moxley RT, 3rd, Ricker K. Proximal myotonic myopathy. Muscle Nerve 1995;18:557–8.
16. Ricker K. Myotonic dystrophy and proximal myotonic myophathy. J Neurol 1999;246:334–8.
17. Liquori CL, Ricker K, Moseley ML, et al. Myotonic dystrophy type 2 caused by a CCTG expansion in intron 1 of ZNF9. Science 2001;293:864–7.
18. Howeler CJ, Busch HF, Geraedts JP, Niermeijer MF, Staal A. Anticipation in myotonic dystrophy: fact or fiction? Brain 1989;112:779–97.
19. Richards RI. Dynamic mutations: a decade of unstable expanded repeats in human genetic disease. Hum Mol Genet 2001;10:2187–94.
20. Harper PS, Harley HG, Reardon W, Shaw DJ. Anticipation in myotonic dystrophy: new light on an old problem. Am J Hum Genet 1992;51:10–6.
21. Lavedan C, Hofmann-Radvanyi H, Shelbourne P, et al. Myotonic dystrophy: size- and sex-dependent dynamics of CTG meiotic instability, and somatic mosaicism. Am J Hum Genet 1993;52:875–83.
22. Hageman AT, Gabreels FJ, Liem KD, Renkawek K, Boon JM. Congenital myotonic dystrophy; a report on thirteen cases and a review of the literature. J Neurol Sci 1993;115:95–101.
23. Martorell L, Monckton DG, Gamez J, et al. Progression of somatic CTG repeat length heterogeneity in the blood cells of myotonic dystrophy patients. Hum Mol Genet 1998; 7:307–12.
24. Tapscott SJ, Thornton CA. Biomedicine. Reconstructing myotonic dystrophy. Science 2001; 293:816–7.
25. Kimura T, Takahashi MP, Okuda Y, et al. The expression of ion channel mRNAs in skeletal muscles from patients with myotonic muscular dystrophy. Neurosci Lett 2000; 295:93–6.
26. Savkur RS, Philips AV, Cooper TA. Aberrant regulation of insulin receptor alternative splicing is associated with insulin resistance in myotonic dystrophy. Nat Genet 2001;29:40–7.
27. Philips AV, Timchenko LT, Cooper TA. Disruption of splicing regulated by a CUG-binding protein in myotonic dystrophy. Science 1998;280:737–41.
28. Winchester CL, Ferrier RK, Sermoni A, Clark BJ, Johnson KJ. Characterization of the expression of DMPK and SIX5 in the human eye and implications for pathogenesis in myotonic dystrophy. Hum Mol Genet 1999;8:481–92.

29. Sarkar PS, Appukuttan B, Han J, et al. Heterozygous loss of Six5 in mice is sufficient to cause ocular cataracts. Nat Genet 2000;25:110–4.
30. Klesert TR, Cho DH, Clark JI, et al. Mice deficient in Six5 develop cataracts: implications for myotonic dystrophy. Nat Genet 2000;25:105–9.
31. Calderon R. Myotonic dystrophy: a neglected cause of mental retardation. J Pediatr 1966;68:423–31.
32. Woodward JB, 3rd, Heaton RK, Simon DB, Ringel SP. Neuropsychological findings in myotonic dystrophy. J Clin Neuropsychol 1982;4:335–42.
33. Bird TD, Follett C, Griep E. Cognitive and personality function in myotonic muscular dystrophy. J Neurol Neurosurg Psychiatry 1983;46:971–80.
34. Portwood MM, Wicks JJ, Lieberman JS, Duveneck MJ. Intellectual and cognitive function in adults with myotonic muscular dystrophy. Arch Phys Med Rehabil 1986;67:299–303.
35. Sinforiani E, Sandrini G, Martelli A, et al. Cognitive and neuroradiological findings in myotonic dystrophy. Funct Neurol 1991;6:377–84.
36. Franzese A, Antonini G, Iannelli M, et al. Intellectual functions and personality in subjects with noncongenital myotonic muscular dystrophy. Psychol Rep 1991;68:723–32.
37. Huber SJ, Kissel JT, Shuttleworth EC, Chakeres DW, Clapp LE, Brogan MA. Magnetic resonance imaging and clinical correlates of intellectual impairment in myotonic dystrophy. Arch Neurol 1989;46:536–40.
38. Turnpenny P, Clark C, Kelly K. Intelligence quotient profile in myotonic dystrophy, intergenerational deficit, and correlation with CTG amplification. J Med Genet 1994;31:300–5.
39. Perini GI, Menegazzo E, Ermani M, et al. Cognitive impairment and (CTG)n expansion in myotonic dystrophy patients. Biol Psychiatry 1999;46:425–31.
40. Aicardi J, Conti D, Goutieres F. [Clinical and genetic aspects of the early form of Steinert's dystrophia myotonica]. J Genet Hum 1975;23(Suppl):146–57.
41. Harper PS. Congenital myotonic dystrophy in Britain. I. Clinical aspects. Arch Dis Child 1975;50:505–13.
42. Tuikka RA, Laaksonen RK, Somer HV. Cognitive function in myotonic dystrophy: a follow-up study. Eur Neurol 1993;33:436–41.
43. Roig M, Balliu PR, Navarro C, Brugera R, Losada M. Presentation, clinical course, and outcome of the congenital form of myotonic dystrophy. Pediatr Neurol 1994;11:208–13.
44. Johnson ER, Abresch RT, Carter GT, et al. Profiles of neuromuscular diseases. Myotonic dystrophy. Am J Phys Med Rehabil 1995;74:S104–16.
45. Goossens E, Steyaert J, De Die-Smulders C, Willekens D, Fryns JP. Emotional and behavioral profile and child psychiatric diagnosis in the childhood type of myotonic dystrophy. Genet Couns 2000;11:317–27.
46. Palmer BW, Boone KB, Chang L, Lee A, Black S. Cognitive deficits and personality patterns in maternally versus paternally inherited myotonic dystrophy. J Clin Exp Neuropsychol 1994;16:784–95.

47. Rubinsztein JS, Rubinsztein DC, McKenna PJ, Goodburn S, Holland AJ. Mild myotonic dystrophy is associated with memory impairment in the context of normal general intelligence. J Med Genet 1997;34:229–33.

48. American Psychiatric Association. Diagnostic and Statistical Manual of Mental Disorders. Washington, DC: American Psychiatric Association, 1994.

49. Faraone SV, Biederman J. Neurobiology of attention-deficit hyperactivity disorder. Biol Psychiatry 1998;44:951–8.

50. Sergeant J. The cognitive-energetic model: an empirical approach to attention-deficit hyperactivity disorder. Neurosci Biobehav Rev 2000;24:7–12.

51. Gilmartin JJ, Cooper BG, Griffiths CJ, et al. Breathing during sleep in patients with myotonic dystrophy and non- myotonic respiratory muscle weakness. Q J Med 1991;78:21–31.

52. van der Meche FG, Bogaard JM, van der Sluys JC, Schimsheimer RJ, Ververs CC, Busch HF. Daytime sleep in myotonic dystrophy is not caused by sleep apnoea. J Neurol Neurosurg Psychiatry 1994;57:626–8.

53. Ververs CC, Van der Meche FG, Verbraak AF, van der Sluys HC, Bogaard JM. Breathing pattern awake and asleep in myotonic dystrophy. Respiration 1996;63:1–7.

54. Rubinsztein JS, Rubinsztein DC, Goodburn S, Holland AJ. Apathy and hypersomnia are common features of myotonic dystrophy. J Neurol Neurosurg Psychiatry 1998;64:510–5.

55. Phillips MF, Steer HM, Soldan JR, Wiles CM, Harper PS. Daytime somnolence in myotonic dystrophy. J Neurol 1999;246:275–82.

56. Ono S, Kurisaki H, Sakuma A, Nagao K. Myotonic dystrophy with alveolar hypoventilation and hypersomnia: a clinicopathological study. J Neurol Sci 1995;128:225–31.

57. Ono S, Takahashi K, Jinnai K, et al. Loss of serotonin-containing neurons in the raphe of patients with myotonic dystrophy: a quantitative immunohistochemical study and relation to hypersomnia. Neurology 1998;50:535–8.

58. Ambrosini PG, Nurnberg HG. Psychopathology: a primary feature of myotonic dystrophy. Psychosomatics 1979;20:393–5, 398–9.

59. Fowler WM Jr, Abresch RT, Koch TR, Brewer ML, Bowden RK, Wanlass RL. Employment profiles in neuromuscular diseases. Am J Phys Med Rehabil 1997;76:26–37.

60. Delaporte C. Personality patterns in patients with myotonic dystrophy. Arch Neurol 1998;55:635–40.

61. Duveneck MJ, Portwood MM, Wicks JJ, Lieberman JS. Depression in myotonic muscular dystrophy. Arch Phys Med Rehabil 1986;67:875–7.

62. Colombo G, Perini GI, Miotti MV, Armani M, Angelini C. Cognitive and psychiatric evaluation of 40 patients with myotonic dystrophy. Ital J Neurol Sci 1992;13:53–8.

63. Bungener C, Jouvent R, Delaporte C. Psychopathological and emotional deficits in myotonic dystrophy. J Neurol Neurosurg Psychiatry 1998;65:353–6.

64. Faulkner CL, Kingston HM. Knowledge, views, and experience of 25 women with myotonic dystrophy. J Med Genet 1998;35:1020–5.
65. Kohen D, Burgess AP, Catalan J, Lant A. The role of anxiety and depression in quality of life and symptom reporting in people with diabetes mellitus. Qual Life Res 1998;7:197–204.
66. Franke P, Maier W, Hautzinger M, et al. Fragile-X carrier females: evidence for a distinct psychopathological phenotype? Am J Med Genet 1996;64:334–9.
67. McConkie-Rosell A, Spiridigliozzi GA, Rounds K, et al. Parental attitudes regarding carrier testing in children at risk for fragile X syndrome. Am J Med Genet 1999;82:206–11.
68. Refsum S, Lonnum A, Sjaastad O, Engeset A. Dystrophia myotonica. Repeated pneumoencephalographic studies in ten patients. Neurology 1967;17:345–8.
69. Glantz RH, Wright RB, Huckman MS, Garron DC, Siegel IM. Central nervous system magnetic resonance imaging findings in myotonic dystrophy. Arch Neurol 1988;45:36–7.
70. Censori B, Provinciali L, Danni M, et al. Brain involvement in myotonic dystrophy: MRI features and their relationship to clinical and cognitive conditions. Acta Neurol Scand 1994;90:211–7.
71. Hashimoto T, Tayama M, Miyazaki M, et al. Neuroimaging study of myotonic dystrophy. I. Magnetic resonance imaging of the brain. Brain Dev 1995; 17:24–7.
72. Giubilei F, Antonini G, Bastianello S, et al. Excessive daytime sleepiness in myotonic dystrophy. J Neurol Sci 1999;164:60–3.
73. Damian MS, Schilling G, Bachmann G, Simon C, Stoppler S, Dorndorf W. White matter lesions and cognitive deficits: relevance of lesion pattern? Acta Neurol Scand 1994;90:430–6.
74. Di Costanzo A, Di Salle F, Santoro L, Bonavita V, Tedeschi G. T2 relaxometry of brain in myotonic dystrophy. Neuroradiology 2001;43:198–204.
75. Abe K, Fujimura H, Toyooka K, et al. Involvement of the central nervous system in myotonic dystrophy. J Neurol Sci 1994;127:179–85.
76. Chang L, Anderson T, Migneco OA, et al. Cerebral abnormalities in myotonic dystrophy. Cerebral blood flow, magnetic resonance imaging, and neuropsychological tests. Arch Neurol 1993;50:917–23.
77. Chang L, Ernst T, Osborn D, Seltzer W, Leonido-Yee M, Poland RE. Proton spectroscopy in myotonic dystrophy: correlations with CTG repeats. Arch Neurol 1998;55:305–11.
78. Kolb B, Whishaw I. Fundamentals of Human Neuropsychology, 4th ed. New York: WH Freeman, 1996:305–33.

III

X-LINKED NONSYNDROMAL DISORDERS AND NEUROBEHAVIORAL DYSFUNCTION

11

Genetics of X-Linked Mental Retardation

Jamel Chelly and Ben C. J. Hamel

1. INTRODUCTION

Mental retardation (MR) is defined as an overall "intelligence quotient" (IQ) <70, associated with functional deficits in adaptive behaviour (such as daily-living skills, social skills and communication), with an onset before 18 years *(1)*. Approximately 2–3% of the population have an intelligence quotient (IQ) <70 *(2,3)* and at least 0.3% of individuals are severely handicapped (IQ < 50) (Table 1), yet a cause for mental retardation is established in less than half of all cases *(4)*. The underlying causes of MR are extremely heterogeneous (Table 2). In addition to multiple nongenetic factors that act prenatally or during early infancy and cause brain injury, chromosomal anomalies, such as aneuploidy syndromes, for example, Down syndrome, the microdeletion syndromes, for example, Prader–Willi, Angelman, Miller–Dieker, Smith–Magenis, and Williams syndromes, represent an important genetic cause of MR. Recent studies suggest that chromosomal rearrangements that affect the telomeric regions of autosomes, not detectable by conventional cytogenetic analysis, may account for up to 7% of moderate to severe MR *(5,6)*. Genetic causes may be involved in one half of severely retarded patients *(7)*. Some disorders for which the gene is identified affect relatively significant numbers of patients and families, such as the fragile X syndrome (which affects approx 1/4000–6000 males) *(8,9)* and Rett syndrome (1/10,000–15,000 girls) *(10)*, but our knowledge of these monogenic causes is still far from complete.

It has been known for many years that among individuals with mental retardation males outnumber females *(11)*. In the early1970s, Lehrke *(12)* was the first to hypothesize that this male excess, which is at present estimated to be about 30%, could be due to mutations in X-linked genes. In recent years, significant progress has been made in the identification of some

From: *Contemporary Clinical Neuroscience:*
Genetics and Genomics of Neurobehavioral Disorders
Edited by: G. S. Fisch © Humana Press Inc., Totowa, NJ

Table 1
Classification of Mental Retardation

Terminology	IQ
Profound	<20
Severe	20–35
Moderate	35–50
Mild	50–70
Borderline	70–85

Table 2
Etiological Classification of Mental Retardation (in %)

IQ	<50 "Severe "MR	>50 "Mild" MR
Chromosomal abnormalities	15	5–10
Monogenic disorders (including fragile X syndrome)	20–25	5–10
CNS malformations; MCA/MR syndromes	10	5
Acquired disorders (pre-, peri-, and postnatal)	30–35	15
Unknown	20	60–65

CNS, central nervous system; MCA, multiple congenital anomalies.

of the X-linked genes involved in MR. Because of the haploid status in males for most genes on the X chromosome and the relative ease of gene mapping on this chromosome, mainly X-linked forms of mental retardation (XLMR) have been mapped *(13,14)*. The observation of large families with a clear X-linked inheritance of MR, and improved epidemiological studies, led to the gradual acceptance that a significant proportion of MR in males might be due to mutations in X-linked genes. In the late 1960s and 1970s, identification of the fragile X syndrome as a distinct clinical entity was an important step in this process *(15,16)*. This syndrome is associated with a specific clinical phenotype and accounts for approx 2–3% of MR in males, and for approx 1 % in females (who are on average less affected than males). The interest in fragile X syndrome led to the description of further X-linked MR (XLMR) syndromes, and identification of an increasing number of large families in which MR is not associated with a specific clinical or metabolic phenotype ("nonsyndromal" XLMR) *(13,14)*. The prevalence of nonsyndromal XLMR has been estimated as 1.8/1000 males with a carrier frequency of 2.4/1000 females *(17)*. It could well be that 20–25% of all male mental retardation and possibly also 10% of mild mental retardation in females is due to mutations in X-linked genes *(8)*. This chapter reviews the development of recent research in XLMR, focusing on the delineation of genetic causes underlying syndromal and nonsyndromal X-linked mental retardation.

2. SYNDROMAL FORMS OF XLMR

The distinction between syndromal and nonsyndromal XLMR is not always clear. In its first description, the Fragile X syndrome was labelled nonsyndromal *(18)*, although it is now the best known and most prevalent example of syndromal XLMR. This strongly argues for standardized clinical evaluation of patients and families. Historically, syndromal XLMR encompasses malformation syndromes, neuromuscular and metabolic disorders, and the X-linked dominant conditions. At present approximately 136 syndromal forms of XLMR are known *(14,19)*; http://xlmr.interfree.it/home.htm). In 58 of these syndromes the genetic defect has been mapped on the X chromosome, while in another 26 the gene and mutations therein are known (Table 3). Most known syndromal forms occur rarely, often in single families. At present it is difficult to say what proportion of XLMR is accounted for by syndromal forms, but it may well be 30–40%, of which somewhat less than half is accounted for by the fragile X syndrome. Some of these syndromal forms are discussed in more detail.

2.1. Fragile X Syndrome

The syndrome derives its name from a fragile site in Xq27.3, FRAXA, which was noted first by Lubs *(15)* in a XLMR family. Cytogenetic expression of the fragile site is best observed when cells are cultured in a folic acid poor medium. Even then it is seen in maximally 30–50% of cells and very often even much lower, particularly among unaffected carriers, in whom the fragile site may well be absent. The first large family in which the fragile X phenotype was segregating was described by Martin and Bell *(18)*. The clinical phenotype varies with age. Usually pregnancy and delivery are uneventful. Early postnatal growth parameters such as weight, length, and head circumference are above average for age. Development is delayed for motor milestones and more so for speech and language. Behavioral characteristics in early childhood such as hyperactivity, attention deficit, temper tantrums, hand flapping, gaze avoidance, and autistic features are more indicative for the diagnosis than physical features, which become more evident as children age. Physical features are exhibited by a prominent forehead, long face,

Table 3
Genes Involved in Syndromal XLMR

Disease	Locus	Gene	Potential function
Syndromes with generally severe MR			
Coffin–Lowry syndrome	Xp22	RPS6KA3/RSK2	Serine/threonine protein kinase
West syndrome (ISSX)	Xp22	ARX	Aristaless-related homeobox gene
Partington syndrome			
Pyruvate dehydrogenase deficiency	Xp22	PDHA1	Pyruvate dehydrogenase
Opitz G/BBB syndrome	Xp22	MID1	Microtubule-associated protein
Hyperglycerolemia	Xp21.3	GK1	Glycerolkinase
OTC deficiency	Xp21.1	OTC	Ornithine transcarbamylase
α-Thalassemia-retardation-X (ATR-X)	Xq13	XNP	DNA-binding helicase
Menkes disease	Xq13	ATP7A	Copper transporting ATPase
PGK1 deficiency	Xq21.1	PGK1	Phosphoglycerate kinase
Pelizaeus–Merzbacher disease	Xq21.33	PLP	Protein component of myelin
Mohr–Tranebjaerg syndrome	Xq22	DDP	Mitochondrial inner membrane transport protein
Lissencephaly	Xq22.3	DCX	Microtubule-associated protein
Lowe syndrome	Xq26.1	OCRL1	Phosphoinositide phosphatase
Lesch–Nyhan disease	Xq26	HPRT	Hypoxanthine–guanine–phosphoribosyltransferase

Fragile X syndrome (FRAXA)	*FMR1*	Xq27.3	mRNA binding protein
Adrenoleucodystrophy	*ABCD1*	Xq28	Peroxisomal ABC transporter
Hunter disease (MPS II)	*IDS*	Xq28	Iduronate sulfatase
Hydrocephalus/MASA syndrome[a]	*L1CAM*	Xq28	Neural cell adhesion molecule
Rett syndrome[a]	*MECP2*	Xq28	Transcriptional silencing

Syndromes with generally inconsistent of mild MR

Duchenne muscular dystrophy	*DMD*	Xp21.2	Component of dystrophin-associated complex
MAO-A deficiency	*MAOA*	Xp11.3	Monoaminooxidase A
Norrie disease	*NDP*	Xp11.3	Secreted protein (?)
Aarskog–Scott syndrome	*FDG1*	Xp11.21	Rho-GEF
Simpson–Golabi–Behmel syndrome	*GPC3*	Xq26	Heparan sulfate proteoglycan
Incontinentia Pigmenti[a]	*NEMO*	Xq28	NF-κB essential modulator
Dyskeratosis congenita	*DKC1*	Xq28	RNA associating protein
Periventricular heterotopia[a]	*FLN1*	Xq28	Actin-binding protein

[a]X-linked dominant

267

large ears with incompletely folded helices, midface hypoplasia, high palate with dental crowding, and prominent chin. Signs of a connective tissue dysplasia are also present: joint laxity, flat feet; less frequently, scoliosis and mitral valve prolapse and rarely aortic dilatation. Testicular enlargement (macroorchidism) is usually seen near or after puberty with testicular volumes in adulthood above 25 mL *(20)*. Mental retardation is commonly moderate, but may vary from mild/borderline to profound depending on the age at which an individual with the full mutation is tested *(21)*. Behavioral problems continue to exist during life. Speech exhibits perseveration and echolalia. Epileptic seizure may occur and usually disappear before puberty. Unusual phenotypes do occur like Sotos and Prader–Willi-like phenotypes. Life expectancy is about normal. More than half of the females with a full mutation show a degree of mental impairment usually without the above-mentioned physical features. Another possible heterozygote manifestation is premature ovarian failure that occurs mainly in daughters of nonmanifesting males with a premutation *(22)*.

In 1991, the Fragile X syndrome gene, *FMR1*, was cloned and identified *(23)*. In almost all cases, the causative mutation is an expansion of a CGG triplet in the 5' untranslated region of the gene. The normal and stably transmitted triplet repeat number is between 6 and about 50. A repeat number between 50 and about 200 is called a premutation. The premutation is generally thought to produce no phenotype, but may increase in size when transmitted by a female carrier to the next generation *(24)*. Inheritance from a female premutation carrier may lead to a full mutation with a repeat number above 200, which, in males, is associated with the clinical picture of the fragile X syndrome and in more than 50% of females, with learning difficulties. A CGG repeat number of more than 200 disrupts the expression of the *FMR1* gene as a consequence of hypermethylation in the promotor region, and inhibits translation of the FMR1 protein. Absence of the FMR1 protein is the actual cause of the mental retardation, not the repeat expansion as such, because unaffected, transmitting males with unmethylated full mutations have been reported *(25)*. The role of the FMR1 protein has not been completely elucidated, but apparently it plays a role in binding mRNAs. Pre- and postnatal diagnosis is routinely performed in most molecular diagnostic laboratories. An elegant and rapid diagnostic method based on antibody detection of the FMR1 protein in blood cells, hair roots, amniocytes, and chorionic villi (but beware of false-negative results!) has been developed *(26)*. Management of patients and families with fragile X syndrome comprise attention for the physical and behavioral problems and genetic counselling, since all mothers of fragile X syndrome patients are carriers of either a pre- or a full mutation *(27)*.

The fragile X syndrome has a prevalence of 1/4000–6000 *(8,9)*, although higher rates have been reported in earlier studies *(28,29)*. At present, screening for female fragile X premutation and full mutation carriers is a frequently debated issue *(30,31)*.

2.2 α-Thalassemia–Retardation–X (ATR-X) Syndrome

The name for this syndrome is derived from the analogy with ATR-16 syndrome: an α-thalassemia-mental retardation syndrome due to deletions involving 16p13.3 and including the α-globin gene. ATR-16 syndrome is less severe compared to ATR-X. In 1990, the first cases of ATR-X were described by Wilkie et al. *(32)*. Classically, ATR-X is characterized by severe mental retardation, hypotonia (in particular of the face), facial dysmorphisms, microcephaly, short stature, genital anomalies, and hemoglobin H inclusions. Facial dysmorphisms consist of telecanthus and hypertelorism, epicanthic folds, low nasal bridge, small triangular nose with anteverted nares, midface hypoplasia, open mouth with prominent lips and often tented upper lip, wide-spaced incisors, and deformed and low-set ears. Facial hypotonia contributes to the facial dysmorphia. Genital anomalies include hypospadias, cryptorchidism, and small penis, and rarely ambiguous genitalia. Minor skeletal abnormalities are seen such as brachydactyly, clinodactyly, and tapering fingers. Short stature originates postnatally and sometimes is not evident until adolescence. Microcephaly is often present at birth. Development is severely delayed from birth. Speech is mostly absent or very limited. Patients with ATR-X do not exhibit a specific behavioral phenotype. Some cases have a mild hypochromic, microcytic anemia due to a mild form of hemoglobin H disease. Staining of erythrocytes with brilliant cresyl blue may reveal hemoglobin H inclusions in a certain percentage (up to 30%) of erythrocytes *(33)*. During infancy, complications such as poor feeding, vomiting, gastroesophageal reflux, respiratory infections, and constipation are frequent. Carrier females rarely show signs and symptoms of ATR-X because carriers typically have a markedly skewed X-inactivation pattern with preferential inactivation of the mutation carrying the X chromosome *(33)*.

ATR-X is caused by mutations in the *XNP* (X-linked nuclear protein) gene in Xq13.3, which was found in 1995 *(34)*. The *XNP* gene belongs to DNA binding helicases and the protein has a function on chromatin remodeling, through which it acts as an transcriptional regulator. Apart from *XNP* mutations in classical ATR-X, *XNP* mutations have also been found in other rare syndromes like Juberg–Marsidi syndrome *(35)*, Carpenter–Waziri syndrome *(36)*, Holmes–Gang syndrome *(37)*, and Smith–Fineman–Myers syndrome *(38)*. These syndromes share with ATR-X the severe mental retardation and the hypotonic facies. Stevenson et al. *(39)* therefore no longer speak about ATR-X, but call this family of syndromes the XLMR-hypotonic facies syndrome. They estimate that no less than 10% of named XLMR syndromes are candidates for allelism with XLMR-hypotonic facies syndrome. Recently, an *XNP* mutation has been found in a family of six patients with mainly mild mental retardation without obvious other features *(40)*. Thus, the clinical variability resulting from *XNP* mutations is enormous, ranging from classical ATR-X syndrome to mild almost nonsyndromal mental retardation.

2.3 Coffin–Lowry Syndrome

The name Coffin–Lowry syndrome was coined by Temtamy et al. *(41)*, who recognized the clinical phenotype independently described by Coffin et al. *(42)* and Lowry et al. *(43)* as one and the same. Coffin–Lowry syndrome is characterized by short stature, facial anomalies, and hyoptonia, features associated with connective tissue dysplasia and skeletal changes. There is a postnatal mild growth deficiency. Facial anomalies are a coarse appearance with down-slanting palpebral fissures, hypertelorism, anteverted nares, tented upper lip, and cupped ears. With age, the face elongates and coarsens with thickening of lips and nose and alae nasi, open mouth with everted lower lip. Large, soft hands, joint hyperextensibility, inguinal hernia, rectal and uterine prolapse, pectus carinatum/excavatum, scoliosis, and flat feet may point to a connective tissue dysplasia. Skeletal features are tapering fingers and X-ray abnormalities such as tufted drumstick appearance to distal phalanges, narrow intervertebral spaces, and notches in the anterior–superior margin of lumbar vertebrae *(44)*. Developmental delay is severe from the outset and is nonprogressive, and leaves the patient usually without speech. As in ATR-X syndrome, there seems to be no common behavorial phenotype. Clinical findings in female carriers are frequent and include short stature, mild facial changes, soft fleshy hands with distal tapering of fingers. X-inactivation in female carriers is not skewed. The frequent and distinctive features that appear in females allow diagnosis of Coffin–Lowry syndrome in females with no affected male relatives.

Coffin–Lowry syndrome is caused by mutations in the *RSK2* (also called *RPS6KA3*) in Xp22 *(45)*. The gene product is a serine/threonine protein kinase, which seemingly plays a role in chromatin-remodeling events and in gene regulation. *RSK2* mutations have also been found in males with mild Coffin–Lowry features *(44)* and even in a family with nonsyndromal XLMR *(46)*. In the latter family, a *RSK2* missense mutation with residual enzymatic RSK2 activity of about 15–20% rescued these patients from the usual severe phenotype, the latter of which is generally due to loss of function mutations in *RSK2*. In a related development, a recently identified other member of the RSK family of protein kinases, *RSK4* (*RPS6KA6*), is also X-linked (Xq21), and therefore an excellent candidate gene for XLMR, but, to date, no mutations in *RSK4* have been found *(47)*. The differential diagnosis of Coffin–Lowry syndrome includes ATR-X syndrome and Williams syndrome. ATR-X syndrome and Coffin–Lowry syndrome are sometimes difficult to distinguish: pictures of two children with proven ATR-X have for years served as examples of Coffin–Lowry syndrome in a famous textbook on malformation syndromes. DNA tests can confirm a clinical diagnosis for either syndrome.

2.4. Rett Syndrome

Andreas Rett, a pediatrician from Vienna, first described Rett syndrome *(48)*, but the syndrome became well known only after Hagberg et al. *(49)* described a series of 35 Rett syndrome female patients. Rett syndrome is characterized by cessation and regression of development in early childhood, ataxia and other neurological features, and acquired microcephaly in females. Essential for the diagnosis of classical Rett syndrome is a normal prenatal and perinatal period with normal development during the first 6–12 (or sometimes 18) mo and normal head circumference at birth. This initial normal period is followed by a gradual regression and loss of acquired motor and cognitive skills, speech, and language. Loss of purposeful hand movements is followed by the development of stereotypic hand movements such as wringing, washing, flapping, patting, pill rolling, and other bizarre movements during waking hours. Other neurological features that evolve over time are hypotonia, jerky truncal and gait ataxia, breathing dysfunction such as hyperventilation, apnea, breath holding, autistic features, seizures and EEG abnormalities, spasticity later with muscle wasting and dystonia, peripheral vasomotor disturbances, and hypotrophic, small and cold feet *(10)*. Cognitive and motor function deterioration continues, until severe mental retardation is evident. Frequently, patients are wheelchair bound. Growth retardation, cachexia, scoliosis, and constipation are frequently seen. Commonly, the clinical course is divided into four stages: stage I is the stagnation in development, stage II devastating regression, stage III partial and minimal recovery of some social and cognitive skills, while in stage IV the disorder reaches a plateau. Lifespan is reduced (75% survival rate by age 35 years; for controls, the survival rate is 98%). Apart from the classical Rett syndrome, several Rett syndrome variants are known, for example, the congenital form (no apparent normal period), the *forme frust* (much milder and protracted form, occurring in about 10% of Rett syndrome cases), and the preserved speech variant. Owing to its evolving nature, the diagnosis often remains tentative during the early years. In the differential diagnosis of Rett syndrome, a broad range of metabolic disorders must be considered, including mitochondrial disorders, and also encephalitis, Angelman syndrome, and XLMR-epilepsy (also occurring only in females) *(10)*.

Rett syndrome occurs almost exclusively in females and the vast majority of these are sporadic. The prevalence among females is about 1/10,000–15,000. Based on rare familial occurrences of Rett syndrome, it was considered an X-linked dominant disorder with prenatal lethality in males *(49)*. Haplotype analysis in these rare families with Rett syndrome suggested a locus in Xq28. In 1999, mutations in the Rett syndrome causative gene *MECP2* in Xq28 were reported. The MECP2 protein acts as a methyl CpG DNA-binding protein and global repressor of transcription *(50)*.

MECP2 mutations were detected in more than 80% of patients with classical and variant forms of Rett syndrome. Mostly, these mutations have a paternal origin *(51)*, thereby explaining the occurrence in females. Later, *MECP2* mutations were also found in boys. The phenotype in these boys varied from Rett syndrome (somatic mosaicism, XXY), severe and fatal neonatal encephalopathy (in families with Rett syndrome girls, mostly as sister, maternal aunt, or cousin), severe mental retardation with progressive spasticity, to Angelman syndrome such as phenotype and nonsyndromal XLMR *(52)*. The real contribution of *MECP2* mutations in cohorts of female and male patients with an Angelman-like phenotype (tested negative for Angelman syndrome), Prader–Willi-like phenotype (tested negative for Prader–Willi syndrome), autistic features *(53)*, nonsyndromal mental retardation (tested negative for fragile X syndrome and with normal cytogenetic analysis) *(54,55)* is at present under investigation. Although rigorous discrimination between polymorphisms and causative mutations is essential in all these studies *(56)*, recurrent mutations such as A140V *(54,57)* associated with MR and psychotic features and inherited mutations that cosegregate with MR phenotypes suggest that MECP2 mutations probably account for a significant proportion of MR.

3. NONSYNDROMAL FORMS OF XLMR

Approximately 78 genetic intervals for nonsyndromal mental retardation (MRX) (http://www.gene.ucl.ac.uk/nomenclature/) corresponding to individual families have been mapped along the X chromosome and can be grouped in 12–15 nonoverlapping regions, suggesting the involvement of a minimum number of 12–15 X-linked genes *(58–60)*. The candidate region for each family is very large, usually in the 20–30 cM range, and might contain 100–200 genes. Therefore, one cannot pool linkage results, even from families in which MRX genes map to overlapping regions, because these families might carry mutations in different genes. Until a recent date only one gene involved in MRX has been identified: loss of expression of *FMR2*, a gene of unknown function adjacent to the fragile X-E (FRAXE) site on Xq28, is consistently correlated with FRAXE expansion in some mild mentally retarded patients *(61)*. Over the past 3 years positional cloning efforts based either on the investigation of balanced X;autosome translocations, deletion mapping or candidate gene strategy allowed to identify, so far, 10 different genes involved in nonsyndromal mental retardation (Table 4).

3.1. FMR2

Some mentally retarded patients present with a fragile site in Xq28, but not with the CGG expansion in the *FMR1* gene that causes the fragile X syndrome. Patients such as these led to the identification of the *FMR2* gene which is the target of a CCG repeat expansion, and is associated with the FRAXE fragile site. Deletion of the *FMR2* gene was also noted in one patient with developmental and speech delay *(61)*. The expansion mutation in *FMR2*, located 600 kb downstream to the *FMR1* gene, is associated with an extinction of transcription of *FMR2*. Male patients with the methylated expansion usually present with mild/borderline nonspecific MR, although cases have been described who are either more severely affected, or within the normal IQ range. The incidence of FRAXE/*FMR2* expansion is about one tenth that of the classic fragile X/*FMR1* expansion. *FMR2* encodes a nuclear protein of unknown function that belongs to a small group of proteins with DNA binding activity and that might function as transcription factors.

3.2. RabGDI1

The Rab GTPases are a subgroup (comprising at least 40 members) of the small Ras-like GTPase family, and are involved in vesicle recycling and neurotransmission *(62)*. In common with most small GTPases, Rabs cycle between an active GTP-bound and an inactive GDP-bound state through the action of regulatory proteins. GDP dissociation inhibitors (GDIs) are required to retrieve from the membrane the GDP-bound form and to maintain a pool of soluble Rab-GDP. In the mammalian brain, αGDI, encoded by the *GDI1* gene, is the most abundant form, and regulates RAB3A and RAB3C, the Rab proteins that participate in synaptic vesicle fusion *(63)*.

The mapping of *GDI1* to Xq28 made the gene an excellent candidate for MRX families showing linkage to this region, and mutations were found in

Table 4
Genes Involved in Nonsyndromal X-Linked Mental Retardation

Gene/location	Cloning strategy	Identified mutations	Frequency of mutations in MR	Potential function
FMR2 Xq28	Deletions and fragile site studies	CGG expansion deletions	?	Transcription factor,
OPHN-1 Xq12	Breakpoint cloning X;12 translocation	One base deletion (MRX60)	<0.5%	Rho GAP (RhoGTPase activation protein) regulation of actin cytoskeleton dynamics/ neuronal morphogenesis
PAK3 Xq22	Candidate gene	Nonsense (MRX30) Missense (MRX47)	0.5–1%	p21 Activating kinase 3 (Rac/ Cdc42 effector) regulation of actin cytoskeleton dynamics/ neuronal morphogenesis
RabGDI1 Xq28	Candidate gene	Nonsense (MRX48) Missense (MRX41, MRXR)	0.5–1%	RabDDI1 (RabGDP-dissocia- tion inhibitor synapticvesicle and activity, neuronal morphogenesis?

Gene / Location	Method of identification	Mutation	Frequency	Protein function
ILIRAPL Xp21.3–22.1	Deletion studies, *in silico* cloning	Deletions Nonsense (1)	0.5–1%	IL-1 receptor accessory protein like, unknown function, synaptic plasticity (?)
TM4SF2 Xp11.4	Breakpoint cloning X;2 translocation	Nonsense (1) Missense (1)	<0.5%	Member of the tetraspanin family, interacts with integrins, regulation of actin cytoskeleton dynamics (?)
ARHGEF6 Xq26	Breakpoint cloning X;21 translocation	Splice mutation (1)	<0.5%	Homologous to RhoGEF, effector of RhoGTPases, regulation of actin cytoskeleton dynamics/neuronal morphogenesis
MECP2 Xq28	Candidate gene	Missense mutations	<1%	Methyl CpG binding protein-1, regulator of gene expression
FACL4 Xq22.3	Deletion studies	Missense mutations	<0.5%	Fatty acid-CoA ligase 4
ARX Xp22.1	Candidate gene	Missense mutations Poly-alanine expansion	<1–1.5%	Aristaless related homeodomain protein

three of seven such families *(64,65)*. One is a nonsense mutation, while the two others are missense mutations that decrease the affinity between RAB3A and GDI *(64)*.

RabGDI α-deficient mice revealed a role for this protein in neurotransmitter release *(66)*. Furthermore, the phenotype of RabGDI α-deficient mice appears opposite to that of Rab3A-deficient mice: RabGDI α-deficiency leads to a sharp increase in facilitation of excitatory transmission during repetitive stimulation, whereas Rab3A deficiency leads to a decrease under the same conditions *(67)*. Recent data reported by Ishizaki et al. *(66)* suggest that RabGDI α has an important role in vivo to suppress hyperexcitability of the pyramidal neurons.

3.3. OPHN1, PAK3, *and* ARHGEF, *Three Genes in the Rho GTPase Pathway*

Three of the newly identified MRX genes, *OPHN1 (68)*, *PAK3 (69,70)*, and *ARHGEF (71)*, encode proteins that interact with Rho GTPases, a family of small Ras-like GTPases that act in signal transduction pathways from extracellular stimuli to the actin cytoskeleton and the nucleus.

OPHN1 is interrupted in a female patient carrying an X;12 balanced translocation associated with MR. A frameshift mutation causing premature termination was identified in one of five families screened. *OPHN1* encodes a protein (oligophrenin) that is similar to Rho GTPase activating proteins (RhoGAP) and stimulates GTPase activity only for members of the Rho family proteins, such as RhoA, Rac, and Cdc42. These proteins are known to play a role in organization of the cytoskeleton, and particularly in growth cone dynamics *(72)*. The transcript and the protein are expressed mainly in fetal and adult brain, in both neurons and glial cells. RhoGAP proteins increase the rate of GTP hydrolysis bound to Rho GTPases, and so loss of function of *OPHN1* may result in constitutively active Rho proteins and alteration of actin cytoskeleton dynamics.

PAK3 is a member of the large family of p21 activating kinase (PAKs), and is highly expressed in developing brain. It was shown to act as a Rac/Cdc42 downstream effector. Mutation screening of this candidate gene showed the presence of a nonsense mutation in one MRX family *(69)*, and a missense mutation cosegregating with MR in another large family *(70)*. PAK proteins have been ascribed roles both in actin cytoskeleton dynamic regulation and in the Rac/Cdc42-induced activation of the Map kinase cascades.

The *ARHGEF6* gene encodes a protein (also known as αPIX or Cool-2) with homology to guanine nucleotide exchange factors for RhoGTPases (Rho GEFs). Molecular analysis of a reciprocal X;21 translocation in a male with MR showed that this gene was disrupted by the rearrangement *(71)*.

Mutation screening of 119 unrelated patients revealed a single intronic mutation in all the affected males in a large MRX family. The mutation causes preferential exon skipping and deletion of 28 amino acids *(71)*. The role of *ARHGEF6* in brain development and neuronal morphogenesis remains to be addressed, but it is required for PAK recruitment to Cdc42- and Rac1-driven actin cytoskeleton rich structures such as focal complexes and lamellipodia.

3.4. TM4SF2

The *TM4SF2* gene that encodes a tetraspanin (also known as TALLA-1/T cell acute lymphoblastic leukaemia antigen; *73*) is inactivated by the Xp11.4 breakpoint of an X;2 balanced translocation in a female patient with MR, and additional point mutations were detected in 2 of 33 MR families *(74)*. Tetraspanins are cell-surface proteins of 200–300 amino acids, that span the membrane four times, and form two extracellular loops. One of the key features of the tetraspanins is their ability to associate with one another, with α_1-integrins and with class I and II HLA proteins. Their interaction with α_1-integrins was suggested to mediate diverse cellular processes such as regulation of actin cytoskeleton dynamics, activation of signaling pathways, proliferation, adhesion, and migration *(75)*. Very little is known about the role of tetraspanins in the physiology of CNS, where *TM4SF2* appears highly expressed, notably in the cerebral cortex and hippocampus *(74)*.

3.5. IL1RAPL

IL1RAPL (IL-1 receptor accessory protein like) was identified through investigation of a 350-kb deletion at Xp22.1–21.3 in an MRX family. The deletion overlapped with independent deletions in MR patients with contiguous gene syndromes that included glycerol kinase (GK) deficiency and adrenal hypoplasia *(76)*. Nonoverlapping deletions and a nonsense mutations in this large gene were identified in patients with cognitive impairment alone. The homologous mouse gene is expressed in the developing and postnatal structures of the hippocampus, which is implicated in learning and memory *(76)*. Recent data suggest that *IL1RAPL* is not involved in the transduction pathway activated by IL1. Although the potential ligand(s) of *IL1RAPL* and downstream effectors remain to be identified, our preliminary data suggest that *IL1RAPL* might be involved in the regulation of exocytosis (Chelly, *personal data*).

3.6. MECP2

Following the recent discovery that the methyl-CpG binding protein 2 (*MECP2*) gene located on Xq28 is involved in Rett syndrome (RTT) *(50)*, a neurodevelopmental disorder that affects almost exclusively young females, a wide spectrum of phenotypes, including severe encephalopathy in males, has been shown to be associated with mutations in the *MECP2* gene. These findings with the compelling genetic evidence suggesting the presence in Xq28 of additional genes, other than *RabGDI1* and *FMR2*, involved in nonsyndromal X-linked mental retardation (MRX) led to the investigation of the *MECP2* gene in MRX families. Two different mutations, not found in Rett syndrome, were identified in two MRX families linked to Xq28. The first mutation, an E137G, was identified in MRX16 family, and the second one, R167W, was identified in a new MR family shown to be linked to Xq28. In both families, polymerase chain reaction-denaturing gradient gel electrophoresis (PCR-DGGE) and sequence analyses revealed that mutations cosegregate with the mental retardation phenotype *(54)*. More recently, a study reported by Klauck et al. *(57)* suggested that the A140V mutation could represent a mutation hotspot for nonspecific X-linked mental retardation associated with psychotic features. In addition to the results demonstrating the involvement of the *MECP2* gene in MRX, convergent data suggest that the frequency of mutations in the *MECP2* gene in the mentally retarded population could account for a significant proportion of MR.

MECP2, implicated in chromatin remodeling *(77)*, seems to represent a major gene for X-linked mental retardation. The gene is ubiquitously expressed and so the particular sensitivity of neurons to its dysfunction remains a mystery. However, new insights should be provided by thorough investigation of recent mouse knockout models that appear to reproduce the human phenotype *(78,79)*.

3.7. FACL4: *Fatty Acid-CoA Ligase 4*

Contiguous gene deletion syndrome ATS-MR characterized by Alport syndrome (ATS) and MR indicated Xq22.3 as a region containing one mental retardation gene *(80)*. Further investigation of the critical region for MR allowed the identification of two point mutations, one missense and one splice site change in the gene *FACL4* in two families with nonspecific MR *(80)*. All carrier females with either point mutations or genomic deletions in *FACL4* showed a completely skewed X-inactivation, suggesting that the gene influences survival advantage. Acyl-CoA synthetases are a family of enzymes that catalyze the formation of acyl-CoA esters from fatty acids, ATP, and coenzyme A. Five forms of fatty acid-CoA ligase have been identified in humans. *FACL4* encodes a protein of 670 amino acids expressed in several tissues, exept liver, the principal tissue of action of both *FACL1* and *FACL2*. In the brain, *FACL4* encodes a longer transcript, resulting from alternative splicing, that produces a brain specific isoform containing 41 additional N-terminal, hydrophobic amino acids. Data reported by Meloni et al. *(80)* suggest that FACL4 protein is specifically expressed in neurons and not in glial cells. Although it is difficult to speculate how the reduced production of arachidonyl-CoA esters could lead to mental retardation, involvement of these molecules in crucial processes such as regulation of Ca^{2+} ions fluxes could *(81)* provide a basis for further investigation to understand mechanisms underlying MR.

3.8. ARX: *Aristaless Related Homeobox Gene*

Investigation of a critical region for an X-linked mental retardation (XLMR) locus led to the identification of a novel Aristaless related homeobox gene *(ARX)*. Inherited and *de novo* ARX mutations, including missense mutations and in-frame duplications/insertions leading to expansions of polyalanine tracts in *ARX*, were found in nine familial and one sporadic case of MR *(82)*. In total, Bienvenu et al. *(82)* identified mutations in ARX in 10 unrelated MRX families (7 out of the 9 families linked to Xp22.1, 2 out of 148 small families and 1 out of the 40 sporadic cases). Almost all available families with genetic intervals encompassing *ARX* were found to be mutated. These findings are interesting *per se* when compared with the very rare mutations (found in one to three families) that have been reported for most of the other known genes involved in MRX. In addition to the involvement of *ARX* in nonspecific MR, further data were reported by Strømme et al. *(83)*, who have identified mutations in *ARX* in families with syndromic forms of mental retardation. These syndromes include: (1) X-linked West syndrome (WS) characterized by the triad of infantile spasms, chaotic electroencephalogram (EEG) patterns termed hypsarrythmia, and mental retardation (ISSX, MIM 308350); (2) Partington syndrome (PRTS, MIM 309510) characterized by MR and dystonic movements of the hands; (3) MR associated with myoclonic epilepsy and spasticity. Phenotype/genotype data concerning *ARX* are particularly striking and uncommon. The spectrum of phenotypes associated with the identical recurrent duplication of the 24 basepairs of exon 2, predicted to cause an expansion of a polyalanine tract from 12 to 20 alanines, include nonspecific forms of mental retardation, West syndrome, and Partington syndrome. Understanding the mechanisms underlying this clinical heterogeneity resulting from the same mutation is a difficult and challenging issue. One potential hypothesis to explain this phenotypic heterogeneity could be differences in genetic and environmental backgrounds that are obviously specific to each family.

In contrast to other genes involved in XLMR, *ARX* expression is specific to the telencephalon and ventral thalamus. Notably there is an absence of expression in the cerebellum throughout development and also in adults *(82)*.

The absence of detectable brain malformations in patients suggests that *ARX* may have an essential role, in mature neurons, required for the development of cognitive abilities.

4. MOLECULAR AND CELLULAR MECHANISMS UNDERLYING MRX

The genetic complexity underlying cognitive function appears enormous. Recent advances in genetics represent an important beginning in our efforts to understand the pathophysiology of MR. Delineation of the monogenic causes of MR and their molecular and cellular consequences will provide insights into the mechanisms required for normal development of cognitive functions in humans.

It is interesting to point out that a significant number of MRX genes (*RhoGAP*, *PAK3*, *RhoGEF*) are directly involved in signal transduction through Rho proteins. These Rho proteins act as molecular switches that integrate extracellular and intracellular signals to regulate rearrangement of the actin cytoskeleton. Because the actin cytoskeleton mediates neuronal motility and morphogenesis, one can envision how mutations in proteins involved in Rho-dependent signaling result in mental retardation by altering neuronal network formation (*see* review in *84*). However, we anticipate that not all forms of nonsyndromal MR can be explained by a direct involvement of the Rho cascades. It is likely that more insights into the understanding of physiopathological mechanisms underlying MR could be provided by the investigation of MR gene-related processes, such as chromatin remodeling, gene expression, and signal transduction mediated by *IL1RAPL*.

5. DIAGNOSTIC APPLICATIONS AND GENETIC AND CLINICAL HETEROGENEITY OF NONSYNDROMAL FORMS OF MENTAL RETARDATION

The identification of a mutation in an MRX gene is in general necessary for accurate diagnosis and counseling for a genetic form of MR. However, given the very low frequency of mutations (<0.5%) in MR patients for most MRX genes and the present technologies, implementation of systematic diagnosis testing in MR patients is all but useless, except perhaps for the *MECP2* and *ARX* genes *(54,57,82,83)*. For these two genes, further and larger studies are required to assess whether implementation of mutation screening of *MECP2* in MR patients, which represent a reasonable task, will result in a relative progress in the field of molecular diagnosis and genetic counseling of mental deficiency or not.

The issue of diagnostic applications is much more complex to address if one considers the real number of genes involved in XMR. If indeed there are 30–50 nonsyndromal MR genes *(59,60)*, their cumulative incidence might account for 5–10% of MR in males. Detection of the mutations in these genes will be necessary if one wants to provide accurate and reliable genetic counseling to parents of MR children. But, how can this be achieved? One possibility may be through methodological improvements in mutation screening using automation, high-density array strategies and/or protein-based assays. Currently, however, these approaches are either not yet applicable for MR genes or have a prohibitive cost. Meanwhile, one could envision a coordinated international effort to study MRX genes systematically in a large number of families with demonstrated or possible XLMR. It would then be possible to assess the numerical contribution of each gene in XLMR, and perhaps identify mutations or rearrangements hotspots not detectable by PCR and sequencing, which could be screened first in MR patients.

Through the analysis of common genetic disorders, it has been shown that mutations in a single gene can produce a remarkably wide range of associated clinical phenotypes. It is therefore reasonable to expect that a proportion of patients with mild or severe, nonsyndromal mental retardation will have mutations in genes already known to cause syndromal forms of mental retardation. We already know that mutations of the *FMR1* gene, which causes fragile X syndrome, may be associated with a very wide spectrum of clinical disorders ranging from the classical syndrome to mild, nonspecific MR *(85)*. A broad phenotypic spectrum was also observed in *XNP*, *RPS6KA3* (also known as *RSK2*), *MECP2*, and *ARX* gene mutations responsible for ATR-X, Coffin–Lowry, Rett, and West syndromes, respectively *(35,45,54,82,83)*. The recent finding in several families including MRX16 and in sporadic cases diagnosed as nonsyndromal mental retardation, of a missense mutation in the *MECP2* gene is a notable example which confirms the extreme clinical heterogeneity in XLMR phenotypes. Clearly these data raise important issues when counseling families at risk and whether mutations in genes involved in syndromal MR might be commonly found in patients with nonsyndromal forms of X-linked MR.

Finally, it should be stressed that genetic counseling and prenatal diagnosis related to mental deficiency raise sensitive ethical issues, especially for the milder forms. Assessment of cognitive functions is a difficult issue and performance can be subjected to profound social and environmental factors in the family and the school, making therefore prediction of the prognosis almost impossible. Also, one should keep in mind that mental deficiency is not the opposite of "intelligence" and genetic causes involved in mental retardation are not necessarily genes that underlie "intelligence," and great caution is required when discussing the controversies regarding the possible genetic basis for difference in IQ.

ACKNOWLEDGMENTS

The authors are grateful to all members of his laboratory and members of the European XLMR Consortium for their helpful comments and participation in studies summarized in this review. Research studies performed by Chelly's group are supported by INSERM, CNRS, Fondation Bettencourt Schuller, Fondation pour la Recherche Médicale (FRM), Association Française du Syndrome de Rett, AFM, Fondation Jérôme Lejeune and European Community (QLG2-CT-1999-00791) and those by Hamel's group are supported by ZorgOnderzoek Nederland, Ter Meulenfonds and de HersenStichting.

REFERENCES

1. American Psychiatric Association. DSM-IV, Diagnostic and Statistical Manual of Mental Disorders, 4th ed. Washington, DC : The American Psychiatric Association, 1994.
2. Birch HG, Richardson SA, Baird D, Horobin G, Ilsley R. Mental subnormality in the community: a clinical and epidemiological study. Baltimore: Williams Wilkins, 1970.
3. Moser HW, Ramey CT, Leonard CO. In: Emery AEH, Rimoin DL, eds. Principles and practice of medical genetics. Edinburgh: Churchill Livingstone, 1983.
4. Crow YJ, Tolmie JL. Recurrence risks in mental retardation. J Med Genet 1998;35:177–82.
5. Knight SJ, Regan R, Nicod A, et al. Subtle chromosomal rearrangements in children with unexplained mental retardation. Lancet 1999;354:1676–81.
6. Knight SJ, Flint J. Perfect endings: a review of subtelomeric probes and their use in clinical diagnosis. J Med Genet 2000;37:401–9.
7. Hagberg B, Kyllerman M. Epidemiology of mental retardation. A Swedish survey. Brain Dev 1983;5:441–9.
8. Turner G. Invited editorial: finding genes on the X chromosome by which homo may have become sapiens. Am J Hum Genet 1996;58:1109–10.
9. De Vries BB, van den Ouweland AM, Mohkamsing S, et al. Screening and diagnosis for the fragile X syndrome among the mentally retarded: an epidemiological and psychological survey. Collaborative Fragile X Study Group. Am J Hum Genet 1997;61:660–7.
10. Ellaway E, Christodoulou J. Rett syndrome: clinical update and review of recent genetic advances. J Paediatr Child Health 1999;35:419–26.
11. Penrose LS. A clinical and genetic study of 1280 cases of mental defect. London: Medical Research Council. Special report series, no. 229, 1938.

12. Lehrke RG. X-linked mental retardation and verbal disability. BD:OAS 1974;X:1–100.
13. Lubs H, Chiurazzi P, Arena J, Schwartz C, Tranebjaerg L, Neri G. XLMR genes: update 1998. Am J Med Genet 1999;83:237–47.
14. Chiurazzi P, Hamel BCJ, Neri G. XLMR genes: update 2000. Eur J Hum Genet 2001;9:71–81.
15. Lubs HA. A marker chromosome. Am J Hum Genet 1969;21:231–44.
16. Sutherland GR. Fragile sites on human chromosomes: demonstration of their dependence on the type of tissue culture medium. Science 1977;197:265–6.
17. Herbst DS, Miller JR. Non-syndromal X-linked mental retardation. II: The frequency in British Columbia. Am J Med Genet 1980;7:461–9.
18. Martin JP, Bell J. A pedigree of mental defect showing sex-linkage. J Neurol Psychiatry 1943;6:154–7.
19. Hamel BCJ, Chiurazzi P, Lubs H. 2000. Syndromic XLMR genes (MRXS): update 2000. Am J Med Genet 2000;94:361–3.
20. Hagerman RJ. Physical and behavioural phenotype. In: Hagerman RJ, Cronister A, eds. Fragile X syndrome: diagnosis, treatment and research, 2nd ed. Baltimore, MD: Johns Hopkins University Press, 1996;3–87.
21. Fisch GS, Simensen R, Tarleton J, et al. Longitudinal study of cognitive abilities and adaptive behavior levels in fragile X males: a prospective multicenter analysis. Am J Med Genet 1996;64:356–61.
22. Hundscheid RD, Sisitermans EA, Thomas CM, et al. Imprinting effect in premature ovarian failure confined to paternally inherited fragile X premutations. Am J Hum Genet 2000;66:413–8.
23. Verkerk AJMH, Pieretti M, Sutcliffe JS, et al. Identification of a gene (FMR-1) containing a CGG repeat coincident with a breakpoint cluster region exhibiting length variations in fragile X syndrome. Cell 1991;65:905–14.
24. Oostra BA, Chiurazzi P. The fragile X gene and its function. Clin Genet 2001;60:399–408.
25. Smeets HJM, Smits APT, Verheij C, et al. Normal phenotype in two brothers with a full FMR1 mutation. Hum Mol Genet 1995;4:2103–8.
26. Willemsen R, Anar B, de Diego Otero Y, et al. Noninvasive test for fragile X syndrome, using hair root analysis. Am J Hum Genet 1999;65:98–103.
27. American Academy of Pediatrics, Committee on Genetics: Health supervision of children with fragile X syndrome. Pediatrics 1996;98:297–300.
28. Sherman SL, Jacobs PA, Morton NE, et al. Further segregation analysis of the fragile X syndrome with special reference to transmitting males. Hum Genet 1985;69:289–99.
29. Webb TP, Bundey SE, Thake AI, Todd J. Population incidence and segregation ratios in the Martin–Bell syndrome. Am J Med Genet 1986;23:573–80.
30. Tejada MI, Duran M. Screening for female fragile X premutation and full mutation carriers. Community Genet 1999;2:49–50.
31. Pembrey ME, Barnicoat AJ, Carmicheal B, Bobrow M, Turner G. An assessment of screening strategies for fragile X syndrome in the UK. Health Technol Assess (Rockv) 2001;5:1–95.

32. Wilkie AO, Zeitlin HC, Lindenbaum RH, et al. Clinical features and molecular analysis of the α-thalassemia/mental retardation syndromes. II. Cases without detectable abnormality of the α globin complex. Am J Hum Genet 1990; 46:1127–40.

33. Gibbons RJ, Brueton L, Buckle VJ, et al. Clinical and hematological aspects of the X-linked α-thalassemia/mental retardation syndrome (ATR-X). Am J Med Genet 1995;55:288–99.

34. Gibbons RJ, Picketts DJ, Villard L, Higgs DR. Mutations in a putative global transcriptional regulator cause X-linked mental retardation with a-thalassemia (ATR-X syndrome). Cell 1995;80:837–45.

35. Villard L, Gécz J, Mattéi JF, Fontes M, Saugier-Veber P, Munnich A, Lyonnet S. XNP mutation in a large family with Juberg–Marsidi syndrome. Nat Genet 1996;12:359–60.

36. Abidi F, Schwartz CE, Carpenter NJ, Villard L, Fontes M, Curtis M. Carpenter–Waziri syndrome results from a mutation in XNP. Am J Med Genet 1999;85:249–51.

37. Stevenson RE, Abidi F, Schwartz CE, Lubs HA, Holmes LB. Holmes–Gang syndrome is allelic with XLMR-hypotonic face syndrome. Am J Med Genet 2000;94:383–5.

38. Villard L, Fontes M, Ades LC, Gecz J. Identification of a mutation in the XNP/ATR-X gene in a family reported as Smith–Fineman–Myers syndrome. Am J Med Genet 2000;91:83–5.

39. Stevenson RE, Schwartz CE, Schroer RJ. X-linked mental retardation. Oxford University Press, 2000:385–8.

40. Yntema HG, Poppelaars FA, Derksen E, et al. The expanding phenotype of XNP mutations: mild to moderate mental retardation. Am J Med Genet 2002;110:243–7.

41. Temtamy SA, Miller JD, Hussels-Maumenee I. The Coffin–Lowry syndrome: an inherited faciodigital mental retardation syndrome. Pediatrics 1975;86: 724–31.

42. Coffin GS, Siris E, Wegienka LC. Mental retardation with osteocartilaginous anomalies. Am J Dis Child 1966;112:205–13.

43. Lowry RB, Miller JR, Fraser FC. A new dominant gene mental retardation syndrome: associated with small stature, tapering fingers, characteristic facies, and possible hydrocephalus. Am J Dis Child 1971;121:496–500.

44. Jacquot S, Zeniou M, Touraine R, Hanauer A. X-linked Coffin–Lowry syndrome (CLS, MIM 303600, *RPS6KA3* gene, protein product known under various names: pp90^{rsk2}, ISPK, MAPKAP1). Eur J Hum Genet 2002;10:2–5.

45. Trivier E, De Cesare D, Jacquot S, et al. Mutations in the kinase Rsk-2 associated with Coffin–Lowry syndrome. Nature 1996;384:567–70.

46. Merienne K, Jacqout S, Pannetier S, et al. A missense mutation in *RSK2* responsible for non-syndromal mental retardation. Nat Genet 1999;22:13–14.

47. Yntema HG, van den Helm B, Kissing J, van Duijnhoven G, Poppelaars F, Chelly J, et al. A novel ribosomal S6-kinase (RSK4) is commonly deleted in patients with complex X-linked mental retardation. Genomics 1999;62:332–43.

48. Rett A. Über ein Eigenartiges hirnatrophisches Syndrome bei Hyper ammonämie in Kindesalter. Wien Mediz Wochenschr 1966;116:723–38.
49. Hagberg B, Aicardi J, Dias K, Ramos O. A progressive syndrome of autism, dementia, ataxia, and loss of purposeful hand use in girls: Rett's syndrome: report of 35 cases. Ann Neurol 1983;14:471–9.
50. Amir RE, Van den Veyver IB, Wan M, Tran CQ, Francke U, Zoghbi HY. Rett syndrome is caused by mutations in X-linked MECP2, encoding methyl-CpG-binding protein 2. Nat Genet 1999;23:185–8.
51. Girard M, Couvert P, Carrié, et al. Parental origin of de novo MECP2 mutations in Rett syndrome. Eur J Hum Genet 2001;9:231–6.
52. Geerdink N, Rotteveel JJ, Lammens M, et al. *MECP2* mutation in a boy with severe neonatal encephalopathy. Clinical, neuropathological and molecular findings. Neuropediatrics 2002;33:33–60.
53. Vourc'h P, Bienvenue T, Beldjord C, et al. No mutations in the coding region of the Rett syndrome gene MECP2 in 59 autistic patients. Eur J Hum Genet 2001;9:556–8.
54. Couvert P, Bienvenu T, Aquaviva C, et al. MECP2 is highly mutated in X-linked mental retardation. Hum Mol Genet. 2001;10:941–6.
55. Yntema HG, Kleefstra T, Oudakker AR, et al. Low frequency of *MECP2*-mutations in mentally retarded males: implications for DNA-diagnostics. Eur J Hum Genet 2002;10:487–90.
56. Moncla A, Kpebe A, Missirian C, Mancici J, Villard L. Polymorphisms in the C-terminal domain of *MECP2* in mentally handicapped boys: implications for genetic counselling. Eur J Hum Genet 2002;10:86–9.
57. Klauck SM, Lindsay S, Beyer KS, Splitt M, Burn J, Poustka A. A mutation hot spot for nonspecific X-linked mental retardation in the MECP2 gene causes the PPM-X syndrome. Am J Hum Genet 2002;70:1034–7
58. The European XLMR Consortium. X-linked nonspecific mental retardation (MRX) linkage studies in 25 unrelated families: The European XLMR consortium. Am J Med Genet 1999;85:263–65.
59. Chelly J. Breakthroughs in molecular and cellular mechanisms underlying X-linked mental retardation. Hum Mol Genet 1999;8:1833–8.
60. Chelly J, Mandel JL. Monogenic causes of X-linked mental retardation. Nat Rev Genet 2001;2:669–80.
61. Gecz J, Gedeon A, Sutherland G, Mulley J. Identification of the gene FMR2, associated with FRAX-E mental retardation. Nat Genet 1996;13:105–8.
62. Novick P, Zerial M. The diversity of Rab proteins in vesicle transport. Curr Opin Cell Biol 1997;9:496–504.
63. Südhof T. Function of Rab3 GDP-GTP exchange. Minireview. Neuron 1997;18:519–22.
64. D'Adamo P, Menegon A, Lo Nigro C, et al. Mutations in GDI1 are responsible for X-linked mental retardation. Nat Genet 1998;19:134–9.
65. Bienvenu T, des Portes V, de Saint Martin A, et al. Non-syndromal X-linked semidominant mental retardation by mutations in a Rab GDP-dissociation inhibitor. Hum Mol Genet 1998;7:1311–5.

66. Ishizaki H, Miyoshi J, Kamiya H, et al. Role of Rab GDP dissociation inhibitor alpha in regulating plasticity of hippocampal neurotransmission. Proc Natl Acad Sci USA 2000;97:11,587–92.
67. Geppert M, Goda Y, Stevens CF, Sudhof TC. The small GTP-binding protein Rab3A regulates a late step in synaptic vesicle fusion. Nature 1997;387:810–14.
68. Billuart P, Bienvenu T, Ronce N, et al. Oligophrenin 1, a novel gene encoding a rho-GAP protein involved in X-linked non-syndromal mental retardation. Nature 1998;392:923–6.
69. Allen KM, Gleeson JG, Bagrodia S, et al. PAK3 mutation in nonsyndromic X-linked mental retardation. Nat Genet 1998;20:25–30.
70. Bienvenu T, des Portes V, McDonell N, et al. Missense mutation in PAK3, R67C, causes X-linked nonspecific mental retardation. Am J Med Genet 2000;93:294–8.
71. Kutsche K, Yntema H, Brandt A, et al. Mutations in ARHGEF6, encoding a guanine nucleotide exchange factor for Rho GTPases, in patients with X-linked mental retardation. Nat Genet 2000;26:247–50.
72. Hall A. RhoGTPases and the actin cytoskeleton. Science 1998;279:509–14.
73. Takagi S. Identification of a highly specific surface marker of T-cell acute lymphoblastic leukemia and neuroblastoma as a new member of the transmembrane 4 superfmily. Int J Cancer 1995;61:706–15.
74. Zemni R, Bienvenu T, Vinet MC, et al. Identification of a novel gene involved in X-linked mental retardation through investigation of an X;2 balanced translocation. Nat Genet 2000;24:167–70.
75. Maecker HT, Todd SC, Levy S. The tetraspanin superfamily: molecular facilitators. FASEB J 1999;11:428–42.
76. Carrié A, Jun L, Bienvenu T, et al. A novel member of the IL-1 receptor family highly expressed in hippocampus and involved in X-linked mental retardation. Nat Genet 1999;23:25–31.
77. Lewis JD, Meehan RR, Henzel WJ, et al. Purification, sequence and cellular localisation of a novel chromosomal protein that binds to methylated DNA. Cell 1992;69:905–14.
78. Guy J, Hendrich B, Holmes M, Martin JE, Bird A. A mouse Mecp2-null mutation causes neurological symptoms that mimic Rett syndrome. Nat Genet 2001;27:322–6.
79. Chen Richard Z, Akbarian S, Tudor M, Jaenisch R. Deficiency of methyl-CpG binding proteins-2 in CNC neurons results in a Rett-like phenotype in mice. Nat Genet 2001;27:327–31.
80. Meloni I, Muscettola M, Raynaud M, et al. FACL4, encoding fatty acid-CoA ligase 4, is mutated in nonspecific X-linked mental retardation. Nat Genet 2002;30:436–40.
81. Knudsen J, Jensen MV, Hansen JK, Faergeman NJ, Neergaard TB, Gaigg B. Role of acylCoA binding protein in acylCoA transport, metabolism and cell signaling. Mol Cell Biochem 1999;192:95–103.
82. Bienvenu T, Poirier K, Friocourt G, et al. *ARX*, a novel prd-class-homeobox gene highly expressed in the telencephalon, is mutated in X-linked mental retardation. Hum Mol Genet 2002;11:1–11.

83. Stromme P, Mangelsdorf ME, Shaw MA, et al. Mutations in the human ortholog of Aristaless cause X-linked mental retardation and epilepsy. Nat Genet 2002;30:441–5.

84. Luo L. Rho GTPAses in neuronal morphogenesis. Nat Rev Neurosci 2000; 1:173–80.

85. Rousseau F, Heitz D, Tarleton J, et al. A multicenter study on genotype-phenotype correlations in the fragile X syndrome, using direct diagnosis with probe StB12.3: the first 2,253 cases. Am J Hum Genet 1994;55:225–37.

12

Nonsyndromal Mental Retardation Associated with the *FRAXE* Fragile Site and the *FMR2* Gene

Jozef Gécz and Gene S. Fisch

1. THE FRAXE PHENOTYPE, HISTORY, AND DESCRIPTION

FRAXE is a folate-sensitive fragile site in Xq28 *(1)*. It lies approximately 600 kb distal to *FRAXA* and approx 1.5 Mb proximal to *FRAXF* (Fig. 1). These three folate-sensitive fragile sites cannot be differentiated by conventional cytogenetic analysis. At the molecular level *FRAXE* was revealed to be an expansion of an unstable CCG repeat *(2)*, similar to that of *FRAXA (3–5)* and *FRAXF (6,7)*.

The *FRAXE* phenotype resulting from a mutation in the *FMR2* gene was initially regarded as a cognitive–behavioral anomaly produced by the *FRAXA* mutation. Romain and Chapman *(8)* cytogenetically identified a male with a fragile site at Xq27.3, presumably the *FRAXF* site, who did not present with mental retardation (MR) or the classic features of fragile X syndrome. Subsequently, Sutherland and Baker (1) examined blood samples from this family, along with a second pedigree, and found fragile sites distal to the *FRAXA* site in members of both families. That these were two novel fragile sites, *FRAXE* (the family of Sutherland and Baker *[1]*) and *FRAXF* (the family of Romain and Chapman *[8]*) was resolved only later. Sutherland and Baker *(2)* also noted that these fragile sites did not segregate with MR in these families. The importance of making a proper differential diagnosis between *FRAXA* and *FRAXE* was underscored by these investigators.

Later studies identified *FRAXE* fragile sites in probands in whom there was mild MR, but without the clinical features associated with Martin–Bell (fragile X) syndrome. That is, there was no macroorchidism nor were there any unusual craniofacial features. Despite reported phenotypic differences

From: *Contemporary Clinical Neuroscience:*
Genetics and Genomics of Neurobehavioral Disorders
Edited by: G. S. Fisch © Humana Press Inc., Totowa, NJ

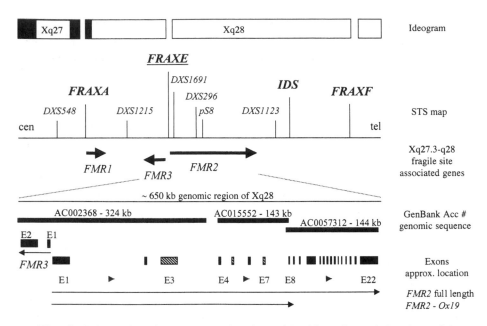

Fig. 1. Schematic of the approx 2-Mb Xq27-q28 region of the three folate sensitive fragile sites *FRAXA*, *FRAXE*, and FRAXF. Position of the fragile site is shown together with framework STS (DXS) markers. Known genes associated with these three fragile sites (*FMR1*, *FMR2*, and *FMR3*) are indicated as *arrows*. **Below**, a more detailed diagram of the approx 650-kb genomic region of the *FRAXE*-associated genes *FMR2* and *FMR3* is shown. Genomic sequences available for this region are shown as *solid bars* with corresponding GenBank accession numbers provided. Exons of the *FMR2* and *FMR3* genes are indicated as *solid rectangles*; alternatively spliced exons of the *FMR2* gene are *hatched*. *Arrows* below the *FMR2* exons represent the two major *FMR2* isoforms, the full length (8.755 kb or 13.7 kb) and the truncated *Ox19* (approx 1.5 kb).

between *FRAXA* and *FRAXE*, genotype–phenotype similarities emerged. In both *FRAXA* and *FRAXE*, the size of the CCG trinucleotide repeat increased in female-to-male transmissions, but decreased in male-to-female transmissions *(2,9)*. Among those individuals with large repeat tracts *(2)* observed that, as with *FRAXA*, hypermethylation at the *FRAXE* site was associated with MR. Curiously, however, they found one male, a methylation mosaic, who exhibited normal intelligence *(2)*.

Of those families examined at the time, description of the clinical features in *FRAXE* was limited. However, 2 years after the discovery of the *FRAXE* site, Hamel and his colleagues *(10)* were able to provide the first comprehensive clinical and psychometric analysis of a large family in which

FRAXE was segregating. Psychometric assessment of four family members revealed IQ scores in the borderline-to-mild MR range. As with *FRAXA*, males with *FRAXE* exhibited lower IQ scores than females. In contrast with *FRAXA*, Hamel et al. *(10)* found that affected males could father affected females.

Later, studies of families, that were cytogenetically positive for a fragile site in distal Xq, but DNA negative for *FRAXA*, brought forth additional similarities with the *FRAXA* mutation. However, inconsistencies with earlier phenotypic results also appeared. As in *FRAXA*, the size of the triplet repeat expansion did not correlate with cognitive impairment *(11,12)*. Unlike previous studies, Knight et al. *(11)* found a decrease in one female-to-male transmission. Moreover, and different from their own earlier findings *(2)* Knight et al. found a carrier male with a hypermethylated repeat expansion associated with a normal phenotype *(11)*. However, no formal psychometric assessments were performed. Mulley et al. *(13)* did employ psychometric procedures to test one of their families, and noted a male with a hypermethylated repeat expansion whose IQ was 104. These researchers also found two normal males in another pedigree in whom hypermethylation was also discovered. Mulley et al. *(13)* concluded that, although this second family did not undergo psychometric evaluation, no obvious correlation between the size of the CCG expansion, methylation status, or degree of cognitive impairment could be established. Using a different probe that could detect both the *FRAXE* site and hypermethylation, Biancalana et al. *(14)* examined four families in which they suspected *FRAXE* was segregating. Once again, although standard psychometric testing was unavailable for all family members, most males whose IQ scores appeared to fall in the borderline-to-mild MR range exhibited fully methylated sites, as did males who were not as affected but displayed language delay only.

Given the relative mild phenotype reported, the prevalence estimate in the population of individuals with mild-to-moderate cognitive impairment and/or developmental delay remained an open question. Allingham-Hawkins and Ray *(15)* examined DNA from 300 males referred but found DNA negative for *FRAXA*. Clinical information was available for only a third of their sample, the majority of whom had been referred on the basis of their developmental delay. None were reportedly severely MR. Allingham-Hawkins and Ray found no males with the *FRAXE* expansion, from which they concluded either the occurrence of the *FRAXE* mutation was rare, or was associated with a phenotype not well represented in the sample tested. Jacobs and her colleagues screened a population of young males 5–18 years of age with a broad range of learning disabilities ("special needs") and were also unable to detect any case of the *FRAXE* full mutation, although they did discover a male with an unstable premutation *(16)*. They, like Allingham-Hawkins and Ray *(15)*, concluded that *FRAXE* full mutations must be uncommon. Knight et al. *(17)* examined 362 males cytogenetically negative for *FRAXA*, found no positive instances of *FRAXE*, and also concluded that the frequency of *FRAXE* was rare, perhaps more than an order of magnitude lower than *FRAXA*. Holden et al. *(18)* examined DNA from 396 males with mild to severe MR who were *FRAXA* negative and also found no instances of the *FRAXE* full mutation. Given the broad range of cognitive abilities observed in *FRAXE*-positive males, individuals who do not present with notable impairment but only language delay may be overlooked. Indeed, as Knight et al. *(17)* note, the target population may be different, that is, language delayed as opposed to MR. Sample sizes used to estimate prevalence might also be an issue. If one assumes the prevalence of the *FRAXE* full mutation is 1/10,000 males and one examines DNA from a sample of 500 normal males, the probability that at least one case of *FRAXE* will be found is about 5%.

2. DISCOVERY OF THE *FMR2* AND *FMR3* GENES ASSOCIATED WITH *FRAXE*

2.1. FMR2

A breakthrough in the pursuit of the *FMR2* gene was made when Gedeon et al. *(19)* identified two patients with MRX and overlapping submicroscopic deletions of Xq28 distal to *FRAXE*. Using the *VK21A (DXS296)* probe (estimated to be about approx 175 kb distal to *FRAXE* fragile site) they detected a large transcript of approx 9.5 kb expressed in placenta and adult brain. Based on these results they hypothesized that this gene might be the *FRAXE* associated *FMR2* gene *(19)*.

Following the work of Gedeon et al. *(19)* the *FMR2* gene was discovered independently by three groups using three different starting points. Gécz et al. *(20)* continued their work using the *VK21A* probe employed by Gedeon et al. *(19)*. Assembled full length cDNA of the *VK21A*-associated gene, and its 5' end in particular, matched the genomic sequence just distal to the *FRAXE* CCG repeat, a fact that clearly suggested that this was indeed the *FRAXE*-associated gene *(20)*. Gu et al. *(21)* took advantage of their genomic sequencing effort in the *FRAXE* region and the fact of the existence of a large gene just distal to *FRAXE* (the *VK21A* gene) to identify the *FRAXE*-associated gene. Both groups *(20,21)* tested fibroblast RNA from *FRAXE* fragile site carrying males. Contemporaneously, they found that when expansion of the CCG repeat at *FRAXE* was present and methylated, it caused transcriptional silencing of the *VK21A*-associated gene. This confirmed the original speculation that the *VK21A*-associated gene was the *FRAXE* associated gene, or *FMR2 (20,21)*. A third group isolated the *FMR2* gene using cross species conservation (ZOO blot) analysis of the region around *FRAXE*. However, they presented only a short, possibly truncated approx 1.5 kb version of the *FMR2* gene (*Ox19*, *see* Subheading 4.) without mRNA expression studies from *FRAXE* individual *(22)*. In summary, these three studies unequivocally demonstrated the existence of the *FMR2* gene, which soon allowed the controversial relationship of the *FRAXE* CCG expansion and mental retardation to be tested.

2.2. FMR3

The search for yet another *FRAXE* fragile site associated gene was prompted by both the existence of a deletion patient *(19)* with apparently normal *FMR2* gene and the identification of deletions of the *FRAXE* CpG island in females with premature ovarian failure (POF) *(23)*. Initially database searches and then reverse transcriptase polymerase chain reaction (RT-PCR) revealed that a transcript of approx 3.8 kb in size is generated from the *FRAXE* CpG island in a direction opposite to that of the *FMR2* gene (Fig. 1) *(24)*. Interestingly, two of the four deletions described so far in POF females would delete part of the exon 1 of the *FMR3* gene. Testing of the RNA from *FRAXE* individuals (with methylated CCG expansions, or full mutations) showed that the *FMR3* gene as well as the *FMR2* gene is transcriptionally silenced by the expansion *(24)*. Apart from this evidence, the *FMR3* gene is a mystery gene in that it does not have any obvious open reading frame (protein coding region). It has unorthodox splice sites and shows no similarity to any previously characterized sequences in public databases. It has been speculated that the *FMR3* gene may represent transcription noise and thus be a nonfunctional gene *(24)*.

Identification of *FMR3* associated with the *FRAXE* fragile site is intriguing, especially to the extent of any contribution this gene might have to *FRAXE* MR. Currently there is only one non-CCG expanded *FMR2* mutation (deletion of exons 2 and 3 *[19]*), which affects only the *FMR2* gene (where a truncated protein of 15 amino acids would be produced) and not the *FMR3*. In all *FRAXE* full mutations so far tested both *FMR2* and *FMR3* transcripts are absent *(24)*. Thus it is currently difficult to estimate the extent of the contribution of *FMR3* to the *FRAXE* MR clinical phenotype and to establish whether the affected phenotype is the outcome of more than one gene.

3. NATURE OF THE *FMR2* MUTATION

Currently there are two different types of *FMR2* mutation described in the literature. The first type is represented by submicroscopic deletions.

Although several deletions (mostly microdeletions) of the *FMR2* gene have been described (for review *see 25*), only one of them (deletion of *FMR2* exons 2 and 3 *[19]*) was demonstrated to cause a mild, developmental delay phenotype *(20)*. The impact of the others *(23,26)* for *FMR2* expression remains to be determined. The second type of *FMR2* gene mutation is represented by *FRAXE* CCG repeat expansions (full mutations). Following the paradigm of the other dynamic mutations of the CCG/GGC type (*FRA11B*, *FRA16A*, *FRAXA*, and *FRAXF*), expansion of the *FRAXE* repeat beyond a threshold (usually >250 repeats) produces hypermethylation which subsequently results in transcription silencing of the *FMR2* gene. To date, no other mutations (point mutations, splice site mutations, etc.) have been reported for the *FMR2* gene. As with the FMR1 gene (point mutations *[27,28]*) mutations other than the *FRAXE* CCG expansion can be expected in the *FMR2* gene. To date, there are no reports of efforts to sequence or otherwise look for point mutations of the *FMR2* gene. Reluctance to do so may have been precipitated by a very low *FRAXE* CCG mutation detection rate among candidate groups of developmentally delayed children (only 7 new *FRAXE* full mutations detected among >13,500 developmentally delayed individuals screened (for review *see 25*); or, by the large size of the gene with 22 exons.

The *FMR2* gene has the unstable *FRAXE* CCG repeat in its 5' end. However, it remains an open question whether the repeat itself is part of the *FMR2* transcript (5' UTR) or not (promoter region). It was originally suggested that it might be transcribed as part of *FMR2*, a speculation based on RT PCR, *FRAXE* CpG island deletion *(26)*, and transcription start site prediction *(29)*. However, irrespective of the position of the *FRAXE* CCG repeat, its effect on *FMR2* (and *FMR3*) transcription has been established. In this regard, recent findings of Tassone et al. *(30)*, showing that more than half of *FRAXA* full mutation males (48 tested) do produce *FMR1* mRNA (at least in the lymphoblastoid cell lines tested), are intriguing. Although the results of Tassone et al. *(30)* need to be confirmed, it is possible to speculate that this phenomenon might be related to the fact that lymphoblastoid cell lines were used. In *FRAXE* the testing is carried out on skin fibroblasts and current experience shows that all *FRAXE* full mutations tested so far do not have detectable levels of *FMR2* mRNA. However, only a few *FRAXE* full mutations (approx 10) have been tested so far.

The *FRAXE* CCG repeat is normally polymorphic with alleles ranging from 3 to 39 CCG repeat units. Copy number and allele frequency are similar for many different populations studied. The major mode is 16–18 CCG repeat units (for review *see 25*). Interestingly, the *FRAXE* CCG repeat when sequenced from different size alleles from individuals of varying ethnic origin did not show the imperfections that are commonly seen in *FRAXA (31)* and some *FRA16A (32)* alleles.

As with *FRAXA*, once the threshold of 200–250 repeats is exceeded (full mutation), the repeat itself together with the surrounding CpG island becomes methylated. However, *FRAXE* premutation alleles appear relatively less frequent in comparison with *FRAXA* premutation alleles *(10)*. Those *FRAXE* premutations found indicate that the critical CCG repeat copy number for the *FRAXE* before the CpG island gets methylated is approx 200 *(33)*. However, the lack of sufficient numbers of *FRAXE* premutations recorded so far preclude definitive conclusions about their size, impact on *FMR2* transcription, translation, and frequency in the population.

The issue of *FRAXE* founder haplotype was addressed by Limprasert et al. *(34)*. They tested 149 unrelated normal X chromosomes with closely linked proximal (<50 kb) and distal (<90 kb) microsatellite markers. *FRAXE* alleles were dissected into three groups (4–15, 16–21, and 22–36) and the hypothesis of allele size vs their stability was formulated (with the largest ones being the most unstable). Surprisingly, while distal microsatellites (*DXS8091* and *DXS1691*) showed significant association with *FRAXE* alleles, the proximal markers (*GT5*, *CA4*, and *CA5*) did not. This was speculated to be a consequence of either higher mutation rate in the proximal microsatellite markers or increased recombination in the region proximal to *FRAXE (34)*. Although no clear founder effects have been formally demonstrated, when CCG alleles were grouped by size, there were significant haplotype associations (haplotype 18–19 and *FRAXE* alleles 23–36). This indicated that there were likely to be founder effects for *FRAXE* alleles *(34)* as there were for *FRAXA* alleles *(35)*.

4. STRUCTURE AND EXPRESSION OF THE *FMR2* GENE

The *FMR2* gene is a large gene spanning more than 600 kb of genomic sequence in Xq28 (Fig. 1) *(20)*. Its size was one of the factors that inhibited *FMR2* gene identification until 1996. Ultimately the combination of (1) description of two patients with genomic deletions distal to *FRAXE* CpG island and mental retardation *(19)* and (2) large-scale genomic sequencing (Baylor College of Medicine) led to the *FMR2* gene discovery *(19,20)*.

The *FMR2* gene is composed of 22 exons (ranging in size from 34 bp for exon 7 to 5.1 kb for exon 22), which are spliced into different size transcripts due to either alternative splicing of internal exons or alternative polyadenylation site usage *(29)*. From among the internal exons, consistent alternative splicing was observed for exon 2 (alternative 5' donor site usage), exon 3 (relatively rarely spliced out), exon 5 (frequently spliced out), exon 7 (alternative 5' donor site usage) and exon 21 (alternative 5' donor site usage). All of these splicing events, except for that of exon 21 (3' UTR region), would result in altered *FMR2* protein. As for the alternative 3' end processing, three major *FMR2* isoforms have been described so far: (1) the 8755-bp isoform *(20)* (GenBank U48436), which is arguably the most abundant one; (2) the 1487-bp *Ox19* isoform *(22)* (GenBank X95463), which is a rare severely truncated isoform; (3) the 13,686-bp isoform *(36)* (GenBank U48436), which is most abundant in fetal brain. Northern blot analysis shows high expression only in adult brain and placenta (only the 8755-bp isoform detected) *(19,20)* and fetal brain (both 8755-bp and 13,868-bp isoforms detected) *(36)*. When various areas of the adult brain were tested, expression was detected in all of them. However, the highest expression levels were in amygdala and hippocampus *(22)*. Evaluation of an additional 50 adult and fetal tissues with both 8755-bp and 13,868-bp isoform specific probes showed significant differences only in fetal brain and adult pituitary gland *(36)*.

Additional information about expression (transcription) of the *FMR2* gene comes from RT PCR studies, express sequence tag (EST) sequencing, and *in situ* hybridization studies in mice. First, for the purpose of testing transcription of the *FMR2* gene various sources of biological material were evaluated including lymphoblasts, fibroblasts, white blood cells, cultured chorionic villi, and amniotic fluid cells, and hair roots *(33)*. Although some expression was detected in white blood cells, the most reliable among these were fibroblasts, cultured chorionic villi, and to a lesser extent hair roots *(33)*. Currently, the material of choice for transcription analysis of *FMR2* is fibroblast RNA. If necessary, however, lymphocytes or white blood cells may be used as an alternative. Second, inspection of the information about *FMR2* transcription as gathered in UNIGENE (EST sequencing and contiging effort; Hs.54472) indicates expression in brain, germ cell, tonsil, whole embryo, colon, head and neck, marrow, placenta, and whole blood. Third, *in situ* hybridization studies of adult mouse brain and early mouse embryos show that the mouse *Fmr2* gene is highly expressed in hippocampus, piriform cortex, Purkinje cells, and the cyngulate gyrus. Expression of the *Fmr2* gene occurs on, or before, d 7 in the embryo and reaches highest levels at 10.5–11.5 d *(37)*. The high expression in the hippocampus in particular is very interesting as this part of the brain plays an important role in processes of learning and memory *(38)*. In concert with these studies on *FMR2/Fmr2* mRNAs, the *FMR2* protein was detected in a subset of neurones in the hippocampus, cerebellum, and neocortex. In particular, the granule cell layer of the dentate gyrus, and the C1, C2, and C3 fields of the hippocampus were stained *(39)*.

5. CHARACTERISTICS OF THE FMR2 PROTEIN

Database searches have shown that the *FMR2* protein is a member of a family of proteins including AF4 *(40)*, LAF4 *(41)*, and AF5q31 *(42)*. Paralogous members of this *AF4/LAF4/*FMR2*/AF5q31* (or ALF) gene family show several similarities: size of transcript(s) at about 1.5 kb, 8.0 kb, and 13 kb; alternative splicing and gene structure conservation *(29,43)*; and protein size of approx 1300 amino acids and nuclear localization of the proteins *(29,41)*.

A limited amount of experimental information is available about the function of the *FMR2* protein. *FMR2* is a large protein of maximum 1231 amino acids, or about 140 kDa (when all alternative splice variants are included; *see* Subheading 4.). It is rich in polar amino acids (30% of the protein), especially serine (11%), threonine (12%), and proline (10%). From previously characterized protein domains there are two bipartite nuclear localization sequences (NLS1 RKEPRPNIPLAPEKKK, and NLS2 KPAPKGKRKHK-PIEVAEKIPEKK) in the *FMR2* protein. That these nuclear localization sequences are functional was demonstrated either by subcellular localization studies using recombinant green fluorescent protein/*FMR2* (GFP-*FMR2*) constructs *(29)*, or more recently using polyclonal antibodies against the *FMR2* protein *(39)*.

Morrissey et al. *(40)* noted (originally for the AF4 protein) many potential phosphorylation sites, some in the vicinity of the NLS1 and 2 sequences. Dephosphorylation of serine may regulate entry of proteins with NLS sequence motifs into the cell nucleus. Moreover, given the large size of the AF4-LAF4-*FMR2*-AF5q31 proteins (approx 130–140 kDa), additional energy might be required for their entry into the nucleus. As a consequence of this Frestedt et al. *(44)* proposed a putative GTP-binding site of the AF4 protein (GNSKPGGKP, position 948–955 of GenBank P51825). However, this sequence is not conserved among the other members of the ALF family.

Nuclear localization of the FMR2 protein is consistent with its speculated *(29)* and experimentally supported role in transcriptional activation *(45)*. The potential of these proteins encoded by the four genes of the ALF gene family to activate transcription was originally shown on AF4 *(46)* and LAF4 *(41)*. To test whether the FMR2 protein is an activator of transcription and to compare its potential to that of the previously tested AF4 and LAF4 proteins Hillman and Gécz *(45)* cloned and tested all three proteins in either yeast and mammalian (HeLa) cells. Their results show that all three proteins tested both activate transcription of the *Gal* reporter gene in yeast and the *CAT* gene in HeLa cells, suggesting an evolutionary conserved function. When comparison of the activation potential was made among the three proteins tested, the *FMR2* activation potential was the highest *(45)*.

For three members of this gene family (*AF4*, *LAF4*, and *FMR2*), similar, severely truncated 1.6–2.8-kb transcripts were reported. These are *FELC* for AF4 *(47)*; *LAF4Δ* for *LAF4 (41)*, and *Ox19* for *FMR2 (22)*. Proteins (if) generated from these short transcripts would retain the activation domain, but not the bipartite NLS1 and 2. Thus it is less likely that these proteins would exert the same function as their full-length counterparts. Nilson et al. *(43)* speculated that these shorter proteins might have different function. However, it is more likely that they might just represent a nonfunctional "noise" of transcription and splicing of large genes (>600 kb) as the members of the ALF gene family are.

In addition to now experimentally tested activation and nuclear localization domains, Nilson et al. *(43)* proposed three new potentially important domains for the members of this family: two terminal, N-terminal and an C-terminal conserved domains (NHD and CHD), and one internal, the most conserved (82%) *(43)* ALF domain (AF4-LAF4-*FMR2* - domain; *see* Fig. 2). The function of these domains remains elusive. Interestingly, recent identification and characterization of the *Drosophila melanogaster* AFL ortholog, *lilli* (*see* Subheading 6.), indicates the highest evolutionary conservation across and thus important role of the CHD domain, respectively. Studies of Ma and Staudt *(41)* show that the CHD domain is not involved in transcription activation and thus must possess another yet to be deciphered, conserved function.

6. RELATED GENES AND PROTEINS

FMR2 belongs to a family of four genes *A̲F4*, *L̲AF4*, *F̲MR2*, and *AF5q31* (or ALF family) *(43)*. The *AF4* gene was originally isolated from t(4;11)(q21;q23) translocation breakpoints in acute lymphoblastic leukemias (ALL) as the trithorax (*MLL*) *(48)* gene translocation partner *(49–52)*. *LAF4* was isolated from a Raji Burkitt's lymphoma cell line cDNA library, which was substracted with K562 erythroleukemia cell line Cdna *(41)*. The human *LAF4* gene maps to chromosome 2q11.2–q12 and its mouse homologue *Laf4* to mouse chromosome 1 *(53)*. The existence of the last member of the family, the *AF5q31* gene, was originally predicted by similarity searches of the dbEST database *(29,44)*. Taki et al. *(42)* ultimately cloned and characterised the *AF5q31* gene. Interestingly, they found the *AF5q31* gene as yet another chromosome rearrangement partner of the trithorax (*MLL*) gene in an infant

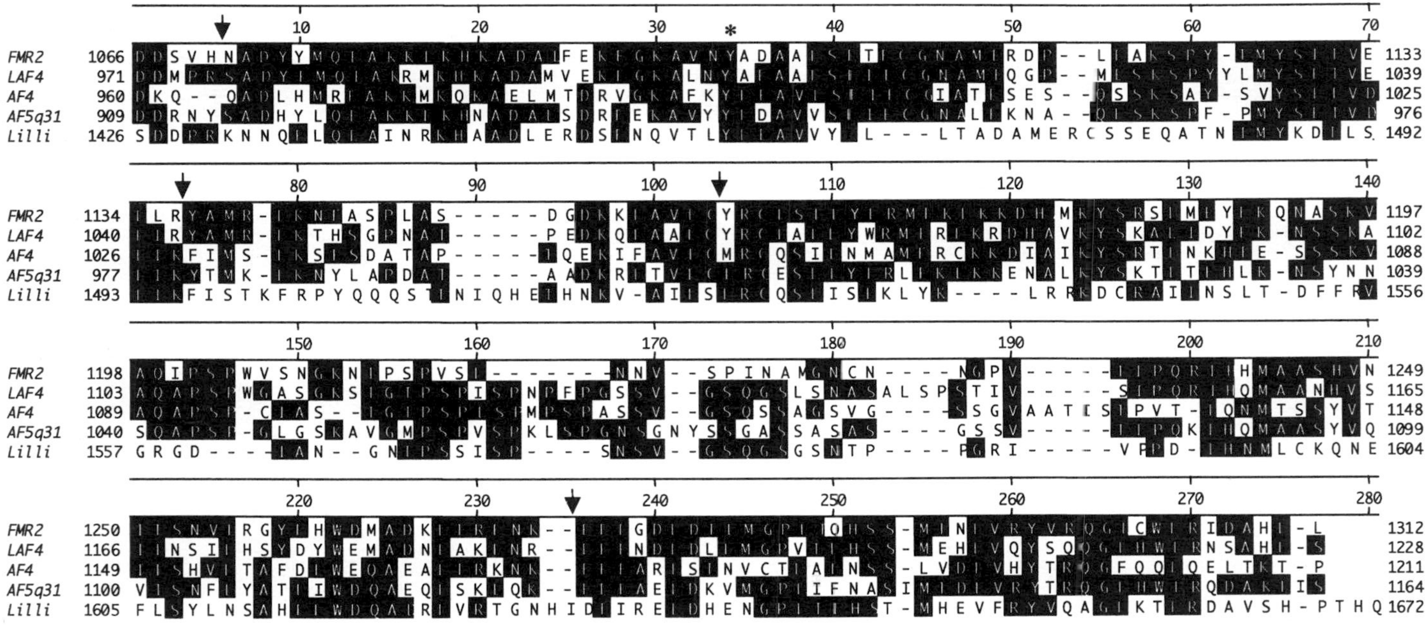

Fig. 2. ClustalW protein alignment of the four members of the human ALF family: *FMR2*, LAF4, AF4, and AF5q31; together with their *Drosophila melanogaster* ortholog Lilli (or Lilliputian). Only the COOH-terminal homologous domain (CHD[43]) is shown. This is also the region of the highest similarity between the ALF proteins and Lilli. Amino acid positions of each protein aligned are shown left and right of the alignment. Conserved exon/exon boundaries are indicated with arrows. The invariable Tyr[1459] (Y), that is mutated in the allele *lilli[16F1]* is marked by an asterisk. (Modified from Wittwer et al., 2001).

299

with acute lymphoblastic leukemia and insertion ins(5;11)(q31;q13q23) *(42)*. It is notable, that two members of the *ALF* gene family have been found involved in either acute myeloid (*AF4*) or lymphoblastoid (*AF5q31*) leukemia. Currently more than 20 partner genes for *MLL* are known *(54)*, which contribute to the "transforming" potential of the MLL fusion product. As far as the AF4 and AF5q31 proteins is concerned, their transcription activation domains fused to the N-end of MLL are speculated to play a role in the initiation of the transformation process due to t(4;11) or ins(5;11) (q31;q13q23) rearrangements *(42,46,55)*.

Recently, three groups independently reported identification of the *Drosophila melanogaster* ortholog of the vertebrate ALF gene family, the *Lilliputian* (or *lilli*) gene *(56–58)*. *Lilli* was originally identified in a screen for dominant suppressors of the rough eye phenotype caused by constitutive activation of Raf during eye development *(59)*. The name *Lilliputian* or *lilli* comes from an observation of a reduced cell size of clones of photoreceptor cells mutant for *lilli* *(60)*. Extensive database searches show that *lilli* is the only *Drosophila melanogaster* ortholog of the ALF gene family. Interestingly, there is no *lilli*/ALF ortholog detected in yet another fully sequenced eukaryotic multicellular genome, that of the roundworm *C. elegans*. Preliminary studies with *lilli* show that it indeed encodes a transcription factor *(56)*.

7. GENOTYPE–PHENOTYPE CORRELATIONS

Isolation and identification of the *FRAXE* gene *FMR2 (19–21)* should permit researchers to more carefully elucidate genotype–phenotype correlations.

To date, several dozen *FRAXE* families have been evaluated, but a neurobehavioral phenotype continues to elude researchers. The *FRAXE* phenotype has often been described in terms of mental retardation *(13,17)*, but it is clear that for many families in which hypermethylated males with the full mutation have been carefully and psychometrically evaluated, there are those whose degree of cognitive impairment is either borderline or absent *(14,61–64)*. This has led Gécz et al. *(33)* to suggest that carriers of the *FRAXE* full mutation may remain undetected in the general population but that extensive psychometric and behavioral evaluations be made to delineate the *FRAXE* phenotype clearly if, in fact, such a phenotype exists.

Two recent studies may prove useful in this regard. Abrams et al. *(65)* examined two unrelated children with the *FRAXE* full mutation. One child was examined at age 1 year, then reassessed 3 years later. The second child was examined initially at the age of 8, then reexamined at ages 10 and 12 years. Although the first child exhibited developmental delays on the Bayley Developmental Scale at age 1, subsequent psychometric testing at age 4 using the Stanford–Binet 4th edition (SBFE) *(66)* yielded a low normal composite IQ score. The second child tested initially in the low-normal range, but later showed a normal full-scale IQ score, that is, 100, on the WISC-R. Using the SBFE, Fisch et al. *(67)* examined three unrelated males ages 4–12 years and found IQ scores in the borderline-to-low normal range. These researchers also noted that the pattern of test–retest IQ scores among these five males differed from that which was observed among young *FRAXA* males of the same age. That is, among *FRAXA* males, IQ scores typically show significant decreases on retesting *(12)*. Among *FRAXE* males, on the other hand, IQ scores remain stable over time, as is the case in children the same age from the general population *(67)*.

Both Abrams et al. *(65)* and Fisch et al. *(67)* observed significantly lower Verbal Reasoning scores in children with *FRAXE*. These results are comparable to the anecdotal reports from Knight et al. *(2,11,17)* and Biancalana et al. *(14)* in which language delay was noted among several young males with the *FRAXE* full mutation. Taken together, these findings suggest that the target population to determine prevalence and identify new cases may not necessarily be those males with MR, but those who present with language delay, as Knight et al. *(17)* proposed earlier. Results from Abrams et al. *(65)* and Fisch et al. *(67)* also support the hypothesis put forth by Lerhke *(68)* in which he argued that verbal deficits were primarily associated with X-linked MR.

REFERENCES

1. Sutherland GR, Baker E. Characterisation of a new rare fragile site easily confused with the fragile X. Hum Mol Genet 1992;1:111–3.
2. Knight SJ, Flannery AV, Hirst MC, et al. Trinucleotide repeat amplification and hypermethylation of a CpG island in *FRAXE* mental retardation. Cell 1993;74:127–34.
3. Kremer EJ, Pritchard M, Lynch M, et al. Mapping of DNA instability at the fragile X to a trinucleotide repeat sequence $p(CCG)_n$. Science 1991;252:1711–4.
4. Oberlé I, Rousseau F, Heitz D, et al. Instability of a 550-base pair DNA segment and abnormal methylation in fragile X syndrome. Science 1991;252:1097–102.
5. Yu S, Pritchard M, Kremer E, et al. Fragile X genotype characterized by an unstable region of DNA. Science 1991;252:1179–81.
6. Parrish JE, Oostra BA, Verkerk AJMH. et al. Isolation of a GCC repeat showing expansion in *FRAXF*, a fragile site distal to *FRAXA* and *FRAXE*. Nat Genet 1994;8:229–35.
7. Ritchie RJ, Knight SJL, Hirst MC, et al. The cloning of *FRAXF*: trinucleotide repeat expansion and methylation at a third fragile site in distal Xqter. Hum Mol Genet 1994;3:2115–21.

8. Romain DR, Chapman CJ. Fragile site Xq27.3 in a family without mental retardation. Clin Genet 1992;41:33–5.

9. Fisch GS, Snow K, Thibodeau SN, et al. The fragile X premutation in carriers and its effect on mutation size inoffspring. Am J Hum Genet 1995;56:1147–55.

10. Hamel BCJ, Smits APT, de Graaff E. et al. Segregation of *FRAXE* in a large family: clinical, psychometric, cytogenetic, and molecular data. Am J Hum Genet 1994;55:923–31.

11. Knight SL, Voelckel MA, Hirst MC, Flannery AV, Moncla A, Davies KE. Triplet repeat expansion at the *FRAXE* locus and X-linked mild mental handicap. Am J Hum Genet 1994;55:81–6.

12. Fisch GS, Carpenter NJ, Simensen R, Smits APT, van Roosmalen T, Hamel BCJ. Longitudinal changes in cognitive–behavioral levels in three children with *FRAXE*. Am J Med Genet 1999;84:291–2.

13. Mulley JC, Yu S, Loesch DZ, et al. *FRAXE* and mental retardation. J Med Genet 1995;32:162–9.

14. Biancalana V, Taine L, Bouix JC, et al. Expansion and methylation status at *FRAXE* can be detected on *Eco*RI blots used for *FRAXA* diagnosis: analysis of four *FRAXE* families with mild mental retardation in males. Am J Hum Genet 1996;59:847–54.

15. Allingham-Hawkins DJ, Ray PN. *FRAXE* expansion is not a common etiological factor among developmentally delayed males. Am J Hum Genet 1995;56:72–6.

16. Murray A, Youings S, Dennis N, et al. Population screening at the *FRAXA* and *FRAXE* loci: molecular analyses of boys with learning difficulties and their mothers. Hum Mol Genet 1996;5:727–35.

17. Knight SJL, Ritchie RJ, Chakrabarti L, et al. A study of *FRAXE* in mentally retarded individuals referred for fragile X syndrome (*FRAXA*) testing in the United Kingdom. Am J Hum Genet 1996;58:906–13.

18. Holden JJA, Julien-Inalsingh C, Chalifoux M, et al. Trinucleotide repeat expansion in the *FRAXE* locus is not common among institutionalized individuals with non-specific developmental disabilities. Am J Med Genet 1996; 64:424–7.

19. Gedeon AK, Keinanen M, Ades LC, et al. Overlapping submicroscopic deletions in Xq28 in two unrelated boys with developmental disorders: identification of a gene near *FRAXE*. Am J Hum Genet 1995;56:907–14.

20. Gécz J, Gedeon AK, Sutherland GR, Mulley JC. Identification of the gene *FMR2*, associated with *FRAXE* mental retardation. Nat Genet 1996;13:105–8.

21. Gu YH, Shen Y, Gibbs RA, Nelson DJ. Identification of *FMR2*, a novel gene associated with the *FRAXE* CCG repeat and CpG island. Nat Genet 1996;13:109–13.

22. Chakrabarti L, Knight SJL, Flannery AV, Davies KE. A Candidate gene for mild mental handicap at the *FRAXE* fragile site. Hum Mol Genet 1996;5: 275–82.

23. Murray A, Webb J, Dennis N, Conway G, Morton N. Microdeletions in *FMR2* may be a significant cause of premature ovarian failure. J Med Genet 1999;36:767–70.

24. Gécz J. *FMR3* is a novel gene associated with *FRAXE* CpG island and transcriptionally silent in *FRAXE* full mutations. J Med Genet 2000a;37:782–4.
25. Gécz J. The *FMR2* gene, *FRAXE* and non-specific X-linked mental retardation: clinical and molecular aspects. Ann Hum Genet 2000b;64:95–106.
26. Brown TC, Tarleton JC, Go RC, Longshore JW, Descartes M. Instability of the *FMR2* trinucleotide repeat region associated with expanded *FMR1* alleles. Am J Med Genet 1997;73: 447–55.
27. De Boulle K, Verkerk AJ, Reyniers E, et al. A point mutation in the *FMR-1* gene associated with fragile X mental retardation. Nat Genet 1993;3:31–5.
28. Lugenbeel KA, Peier AM, Carson NL, Chudley AE, Nelson DL. Intragenic loss of function mutations demonstrate the primary role of *FMR1* in fragile X syndrome. Nat Genet 1995;10:483–5.
29. Gécz J, Bielby S, Sutherland GR, Mulley JC. Gene structure and subcellular localization of *FMR2*, a member of a new family of putative transcription activators. Genomics 1997;44:201–13.
30. Tassone F, Hagerman RJ, Taylor AK, Hagerman PJ. A majority of fragile X males with methylated, full mutation alleles have significant levels of *FMR1* messenger RNA. J Med Genet 2001;38:453–6.
31. Zhong N, Ju W, Curley D, et al. A survey of *FRAXE* allele sizes in three populations. Am J Med Genet 1996;64:415–9.
32. Nancarrow JL, Holman K, Mangelsdorf M, et al. Molecular basis of p(CCG) repeat instability at the *FRA16A* fragile site locus. Hum Mol Genet 1995;4:367–72.
33. Gécz J, Oostra BA, Hockey A, et al. *FMR2* expression in families with *FRAXE* mental retardation. Hum Mol Genet 1997;6:435–41.
34. Limprasert P, Zhong N, Currie JR, Brown WT. Possible founder effects for *FRAXE* alleles. Am J Med Genet 1999;84:286–90.
35. Richards RI, Crawford J, Narahara K, et al. Dynamic mutation loci: allele distributions in different populations. Ann Hum Genet 1996;60:391–400.
36. Gécz J, Mulley JC. Characterisation and expression of a large, 13.7 kb *FMR2* isoform. Eur J Hum Genet 1999;7:157–62.
37. Chakrabarti L, Bristulf J, Foss GS, Davies KE. Expression of the murine homologue of *FMR2* in mouse brain and during development. Hum Mol Genet 1998;7:441–8.
38. Bliss TVP, Collingridge GL. A synaptic model of memory: long-term potentiation in the hippocampus. Nature 1993;361:31–9.
39. Miller WJ, Skinner JA, Foss GS, Davies KE. Localization of the fragile X mental retardation 2 (*FMR2*) protein in mammalian brain. Eur J Neurosci 2000;12:381–4.
40. Morrissey J, Tkachuk DC, Milatovich A, Francke U, Link M, Cleary ML. A serine/proline-rich protein is fused to HRX in t(4;11) acute leukemias. Blood 1993;81:1124–31.
41. Ma C, Staudt LM. LAF-4 encodes a lymphoid nuclear protein with transactivation potential that is homologous to AF-4, the gene fused to MLL in t(4;11) leukemias. Blood 1996;87:734–45.
42. Taki T, Kano H, Taniwaki M, Sako M, Yanagisawa M, Hayashi Y. AF5q31, a newly identified AF4-related gene, is fused to MLL in infant acute lympho-

blastic leukemia with ins(5;11)(q31;q13q23). Proc Natl Acad Sci USA 1999;96:14,535–40.

43. Nilson I, Reichel M, Ennas MG, et al. Exon/intron structure of the human *AF-4* gene, a member of the *AF-4/LAF-4/FMR-2* gene family coding for a nuclear protein with structural alterations in acute leukaemia. Br J Haematol 1997;98:157–69.

44. Frestedt JL, Hilden JM, Kersey JH. *AF4/FEL*, a gene involved in infant leukemia: sequence variations, gene structure, and possible homology with a genomic sequence on 5q31. DNA Cell Biol 1996;15:669–78.

45. Hillman M, Gécz J. Fragile XE associated familial mental retardation protein 2 (FMR2) acts as a potent transcription activator. J Hum Genet 2001;46:251–9.

46. Prasad R, Yano T, Sorio C, et al. Domains with transcriptional regulatory activity within the ALL1 and AF4 proteins involved in acute leukemia. Proc Natl Acad Sci USA 1995;92:12,160–4.

47. Marschalek R, Greil J, Lochner K, et al. Molecular analysis of the chromosomal breakpoints and fusion transcripts in the acute lymphoblastic SEM cell line with chromosomal translocation t(4;11). Br J Haematol 1995;90:308–20.

48. McCabe NR, Burnett RC, Gill HJ, et al. Cloning of cDNAs of the MLL gene that detect DNA rearrangements and altered RNA transcripts in human leukemic cells with 11q23 translocations. Proc Natl Acad Sci USA 1992;89:11794–8.

49. Gu Y, Nakamura T, Alder H, et al. The t(4;11) chromosome translocations of human acute leukemias fuses the *ALL-1* gene, related to *Drosophila* trithorax, to the *AF-4* gene. Cell 1992;71:701–8.

50. Domer PH, Fakharzadeh SS, Chen CH, et al. Acute mixed-lineage leukemia t(4;11)(q21;q23) generates an MLL-AF4 fusion product. Proc Natl Acad Sci USA 1993;90:7884–8.

51. Parry P, Djabali M, Bower M, et al. Structure and expression of the human trithorax-like gene 1 involved in acute leukemias. Proc Natl Acad Sci USA 1993;90:4738–42.

52. Tkachuk DC, Kohler S, and Cleary M. Involvement of a homolog of *Drosophila* Trithorax by 11q23 chromosomal translocations in acute leukemias. Cell 1992;71:691–700.

53. Liao X, Ma C, Trask B, et al. *LAF4* maps to mouse chromosome 1 and human chromosome 2q11.2-q12. Mammal Genome 1996;7:467–8.

54. Rubnitz JE, Behm FG, Downing JR. 11q23 rearrangements in acute leukemia. Leukemia 1996;10:74–82.

55. Morrissey JJ, Raney S, Cleary ML. The FEL (AF-4) protein donates transcriptional activation sequences to Hrx-Fel fusion proteins in leukemias containing t(4;11)(q21;q23) chromosomal translocations. Leuk Res 1997;21:911–7.

56. Su MA, Wisotzkey RG, Newfeld SJ. A screen for modifiers of *decapentaplegic* mutant phenotypes identifies *lilliputioan*, the only member of the fragile-X/ Burkitt's lymphoma family of transcription factors in *Drosophila melanogaster*. Genetics 2001;157:717–25.

57. Tang AH, Neufeld TP, Rubin GM, Muller HAJ. Transcriptional regulation of cytoskeletal functions and segmentation by a novel paired-rule gene, *Lilliputian*. Development 2001;128:801–13.

58. Wittwer F, van der Straten A, Keleman K, Dickson BJ, Hafen E. Lilliputian: an AF4/*FMR2*-related protein that controls cell identity and cell growth. Development 2001;128:791–800.

59. Dickson BJ, van der Straten A, Dominguez M, and Hafen E. Mutations modulating Raf signaling in *Drosophila melanogaster* eye development. Genetics 1996;142:163–71.

60. Neufeld TP, Tang AH, Rubin GM. A genetic screen to identify components of the sina signaling pathway in *Drosophila* eye development. Genetics 1998;148:277–86.

61. Barnicoat AJ, Wang Q, Turk J, et al. Clinical, cytogenetic, and molecular analysis of three families with *FRAXE*. J Med Genet 1997;34:13–7.

62. Murgia A, Polli R, Vinanzi C, et al. Amplification of the Xq28 *FRAXE* repeats: extreme phenotype variability? Am J Med Genet 1996;64:441–5.

63. Carbonell P, Lopez I, Gabarron J, et al. *FRAXE* mutation analysis in three Spanish families. Am J Med Genet 1996;64:434–40.

64. Lo Nigro C, Faravelli F, Cavani S, et al. *FRAXE* mutation in a mentally retarded subject and in his phenotypically normal twin brother. Eur J Hum Genet 2000;8:157–62.

65. Abrams MT, Doheny KF, Mazzocco MMM, et al. Cognitive, behavioral, and neuroanatomical assessment of two unrelated male children expressing *FRAXE*. Am J Med Genet (Neuropsych Genet) 1997;74:73–81.

66. Thorndike RL, Hagen EP, Sattler JM. The Stanford–Binet Intelligence Scale, 4th ed.Chicago: Riverside, 1986.

67. Fisch GS, Carpenter N, Howard-Peebles PN, et al. Lack of association between mutation size cognitive/behavior deficits in fragile X males: a brief report. Am J Med Genet 1996;64:362–4.

68. Lehrke R. A theory of X-linkage of major intellectual traits. Am J Ment Defic 1972;6:611–9.

IV

X-Linked Syndromal Disorders and Neurobehavioral Dysfunction

13

ATR-X Syndrome

Takahito Wada and Richard J. Gibbons

1. BACKGROUND AND HISTORY OF ATR-X

The rare association of α-thalassemia and mental retardation was recognized 20 years ago by Weatherall and colleagues *(1)*. It was known that α-thalassemia arises when there is a defect in the synthesis of the α-globin chains of adult hemoglobin (HbA, $\alpha2\beta2$). When they described three mentally retarded children with α-thalassemia and a variety of developmental abnormalities, their interest was stimulated by the unusual nature of the α-thalassemia. The children were of North European origin, where α-thalassemia is uncommon and although one would have expected to find clear signs of this inherited anemia in their parents, it appeared to have arisen *de novo* in the affected offspring. It was concluded that the combination of α-thalassemia, mental retardation (ATR), and the associated developmental abnormalities represented a new syndrome and that a common genetic defect might be responsible for the diverse clinical manifestations. This conjecture has been confirmed, and what has emerged is the identification of two quite distinct syndromes: ATR-16, a contiguous gene syndrome and ATR-X, which results from mutation of a putative chromatin remodelling factor.

In the first syndrome, ATR-16, there are large (1–2 Mb) chromosomal rearrangements that delete many genes, including the α-globin genes from the tip of the short arm of chromosome 16 *(2)*. The mental retardation is in the mild to moderate range and there is considerable variation in the phenotype which has been ascribed in part to differences in the size of the 16p deletion. In many cases it has been shown that the deletion has resulted from an unbalanced chromosome translocation and hence aneuploidy of a second chromosome is present and probably contributes to the clinical picture.

In the second syndrome, intially called nondeletional α-thalassemia/MR syndrome and subsequently ATR-X, Wilkie et al. demonstrated that there

From: *Contemporary Clinical Neuroscience:*
Genetics and Genomics of Neurobehavioral Disorders
Edited by: G. S. Fisch © Humana Press Inc., Totowa, NJ

were no structural abnormalities in the α-globin cluster *(3)*. This group of patients presented with a much more uniform phenotype and a recognizable facial dysmorphism (*see* Subheading 2.4.). Recognition of characteristic facial features by Wilkie in previously published case reports of X-linked mental retardation indicated that this syndrome results from mutations in an X-encoded factor that is a putative regulator of gene expression.

Since the identification of the *ATRX* gene, numerous other forms of syndromal X-linked mental retardation (often representing single family reports) have been identified as resulting from *ATRX* mutations: Juberg–Marsidi *(4)*, X-linked mental retardation with spastic paraplegia *(5)*, Carpenter *(6)*, Holmes-Gang *(7)*, and Smith–Fineman–Myers *(8)* syndromes. As will be discussed there is little rational for splitting these into distinct conditions and for the purpose of this article, these conditions have been amalgamated under the term ATR-X syndrome.

2. CLINICAL AND HEMATOLOGIC FINDINGS IN ATR-X SYNDROME

A total of 165 cases of the ATR-X syndrome from more than 90 families have now been characterised and a definite phenotype is emerging (Table 1).

2.1. Neonatal Period

Pregnancy is usually uneventful, proceeds to term and in 90% of cases birth weight is normal. Affected neonates usually have marked hypotonia and associated feeding difficulties. Poor temperature control, hypoglycemia, apneic episodes, abnormal movements, and seizures have been also been noted on a number of occasions.

2.2. Psychomotor Retardation and the Central Nervous System

In early childhood, all milestones are delayed. Many patients do not walk until later in childhood and some are never ambulant. Most have no speech with a few limited to a handful of words or signs. They frequently have only situational understanding, and are dependent for almost all activities of daily living. More recent reports, however point to a wider spectrum of intellectual handicap than previously thought. A mutation in the *ATRX* gene has recently been identified in family originally described by Carpenter and colleagues *(9)*. All the affected males have moderate mental retardation and exhibit expressive launguage delay though no psychometric evaluation is available. Guerrini and colleagues have reported a mutation in an Italian family with four affected male cousins, one has profound mental retardation, whereas the others have IQs of 41, 56, and 58 *(10)*. The basis for this

Table 1
Clinical Findings in 165 ATR-X Syndrome Patients

Clinical finding	Total[a]	%
Profound mental retardation	157/164[b]	96
Characteristic face	136/144	94
Skeletal abnormalities	125/139	90
HbH inclusions	120/139	86
Neonatal hypotonia	85/102	83
Genital abnormalities	116/147	80
Microcephaly	100/131	76
Gut dysmotility	87/115	76
Short stature	71/109	65
Seizures	51/151	34
Cardiac defects	31/146	21
Renal/urinary abnormalities	22/148	15

[a]Total represents the number of patients on whom appropriate information is available and includes patients who do not have α-thalassemia but in whom *ATRX* mutations have been identified.
[b]One patient too young (<1 year) to assess degree of mental retardation.

marked variation is unknown. Generally, affected individuals continue to acquire new skills though a brief period of neurological deterioration has been reported in 3 cases, in one of which EEG changes were consistent with encephalitis *(11)*. In the family originally reported by Holmes and Gang *(12)* [subsequently shown to have a *ATRX* mutation *(7)*], all three affected males died in chilhood and the death of one was attributed to encephalitis.

As the affected individuals grow older there is often a tendency toward spasticity. A recent report described a family with an *ATRX* mutation where affected members had spastic paraplegia from birth *(5)*.

Seizures occur in approximately one third of cases and most frequently are clonic/tonic or myoclonic in nature. A number of parents have reported jerking movements that are not associated with epileptiform activity on EEG.

Assessment of vision and hearing is difficult. Vision usually appears normal although 2 cases have been reported as blind. Optic atrophy or pale discs are commonly noted as are refractive errors (especially myopia). Sensorineural deafness has previously been considered a feature that distinguishes ATR-X syndrome from the allelic condition Juberg–Marsidi syndrome *(13)*. However, of the 12 cases with a documented sensorineural hearing deficit 6 have ATR-X syndrome as determined by the presence of α-thalassemia.

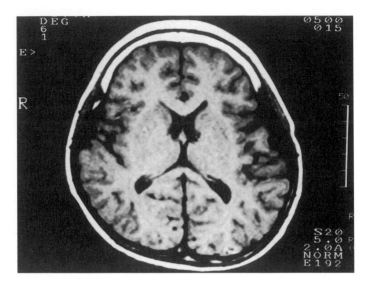

Fig. 1. The brain MRI (axial,T1-weighted) of a Japanese ATR-X patient shows mild brain atrophy but no abnormal myelination or structural abnormalities. (Reproduced from Wada T, Nakamura M, Matsushita Y, et al. Three Japanese children with X-linked alpha-thalassemia/mental retardation syndrome (ATR-X). No To Hattatsu 1998;30:283–9. With permission.)

Although the head circumference is usually normal at birth, postnatal microcephaly usually develops. Macrocephaly has not been reported.

Computed tomography (CT) or magnetic resonance (MR) brain imaging frequently shows no abnormality though mild cerebral atrophy may be seen (Fig. 1) and in two cases partial or complete agenesis of the corpus callosum has been reported. There have been autopsy reports in just 3 cases; the brain was small in each case, in 2 the morphology was normal in 1 the temporal gyri on the right were indistinct and there was hypoplasia of the cerebral white matter.

2.3. Behavioral Phenotype

Curiously, no systematic study of behaviour has been carried out in ATR-X syndrome. Consequently most reports of behavioural characteristics are rather anecdotal and ascertainment is poor. Nevertheless a thumbnail sketch of the mannerisms of this condition is slowly emerging *(14,15)*, and this may be diagnostic (Table 2).

The subjects are usually described by their parents as content and of a happy disposition. They exhibit a wide range of emotions which are usually appropriate to their circumstances. There have been reports, however, of unprovoked emotional outbursts with sustained laughing or crying. There

Table 2
Behavioural Characteristics Reported
in 73 ATR-X Syndrome Patients

Behavioural characteristic	Cases[a]
Putting hand into mouth	26
Happy disposition	22
Autistic-like	20
Self injury	20
Unprovoked laughter/crying	17
Breath holding	17
Emotional fluctuation	16
Hyperkinetic movement	10
Self-induced vomiting	9
Pushing throat with hand	8
Repetitive movement	8
Total[b]	73

[a]Represents the number of patients reported to exhibit this behavior
[b]Represents the total number of patients on whom behavioral information is available

may be emotional fluctuation with sudden switches between almost manic-like excitement or agitation to withdrawal and depression.

Whereas many of the individuals are affectionate to their carers and appreciate physical contact, in some cases there is autistic-like behaviour with the subjects apparently in a world of their own, showing little interest or even recognition of those around them and avoiding eye contact. The latter behaviour may be associated with an unusual and persistent posture such as sitting with the head tilted, gazing upways.

They may be restless, exhibiting choreoathetoic-like movements; continously putting their hands into their mouths by which they may induce vomiting; causing self-injury through biting or hitting themselves; they may hit, push or squeeze their necks with their hands to the point of cyanosis, a state they may also achieve through breath-holding. Repetitive stereotypic movements may be exhibited, these may vary from pill-rolling or hand flapping to spinning around on one spot while gazing into a light. These characteristic behaviours which are reminiscent of Angelman syndrome may lead to diagnostic confusion.

Autism occurs more often in some genetic abnormalities producing MR (e.g., fragile X syndrome, Rett syndrome, or tuberous sclerosis) than in others (e.g., Down syndrome or Prader–Willi syndrome) *(16)*. It is possible that

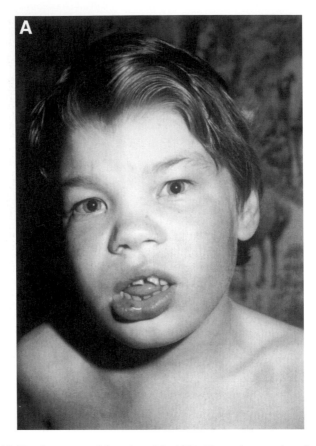

Fig. 2. (A) Twelve-year-old male with ATR-X syndrome showing the typical facial appearance. (Reproduced from Wilkie AOM, Zeitlin HC, Lindenbaum RH, et al. Clinical features and molecular analysis of the α-thalassemia/mental retardation syndromes. II. Cases without detectable abnormality of the α globin complex. Am J Hum Genet 1990;46:1127–40.)

some neurobiological mechanisms that produce MR place the developing organism at greater risk for autism than do others and ATRX may have a role in such a pathway.

A better appreciation of the behavioural phenotype in ATR-X is important to facilitate counselling, to aid diagnosis and inform research.

2.4. Facial Anomalies

Distinctive facial traits are most readily recognised in early childhood and the gestalt is probably secondary to facial hypotonia (Figs. 2a and 2b). The frontal hair is often upswept; there is telecanthus, epicanthic folds, flat

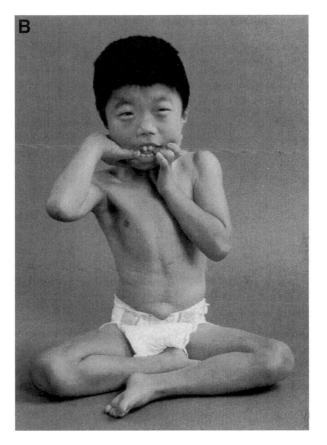

Fig. 2. (B) Nine-year-old Japanese male with ATR-X syndrome and characteristic facial features exhibiting typical behavior: avoidance of eye contact, one hand in his mouth and the other pressed against his neck. (Reproduced from Wada T, Nakamura M, Matsushita Y, et al. Three Japanese children with X-linked alpha-thalassemia/mental retardation syndrome (ATR-X). No To Hattatsu 1998;30:283–9.)

nasal bridge and mid-face hypoplasia, and a small triangular upturned nose with the alae nasi extending below the columella and septum. The upper lip is tented, the lower lip full and everted, giving the mouth a "carp-like" appearance. The frontal incisors are frequently widely spaced, the tongue protrudes, and there is prodigious dribbling. The ears may be simple, slightly low set and posteriorly rotated.

2.5. Genital Abnormalities

Genital abnormalities are seen in 80% children. These may be very mild, for example, undescended testes or deficient prepuce, but the spectrum of abnormality extends through hypospadias, micropenis to external female genitalia with the affected children being defined as male pseudohermaphrodites. In these most extreme cases dysgenetic testes or streak gonads have been found intraabdominally. Of particular interest is the finding that these abnormalities breed true within families *(17)*. Puberty is frequently delayed and in a few cases appears to be arrested. Curiously, premature adrenarche has been noted in two children.

2.6. Skeletal Abnormalities

A wide range of relatively mild skeletal abnormalities have been noted, some of which are probably secondary to hypotonia and immobility *(18)*. Fixed flexion deformities, particularly of the fingers, are common. Other abnormalities of the fingers and toes that have been observed are clinodactyly, brachydactyly, tapering of the fingers, drum stick phalanges, cutaneous syndactyly, overlapping of the digits, and a single case with a bifid thumb. Foot deformities occur in 29% and include pes planus, talipes equinovarus, and talipes calcaneovalgus. Almost a third of the cases have kyphosis and/or scoliosis and chest wall deformity has been seen in 10 cases. Sacral dimples were present in three cases, radiological spina bifida in two and other abnormalities of the vertebrae in five cases. Only a few of the cases have had thorough radiological investigation. In those who have, the most common findings were delayed bone age and coxa valga. Short stature was seen in two thirds of cases. Longitudinal data are available in only a few cases. As has been noted previously, in some patients growth retardation is apparent throughout life whereas in others it has become manifest at a later stage, for example, around the time of the pubertal growth spurt.

2.7. Miscellaneous Abnormalities

Recurrent vomiting or regurgitation, particularly in early childhood, is a common finding and seems likely to be a manifestation of a more generalized dysmotility of the gut. In severe cases surgical treatment by fundoplication has been undertaken as have feeding gastrostomies. An apparent reluctance to swallow reported by a number of parents, probably reflects the dyscoordinated swallowing that has been observed radiologically in one or two well studied cases. The tendency to aspiration is commonly implicated as a cause of death in early childhood. Excessive drooling is very common, as is frequent eructation. Constipation is common and in some individuals is a major management problem. Hospital admissions for recurrent ileus have been reported in two cases and reduced intestinal mobility has been observed radiologically in four cases.

A wide range of cardiac abnormalities have been noted: septal defects (10 cases); patent ductus arteriosus (6); pulmonary stenosis (3); aortic steno-

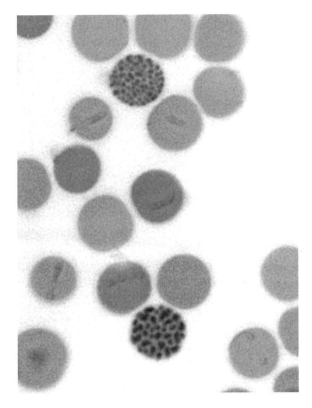

Fig. 3. Photomicrograph of the peripheral blood of a patient with ATR-X syndrome showing two cells containing HbH inclusions.

sis (2); tetralogy of Fallot (2); and single cases of transposition of the great arteries, dextracardia with situs solitus and aortic regurgitation.

Renal abnormalities (hydronephrosis, renal hypoplasia or agenesis, polycystic kidney, vesico–ureteric reflux) may present with recurrent urinary tract infections.

2.8. Hematology

Although initially the presence of α-thalassemia was one of the defining elements of the syndrome, it is clear that there is considerable variation in the hematological manifestations associated with *ATRX* mutations. A number of families have been identified in which some or all of the affected members have no signs of α-thalassemia (*19* and Table 2). Nevertheless, the test for α-thalassemia is a simple investigation and when positive quickly establishes the diagnosis. The most sensitive test is to look by light microscopy for red cells containing HbH inclusions (Fig. 3) after incubation, at room temperature, of venous blood with 1% brilliant cresyl blue for 4–24 h.

HbH is unstable and cells with inclusions may be more difficult to find in older blood samples. Where there is a high index of suspicion from the family history and phenotype, a careful search for inclusions should be made in all the affected individuals and repeated if necessary. The hematology is often surprisingly normal considering the presence of α-thalassemia. Neither the hemoglobin concentration nor mean cell hemoglobin are as severely affected as in the classical forms of α-thalassemia, and this probably reflects the different pathophysiology of the conditions.

2.9. Phenotype of Carriers

Female carriers are intellectually normal and no consistent physical manifestations have been recognised. Rare cells with HbH inclusions may be found in about a quarter of obligate carriers *(18)*. Studies of the pattern of X inactivation in carriers for ATR-X syndrome show that in most of them the abnormal X chromosome is predominantly inactivated in cells from a variety of tissues thus explaining the scarcity of cells with HbH inclusions in these individuals *(20)*. Since the identification of the *ATRX* gene, mutation detection has become the mainstay of carrier identification. Nevertheless it has recently been shown that germline mosaicism can occur and that despite a negative mutation test a mother of an ATR-X case may still be at risk of further affected offspring *(21)*.

2.10. Differential Diagnosis

The diagnosis of ATR-X syndrome presents little difficulty in the patient with typical clinical features and the presence of HbH inclusions. However, where the hematology has not been checked or HbH inclusions are absent, diagnostic difficulty may arise. Coffin–Lowry syndrome may be confused with ATR-X syndrome particularly in early childhood. Distinguishing features are the down-slanting palpebral fissures, broad nose, pudgy tapering digits, absence of genital abnormalities, and the frequent presence of carrier manifestations in Coffin–Lowry syndrome. There is phenotypic overlap with Angelman syndrome (profound MR with absent speech and walking, seizures, happy disposition, emotional lability) and Smith–Lemli–Opitz (facial dysmorphism, skeletal and genital abnormalities); diagnostic testing or mutational analysis should allow these conditions to be excluded in most cases.

3. GENETICS AND GENOMICS OF ATRX

The five original "nondeletion" cases described by Wilkie et al. were sporadic cases and apart from all being male there were no immediate clues to the genetic etiology. Somatic cell hybrids composed of a mouse erythroleukemia cell line containing the chromosome 16 (wherein the α-globin gene lies) derived from an affected boy produced human α-globin in a manner indistinguishable from a similar hybrid containing chromosome 16 from a normal individual *(3)*. It seemed likely that the defect in globin synthesis lay *in trans* to the globin cluster. This was confirmed in a family with four affected sibs in whom the condition segregated independently of the α-globin cluster. In more extended families affected individuals were always related via the female line suggesting an X-linked pattern of inheritance. Consistent with this was the normal phenotype of obligate females associated with a highly skewed pattern of X-inactivation *(20)*.

Linkage analysis in 16 families mapped the disease interval to Xq13.1–q21.1. No cases had visible cytogenetic abnormality and initially no molecular rearrangements were found in a panel of over 20 affected individuals.

A candidate gene approach was taken capitalizing on advances in gene trap techniques. Fontès and colleagues developed a strategy for isolating cDNA fragments by hybridization to cloned DNA from Xq13.3. A number of these cDNA fragments were hybridized to DNA from a panel of affected individuals. An absent hybridization signal was noted in 1 patient when an 84bp cDNA fragment, E4, was used. E4 was shown to be part of a gene known as *XH2/XNP (22)*. Subsequently a 2-kb genomic deletion was demonstrated in this individual..

We now know that the *ATRX* gene spans about 300 kb of genomic DNA and contains 36 exons *(23)*. It encodes at least two alternatively spliced approx 10.5-kb mRNA transcripts that differ at their 5' ends and are predicted to give rise to slightly different proteins of 265 and 280 kDa, respectively.

Within the N-terminal region lies a complex cysteine-rich segment (ADD, Fig. 4), part of which shows striking similarity to a PHD finger domain *(24)*. The PHD finger is a putative zinc-binding domain (Cys_4-His-Cys_3) 50–80 amino acids in length that has been identified in a growing number of proteins, many of which are thought to be involved in chromatin-mediated transcriptional regulation *(25)*. The functional significance of this segment is demonstrated by the high degree of conservation between human and mouse (97 of 98 amino acids) and the fact that it represents a major site of mutations in patients with ATR-X syndrome containing more than 60% of all mutations (Fig. 4 and *see* Subheading 5.2.).

The central and C-terminal regions show the greatest conservation between murine and human sequences (94%) *(26)*. The central portion of the molecule contains motifs that identify ATRX as a novel member of the SNF2

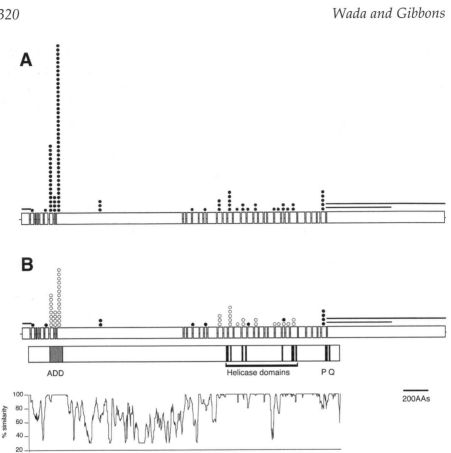

Fig. 4. (A) Distribution of 94 published *ATRX* mutations from Table 3. Schematic diagram of the complete *ATRX* cDNA, the boxes represent the 35 exons (excluding the alternatively spliced exon 7), thin horizontal lines represent the introns (not to scale). The positions of the mutations are shown by *filled circles*; deletions are indicated by *horizontal dashed lines*. **(B)** Characterization of 58 different *ATRX* mutations from Table 3. *Circles* represent mutations; *filled circles* represent mutations (nonsense or leading to a frameshift) that would cause protein truncation. The largest ORF is shown as an *open box*. The principal domains, the zinc finger motif (ADD) and the highly conserved helicase motif are indicated as are the P box (P) and a glutamine-rich region (Q). In the lower part of the figure is a graphical representation of the amino acid similarity between human and mouse ATRX proteins.

subgroup of a superfamily of proteins. This group of proteins are characterised by the presence of seven highly conserved colinear helicase motifs. Other members of this subfamily are involved in a wide variety of cellular functions including the regulation of transcription (SNF2, MOT1, and brahma), control of the cell cycle (NPS1), DNA repair (RAD16, RAD54, and ERCC6) and mitotic chromosome segregation (lodestar). An interaction with chromatin has been shown for SNF2 and brahma and may be a common theme for all this group (reviewed in *27*). The ATRX protein, although showing marginally higher sequence homology to RAD54 than other members of this group, does not obviously fall into a particular functional category by virtue of homology in these flanking segments. There is no clinical evidence for ultraviolet sensitivity or the premature development of malignancy in the ATR-X syndrome that might point to this being a defect in DNA repair. Furthermore, cytogenetic analysis has not demonstrated any evidence of abnormal chromosome breakage or segregation. Rather, the consistent association of ATR-X with α-thalassemia suggests that the protein normally exerts its effect at one or more of the many stages involved in gene expression.

The extreme C-terminus of ATRX encodes two additional domains of potential functional importance which are highly conserved in mouse. The P-box (Fig. 4) is an element conserved among other SNF-2-like family members involved in transcriptional regulation, and a stretch of glutamine residues (Q-box) represents a potential protein interaction domain.

4. STUDIES OF ATRX FUNCTION

4.1. Cellular Localization

A panel of antibodies have now been developed against the ATRX protein and by Western blot analysis in normal individuals these all detect a approx 280-kDa fragment consistent with the predicted size of the ATRX protein *(28)*. Immunocytochemical analysis and indirect immunolocalisation demonstrate that ATRX is a nuclear protein with a punctate staining pattern. In mouse cells at interphase, >90% ATRX protein colocalizes with DAPI bright regions of the nucleus, which are known to represent pericentromeric heterochromatin and this association is maintained in metaphase. In human cells at interphase the pattern of staining is similarly punctate but the relationship to pericentromeric heterochromatin is less clear cut and in unsynchronised HeLa cells there is a considerable variation from cell in the proportion of ATRX colocalizing with centromeric signals. Bérubé et al. used sequential extraction of HeLa and 293 cells to demonstrate that in interphase the majority of ATRX is tightly associated with the nuclear matrix *(29)*. In metaphase, ATRX is associated with the centromeres and this is concomitant with phosphorylation of ATRX and it is possible that the distribution of ATRX during the cell cycle in human cells is phosphorylation dependent. An additional striking finding in human metaphase preparations is that ATRX antibodies consistently localise to the short arms of acrocentric chromosomes and colocalises with a transcription factor, upstream binding factor, which is known to bind the rDNA arrays in nucleolar organiser regions.

4.2. Functional Consequences of Mutations

The effects of ATRX mutations on the chromatin structure of the rDNA arrays located in these regions has been studied. Although no gross changes in DNase1, micrococcal nuclease, or endonuclease accessibility was detected, striking differences were noted in the pattern of rDNA methylation between normal controls and patients with ATR-X syndrome *(30)*. Whereas in normal individuals approx 20% of the transcribed units were methylated, in ATR-X patients rDNA genes were substantially unmethylated. The hypomethylated regions in ATR-X individuals localised within the CpG-rich region of the rDNA repeat which contains the transcribed 28S, 18S, and 5.8S genes and resembles a large CpG island.

Because ATRX is also associated with heterochromatin which contains a substantial proportion of the highly repetitive DNA in mammalian genomes, these methylation studies were extended to other repetitive sequences containing CpG dinucleotides which are known to be epigenetically modified by methylation. In this way, two additional sequences were identified that were abnormally methylated in ATR-X patients. The Y-specific repeats (DYZ2) were almost all methylated in ATR-X patients, whereas approx 6% were unmethylated in peripheral blood of normal individuals. Subtle changes in the pattern of methylation were also observed in the TelBam3.4 family of repeats which are mainly found in the subtelomeric regions. To date, no change in the pattern of methylation has been detected in the α-globin gene cluster that might explain the reduced expression of the α-globin genes. However, the subtle changes in methylation seen in the repetitive sequences of rDNA and DYZ2 are probably below the level of detection at single copy loci.

These findings can be most clearly be related to the effects of mutations of the DDM1 gene of *Arabidopsis thaliana*, which, like *ATRX*, encodes a SWI/SNF protein *(31)*. Mutations of DDM1 display a number of developmental defects and are hypomethylated at a variety of CpG-rich repetitive elements including rDNA, centromeric repeats, and telomere-associated sequences *(32–34)*. These observations raise the possibility that ATRX in mammalian cells and DDM1 in plants provide the ATPase-dependent chromatin remodeling activity to a complex involved in the establishment or maintenance of DNA methylation.

Interestingly, the ADD domain of ATRX, is most closely related to that found in the recently characterised human DNMT3 family of *de novo* methyltransferases, providing one possible link between ATRX and the methylation machinery *(35)*. Of note, putative ATRX orthologues in *C. elegans* and *D. melanogaster*, organisms that do not have DNA methylation, are lacking the ADD motif seen in mammalian ATRX protein and in a putative plant orthologue *(36)*. One possibility is that ATRX protein is involved in facilitating access of the DNA methyltransferases to chromatin.

4.3. Protein Interactions

Like other members of the SNF2 family, ATRX appears to to be part of a multiprotein complex. Preliminary experiments show that ATRX fractionates as a very large complex (>1 Md) by Superose 6 gel filtration. One of the proteins with which ATRX has been shown to interact is the heterochromatin protein HP1. Analysis of ATRX in a yeast two-hybrid screen has shown that it interacts with a murine homologue (mHP1α) of the *Drosophila* heterochromatic protein HP1 via an N-terminal region (326–1196) that lies outside the cysteine rich domain *(37)*. This region is poorly conserved between mouse and man but includes the coiled-coil motif that could mediate the interaction. Further evidence comes from indirect immunoflourescence, where it has been shown in mouse cells that ATRX protein, colocalizes with mHP1α at pericentromeric heterochromatin during interphase and mitosis *(28)*. Finally ATRX and HP1 coimmunoprecipitate using either anti-ATRX or anti-HP1 antibodies *(29)*. Emerging evidence suggests that HP1, a known chromatin-binding protein, is a structural adapter whose role is to assemble macromolecular complexes in chromatin. HP1-like proteins interact with many nuclear proteins, including the lamin B receptor (an integral protein of the nuclear envelope) components of the SWI/SNF complex; the nuclear receptor cofactor TIF1-α; the product of Su(var)3-7, Orc1 and Orc2 (two members of the origin recognition complex); SP100 (a component of PML bodies, nuclear structures that are disrupted in promyelocytic leukemia); and transcriptional regulators such as Ikaros *(38,39)*. Therefore, an interaction between ATRX and HP1 may be sufficient to colocalize ATRX within heterochromatin via a protein–protein interaction.

In a more directed use of the yeast two-hybrid system, Fontès and colleagues investigated the interaction of ATRX with a variety of heterochromatin-associated proteins. An interaction was demonstrated between ATRX (475–734) and the SET domain of polycomb group protein EZH2 *(40)*.

In the future, a considerable amount of work will be necessary to integrate the phenotype of ATR-X syndrome with the molecular mechanisms responsible. Important areas for future work are the identification of "target" genes whose expression is directly influenced by ATRX; determination of how ATRX is directed within the nucleus to its target sites; characterization of the multiprotein complex of which ATRX is a component; analysis of the biochemical properties of ATRX; and resolution of the direct and indirect consequences of ATRX mutations.

5. MUTATIONS OF THE *ATRX* GENE AND THEIR ASSOCIATED PHENOTYPE

5.1. Allelic Conditions

Since the identification of the *ATRX* gene in 1995 it has been shown to be the disease gene for numerous forms of syndromal X-linked mental retardation (X-linked α-thalassemia/mental retardation (ATR-X) *(22)*, Carpenter *(6)*, Holmes–Gang *(7)*, Juberg–Marsidi *(4)* and Smith–Fineman–Myers *(8)* syndromes as well as X-linked mental retardation with spastic paraplegia *(5)*. It has been estimated that approx 10% of named X-linked mental retardation syndromes are candidates for allelism based on phenotypic findings. These include XLMR-arch fingerprints-hypotonia, Brooks, Chudley–Lowry, Miles-Carpenter, Proud, Vasquez, Young–Hughes, and XLMR-psoriasis syndromes *(41)*. It is now important to establish the full range of disease causing mutations to facilitate genetic counselling and to elucidate functionally important aspects of the protein.

5.2. Distribution of Mutations

To date 58 different mutations have been documented in 94 separate families (Table 3 and Fig. 4). The missense mutations, in particular, are clustered in two regions, the ADD domain and the helicase domain. Analysis of the mutations and their resulting phenotypes allow important conclusions to be drawn.

5.3. Mutations of ATRX Probably Cause Reduced Function

A number of mutations predicted to cause protein truncation are scattered throughout the gene (Table 3). Such mutations would be expected to result in loss of function if critical domains are removed. It is clear, however, that these mutations are not lethal. Furthermore the resulting phenotype is similar to that seen for the other mutations. Using the monoclonal antibodies against ATRX and Western blot analysis, it has been possible to look at ATRX protein in patients with mutations predicted to cause protein truncations. A curious observation is that not only is the predicted truncated product observed but a small amount of full-length product is also observed *(28)*. The reason for full-length product is as yet unexplained, although alternate splicing has been excluded. It is possible that complete absence of ATRX, a true null, may be lethal but a comprehensive analysis of ATRX protein in many different patients will be needed to address this. Levels of ATRX protein were found to be substantially reduced in patients with missense mutations involving the ADD domain, possibly because the resulting incorrect folding of the zinc finger motif leads to protein degradation. *(28,42).* A patient with a mutation in the helicase domain, however, was found to have normal levels of the ATRX protein suggesting that such a mutation affects function rather than structure *(unpublished observation).* An intriguing finding is that all the helicase mutations so far described are located adjacent to, rather than within, the seven highly conserved motifs that characterise the SNF2 helicase/ATPase proteins. It is known that in other SNF2 proteins mutations that fall in the motifs completely abolish activity. It is possible that the ATRX mutations alter rather than abolish the protein's activity. These findings are consistent with the view that the common final pathway of ATRX mutations is a decrease in ATRX activity.

5.4. Genotype–Phenotype Correlations

Since the discovery of the *ATRX* gene, most new cases have been defined on the basis of severe MR with the typical facial appearance associated with a mutation in the *ATRX* gene. This allows a less biased evaluation of the effect of ATRX mutations on the commonly associated clinical manifestations. The severity of three aspects of the phenotype, mental retardation, genital abnormality and α-thalassemia, are quantifiable to some degree.

The greatest variation in intellectual handicap is associated with a truncating mutation at the N-terminal of the protein *(10).* Analysis of the RNA derived from patient cell lines showed no alternate splicing that might be associated with skipping of the mutation and degrees of phenotypic rescue. As discussed above, protein analysis by Western blotting has shown small amounts of full-length protein for each patient. This may be associated with inefficient recognition of the premature stop codon. Nevertheless there is no obvious correlation between the degree of retardation and the amount of full-length protein.

There are now 8 different mutations associated with the most severe urogenital abnormalities (Table 3). In five, the protein is truncated resulting in the loss of the C-terminal domain including a conserved element (P in Fig. 4) and polyglutamine tract (Q in Fig. 4). From the available data it appears that in the absence of the C-terminal domain, severe urogenital abnormalities are likely (although not inevitable as one mutation in this region was associated with cryptorchidism), suggesting that this region may play a specific role in urogenital development. Consistent with this, in families with such muta-

Table 3
Summary of ATRX Mutations[a]

No.	Exon /intron[b]	Mutation[c]	De novo mutation[d]	No. of peds	No of cases	Genital abnormality[e]	HbH inc cells %[f]	Reference
1[a]	1	EX1_2del		1	2	+ to ++	0	46
2	2	324C>T; R37X		1	4	n to ++	0 to 0.006	10
3	6	628_629delAA; K138fs		1	1	+	0	46
4	8	739G>A; G175E		1	1	+	+	47
5	8	743_744insCAA; 176_177insQ		1	3	+	0.003 to 0.12	24
6	8	751A>G; S c747-809del; V178_K198del	+	8	9	n to ++	0 to 1.5	23
								24
								47
								48
								46
7	8	783C>G; P190A		1	1	++	4.8	24
8	8	783C>T; P190S		2	2	n	+ to 5	46
								47
9	8	784C>T; P190L	+	1	1	+	+	48
10	8	791G>C; L192F		1	1	n	<0.01	24
11	8	795G>A; V194I	+	1	1	+	11.6	48
12	9	814G>C; C200S	+	1	1	++	31.5	24
13	9	871A>C; Q219P		1	1	n	+	47
14	9	873T>C; C220R		1	1	++	0.01	24
15	9	874G>A; C220Y		1	3	n	nd	7
16	10	880G>C; W222S		1	1	++	0.003	24
17	10	881G>T; W222C		1	1	++	4	unpublished

No.	Exon	Mutation		n	n	Activity	Value	Ref.
18	10	932C>A; F239L		1	1	U	2	46
19	10	934G>T; C240F	+	1	1	++	6	24
20	10	946T>A; I244N	+	1	1	+	16	46
21	10	951C>T; R246C	+	26	32	n to ++++	0 to 14	24, 46, 48
22	10	952G>T; R246L		2	2	n to +	+ to 1.0	unpublished, 49
23	10	954A>G; N247D		1	1	++	+	47
24	10	960G>T; G249C	+	1	1	+	+	46
25	10	961G>A; G249D	+	1	2	++	2.5 to 3.9	47
26	10	1002T>C; W263R		1	1	n	0.4	24
27	10	1012A>G; Y266C		1	1	++	10	46
28	10	1942C>A; S576X		2	6	n to +++	1.4 to 10	46
29	10	1963delC; T583fs		1	1	n	0	46
30	int12	4159-2A>G; 4532G>A;		1	1	++	3.7	46
31	15	S insertion 86bp (fs)		1	2	++ to +++	0.9 to 3.6	49
32	17	S insertion 53bp (fs)		1	1	+++	11	23
33	17	4828T>G; V1538G; 4832_4837del; 1540_1541delIDE		1	2	n to +++	0.9 to 1.0	23
34	17	4869G>T; V1552F		1	2	+ to +++	41 to 56	46
35	19	5041A>G; H1609R		1	1	+++	1.6	48
36	19	5055T>C; C1614R		1	1	+++++	>5	22
37	19	5079G>A; A1622T	+	1	1	++	18.2	22, 46

(continued)

Table 3 (*continued*)
Summary of ATRX Mutations

No.	Exon /intron[b]	Mutation[c]	De novo mutation[d]	No. of peds	No. of cases	Genital abnormality[e]	HbH inc cells %[f]	Reference
38	19	5149T>C; K1645S		1	1	n	0.2	48
39	19	5165G>T; K1650N		1	2	n	0.4 to 0.6	22
40	20	5254T>C; I1680T		1	1	+++++	+	4
41	21	5352C>T; P1713S		1	1	n	0	43
42[a]	21	5440G>A; R1742K	+	1	3	++	3	5
43	int 21	5488-10T>A;S c5488-5663del; Y1758X		1	3	n to +++	>0.001 to 30	19
44	23	5713A>G; Y1833C		1	1	++	0.2	46
45	23	5755A>G; Y1847C		1	1	+	+	48
46	int 26	6172-2A>G; S c6172_6237del; p1986_2007del	+	1	1	+	+	46
47	27	6319A>T; D2035V		1	2	+++	7 to 27	22
48	28	6364T>C; I2050T		1	4	n	U	6
49	int 28	6433-12574G>A; S insertion 124bp (fs)	+	1	1	++	1.4	23
50	29	6465T>C; Y2084H		1	1	++	>5	22
51	30	6607G>A; R2131Q		1	3	+++	U	4
52	30	6703A>G; Y2163C	+	1	1	+	12	22
53	35	7371C>T; R2386X	+	2	3	++++ to +++++	v.rare to 0.02	22
54	35	7377G>T; E2388X		1	2	+++++	0.03	22

55	int 35	7416-2A>G; S c7416_7423del; L2401fs	1		++	0		8
56	int 35	7416-2delCTAA; S c7416_7423del; L2401fs	2		+++++			50
57	36	IVS35_9004del	5	1	+++++	0§	0.03 to 1.1	22
58	36	EX36del	3	2	+++++	6.5		46

[a] Mental retardation was profound (severity as defined in ICD-10 classification [52]), except for No. 2, where retardation was mild to profound, and No. 42, where retardation was moderate.

[b] Exon or intron in which mutation lies; numbering based on a total of 36 exons with exon 7 spliced out (accession no. U72937).

[c] Nomenclature of mutations as recommended (51). For base substitutions the DNA mutation is followed by the amino acid change; for splicing abnormalities (S) the resulting principal cDNA is given (preceded by c); mutations leading to frameshift are indicate by fs and where appropriate the first affected amino acid is given; where the precise extent of a deletion is not determined the deleted exons are indicated. All amino acid substitutions occur at residues conserved in the predicted human and mouse protein sequences.

[d] + indicates that this mutation arises de novo in a member of the family.

[e] For a given mutation the range of genital abnormality present is shown: n, normal; +, very mild, e.g. high lying testes; ++, cryptorchidism; +++, hypospadias; ++++, micropenis; +++++, ambiguous genitalia or male pseudohermaphrodite.

[f] For a given mutation the proportion of cells with HbH inclusions is shown. Where values from more than one individual are available, a range is shown. + indicates when inclusions were observed but not quantified. §, 0/5000 red cells had HbH inclusions but α/β globin chain ratio = 0.85, 15% below control samples.

U, not determined.

tions severe urogenital abnormalities breed true *(17)* and an identical, independently arising nonsense mutation (no. 53, Table 3) gives rise to a similar phenotype. At other sites however there is no obvious link between phenotype and genotype and there is considerable variation in the degree of abnormality seen in individuals with identical mutations.

The relationship between *ATRX* mutations and α-thalassemia is unclear. Since the presence of excess β chains (HbH inclusions) was originally used to define the ATR-X syndrome, current observations are inevitably biased. Nevertheless, there is considerable variability in the degree to which α-globin synthesis is affected by these mutations as judged by the frequency of cells with HbH inclusions. Some patients do not have HbH inclusions *(4,19,43)*, although this does not rule out down-regulation of α-globin expression, as inclusions may not appear until there is 30–40% reduction in α chain synthesis *(44)*. It is interesting that patients with identical mutations may have very different, albeit stable, degrees of α-thalassemia suggesting that the effect of ATRX protein on α-globin expression may be modified by other genetic factors. This is most clearly illustrated by comparing the hematology of cases with identical mutations (Table 3). In the 5' splicing mutation (mutation no. 6, Table 3) there are nine affected individuals from eight different families and frequency of cells with HbH inclusions varies from 0 to 1.5%. Furthermore, comparison of the 32 cases from 26 pedigrees with the common 951C>T mutation (no. 21, Table 3) shows an even greater variation in the frequency of HbH inclusions (0–14%). This may be analogous to mutations of other members of the SNF2 family, whose effects are known to be modified by a variation in many genes encoding proteins that interact with SNF2-like proteins *(27,45)*.

In conclusion, it is clear that there is a broad phenotypic spectrum associated not only with different *ATRX* mutations, but also identical mutations. In different reports the presence or absence of certain findings has been emphasized but the case for phenotype splitting is not persuasive. Systematic mutation analysis of a broad population of patients with learning difficulties should help determine the extent of the phenotypic spectrum associated with *ATRX* mutations and their prevalence.

ACKNOWLEDGMENTS

We thank the families and their clinicians for their invaluable information; Liz Rose for typing of the manuscript; Vina Bachoo and Jennifer Shanahan for technical assistance; and Professor D. R. Higgs for his continued support and encouragement. Work on ATR-X syndrome is supported by the MRC and by grants (053014—RG; 061984—TW) from the Wellcome Trust.

REFERENCES

1. Weatherall DJ, Higgs DR, Bunch C, et al. Hemoglobin H disease and mental retardation. A new syndrome or a remarkable coincidence? N Engl J Med 1981;305:607–12.
2. Wilkie AOM, Buckle VJ, Harris PC, et al. (1990) Clinical features and molecular analysis of the α-thalassaemia/mental retardation syndromes. I. Cases due to deletions involving chromosome band 16p13.3. Am J Hum Genet 1990;46:1112–26.
3. Wilkie AOM, Zeitlin HC, Lindenbaum RH, et al. Clinical features and molecular analysis of the α-thalassemia/mental retardation syndromes. II. Cases without detectable abnormality of the α globin complex. Am J Hum Genet 1990;46:1127–40.
4. Villard L, Gecz J, Mattéi JF, et al. XNP mutation in a large family with Juberg–Marsidi syndrome. Nat Genet 1996;12:359–60.
5. Lossi AM, Millan JM, Villard L, et al. Mutation of the XNP/ATR-X gene in a family with severe mental retardation, spastic paraplegia and skewed pattern of X inactivation: demonstration that the mutation is involved in the inactivation bias. Am J Hum Genet 1999;65:558–62.
6. Abidi F, Schwartz CE, Carpenter NJ, Villard L, Fontes M, Curtis M. Carpenter-Waziri syndrome results from a mutation in XNP. Am J Med Genet 1999;85:249–51.
7. Stevenson RE, Abidi F, Schwartz CE, Lubs HA, Holmes LB. Holmes-Gang syndrome is allelic with XLMR-hypotonic face syndrome. Am J Med Genet 2000;94:383–5.
8. Villard L, Fontes M, Ades LC, Gecz J. Identification of a mutation in the XNP/ATR-X gene in a family reported as Smith–Fineman–Myers syndrome. Am J Med Genet 2000;91:83–5.
9. Carpenter NJ, Qu Y, Curtis M, Patil SR. X-linked mental retardation syndrome with characteristic "coarse" facial appearance, brachydactyly, and short stature maps to proximal Xq. Am J Med Genet 1999;85:230–5.
10. Guerrini R, Shanahan JL, Carrozzo R, Bonanni P, Higgs DR, Gibbons RJ. A nonsense mutation of the ATRX gene causing mild mental retardation and epilepsy. Ann Neurol 2000;47:117–21.
11. Donnai D, Clayton-Smith J, Gibbons RJ, Higgs DR. The non-deletion α-thalassaemia/mental retardation syndrome. Further support for X linkage. J Med Genet 1991;28:742–5.
12. Holmes LB, Gang DL. Brief clinical report: an X-linked mental retardation syndrome with craniofacial abnormalities, microcephaly and club foot. Am J Med Genet 1984;17:375–82.
13. Saugier-Veber P, Munnich A, Lyonnet S, et al. Letter to the Editor: Lumping Juberg-Marsidi syndrome and X-linked α-thalassemia/mental retardation syndrome? Am J Med Genet 1995;55:300–1.
14. Kurosawa K, Akatsuka A, Ochiai Y, Ikeda J, Maekawa K. Self-induced vomiting in X-linked α-thalassemia/mental retardation syndrome. Am J Med Genet 1996;63:505–6.

15. Wada T, Nakamura M, Matsushita Y, et al. Three Japanese children with X-linked alpha-thalassemia/mental retardation syndrome (ATR-X). No To Hattatsu 1998;30:283–9.
16. Dykens EM, Volkmar FR. Medical conditions associated with autism. In: Cohen DJ, Volkmar FR, eds. Handbook of autism and pervasive developmental disorders, 2nd ed. New York: Wiley, 1997;388–410.
17. McPherson E, Clemens M, Gibbons RJ, Higgs DR. X-linked alpha-thalassemia/mental retardation (ATR-X) syndrome. A new kindred with severe genital anomalies and mild hematologic expression. Am J Med Genet 1995; 55:302–6.
18. Gibbons RJ, Brueton L, Buckle VJ, et al. The clinical and hematological features of the X-linked α-thalassemia/mental retardation syndrome (ATR-X). Am J Med Genet 1995;55:288–99.
19. Villard L, Toutain A, Lossi A-M, et al. Splicing mutation in the ATR-X gene can lead to a dysmorphic mental retardation phenotype without α-thalassemia. Am J Hum Genet 1996;58:499–505.
20. Gibbons RJ, Suthers GK, Wilkie AOM, Buckle VJ, Higgs DR. X-linked α-thalassemia/mental retardation (ATR-X) syndrome: localisation to Xq12-21.31 by X-inactivation and linkage analysis. Am J Hum Genet 1992;51:1136–49.
21. Bachoo S, Gibbons RJ. Germline and gonosomal mosaicism in the ATR-X syndrome. Eur J Hum Genet 1999;7:933–6.
22. Gibbons RJ, Picketts DJ, Villard L, Higgs DR. Mutations in a putative global transcriptional regulator cause X-linked mental retardation with α-thalassemia (ATR-X syndrome). Cell 1995;80:837–45.
23. Picketts DJ, Higgs DR, Bachoo S, Blake DJ, Quarrell OWJ, Gibbons RJ. *ATRX* encodes a novel member of the SNF2 family of proteins: mutations point to a common mechanism underlying the ATR-X syndrome. Hum Mol Genet 1996;5:1899–1907.
24. Gibbons RJ, Bachoo S, Picketts DJ, et al. (1997) Mutations in a transcriptional regulator (hATRX) establish the functional significance of a PHD-like domain. Nat Genet 1997;17:146–8.
25. Aasland R, Gibson TJ, Stewart AF. The PHD finger: implications for chromatin-mediated transcriptional regulation. TIBS 1995;20:56–9.
26. Picketts DJ, Tastan AO, Higgs DR, Gibbons RJ. Comparison of the human and murine ATRX gene identifies highly conserved, functionally important domains. Mammal Genome 1998;9:400–3.
27. Carlson M, Laurent BC. The SNF/SWI family of global transcriptional activators. Curr Opin Cell Biol 1994;6:396–402.
28. McDowell TL, Gibbons RJ, Sutherland H, et al. Localization of a putative transcriptional regulator (ATRX) at pericentromeric heterochromatin and the short arms of acrocentric chromosomes. Proc Natl Acad Sci USA 1999;96:13,983–8.
29. Berube NG, Smeenk CA, Picketts DJ. Cell cycle-dependent phosphorylation of the ATRX protein correlates with changes in nuclear matrix and chromatin association. Hum Mol Genet 2000;9:539–47.
30. Gibbons RJ, McDowell TL, Raman S, et al. Mutations in ATRX, encoding a SWI/SNF-like protein, cause diverse changes in the pattern of DNA methylation. Nat Genet 2000;24:368–71.

31. Jeddeloh JA, Stokes TL, Richards EJ. Maintenance of genomic methylation requires a SWI2/SNF2-like protein [see comments]. Nat Genet 1999;22:94–7.
32. Vongs A, Kakutani T, Martienssen RA, Richards EJ. Arabidopsis thaliana DNA methylation mutants. Science 1993;260:1926–8.
33. Kakutani T, Jeddeloh JA, Richards EJ. Characterization of an *Arabidopsis thaliana* DNA hypomethylation mutant. Nucleic Acids Res 1995;23:130–7.
34. Jacobsen SE. Gene silencing: maintaining methylation patterns. Curr Biol 1999;9:R617–9.
35. Xie S, Wang Z, Okano M, et al. Cloning, expression and chromosome locations of the human DNMT3 gene family. Gene 1999;236:87–95
36. Villard L, Fontes M, Ewbank JJ. Characterization of xnp-1, a *Caenorhabditis elegans* gene similar to the human XNP/ATR-X gene. Gene 1999;236:13–9.
37. Le Douarin B, Nielsen AL, Garnier J-M, et al. A possible involvement of TIF1α and TIF1β in the epigenetic control of transcription by nuclear receptors. EMBO J 1996;15:6701–15.
38. Brown KE, Guest SS, Smale ST, Hahm K, Merkenschlager M, Fisher AG. Association of transcriptionally silent genes with Ikaros complexes at centromeric heterochromatin. Cell 1997;91:845–54.
39. Lamond AI, Earnshaw WC. Structure and function in the nucleus. Science 1998;280:547–53.
40. Cardoso C, Timsit S, Villard L, Khrestchatisky M, Fontès M, Colleaux L. Specific interaction between the *XNP/ATR-X* gene product and the SET domain of the human EZH2 protein. Hum Mol Genet 1998;7:679–84.
41. Stevenson RE, Schwartz CE, Schroer RJ. X-linked mental retardation. Oxford: Oxford UniversityPress, 2000.
42. Cardoso C, Lutz Y, Mignon C, et al. ATR-X mutations cause impaired nuclear location and altered DNA binding properties of the *XNP/ATR-X* protein. J Med Genet 2000;37:746–51.
43. Villard L, Lacombe D, Fontés M. A point mutation in the XNP gene, associated with an ATR-X phenotype without α-thalassemia. Eur J Hum Genet 1996;4:316–20.
44. Higgs DR, Vickers MA, Wilkie AOM, Pretorius I-M, Jarman AP, Weatherall DJ. (1989) A review of the molecular genetics of the human α-globin gene cluster. Blood 1989;73:1081–104.
45. Hirschhorn JN, Brown SA, Clark CD, Winston F. Evidence that SNF2/SWI2 and SNF5 activate transcription in yeast by altering chromatin structure. Genes Dev 1992;6:2288–98.
46. Gibbons RJ, Higgs DR. The molecular–clinical spectrum of the ATR-X syndrome. Am J Med Genet (Semin Med Genet) 2000;97:204–12.
47. Villard L, Bonino MC, Abidi F, et al. Evaluation of a mutation screening strategy for sporadic cases of ATR-X syndrome. J Med Genet 1999;36:183–6.
48. Wada T, Kubota T, Fukushima Y, Saitoh S. Molecular genetic study of japanese patients with X-linked alpha- thalassemia/mental retardation syndrome (ATR-X). Am J Med Genet 2000;94:242–8.
49. Fichera M, Romano C, Castiglia L, et al. New mutations in XNP/ATR-X gene: a further contribution to genotype/phenotype relationship in ATR/X syndrome. Mutations in brief no. 176. Online. Hum Mutat 1998;12:214.

50. Ion A, Telvi L, Chaussain JL, et al. (1996) A novel mutation in the putative DNA Helicase *XH2* is responsible for male-to-female sex reversal associated with an atypical form of the ATR-X syndrome. Am J Hum Genet 1996;58:1185–91.
51. Dunnen JT, Antonarakis SE. Mutation nomenclature extensions and suggestions to describe complex mutations: a discussion. Hum Mutat 2000;15:7–12.
52. ICD-10. The ICD-10 Classification of Mental and Behavioural Disorders. Clinical description and diagnostic guidelines. Geneva, WHO, 1992.

Brown et al. *(31)* and Meryash et al. *(32)* were the first to find cytogenetically positive cases of fragile X in autistic males, and several other investigators found children who were positive for *FRAXA* were also autistic *(11,12,33)*. However, several researchers found relatively few *FRAXA*-positive individuals among the autistic males they examined—three of 131 autistic males or 2% *(28)*. Studies of fragile X among autistic males were undertaken over the following years with widely varying outcomes. Venter et al. found 0/40 (0%) of autistic males with fragile X *(34)*, while Blomquist et al. found 11/81 (14%) *(35)*. To determine whether there was a relationship between fragile X and autism as opposed to MR only, Fisch performed a meta-analysis of all 59 published studies of males diagnosed with MR only, or diagnosed as autistic and MR *(36)*. He found the prevalences of fragile X in the two different populations were not significantly different from one another. He concluded that there was likely no relationship between FXS and autism, other than the increased risk associated with MR.

Early cases of speech and language difficulties were reported by Newall et al. *(37)* and Paul et al. *(38)*. As mentioned earlier, a lack of content and grammatical structure was observed by Chudley et al. *(28)*. Also noted were rapid speech *(37)*, stuttering *(28)*, repetitive speech, perseveration, and echolalia *(12,39)*. Sudhalter et al. compared young fragile X males to age-equivalent matched controls and found fragile X individuals exhibited significantly greater semantic deficits *(40)*. Fryns et al. noted that vocabulary and expressive speech appeared to level off at age equivalents of 5–6 years *(12)*, while Fisch et al. noted that age equivalent scores plateaued at between 3–4 years *(41)*.

Age-related features of speech and language were recently examined in detail by Roberts et al. *(42)*. Using the Reynell Developmental Language Scales (RDLS), these researchers examined 39 children with the fragile X mutation, ages 1.5–7 years. Their results show that both receptive and expressive language skills develop more slowly than in same-aged children in the general population. In addition, Roberts et al. note that expressive language skills progress more slowly than receptive language, and that both were related to cognitive ability. Although they did not observe a plateauing of language skills as noted by Fryns et al. *(12)* and Fisch et al. *(41)*, they did note that older children may need to be retested three or more times to determine whether or not this is the case.

1.2. Adaptive and Maladaptive Behavior in FXS

As stated earlier, anecdotal reports describe affected males as socially adept; however, behavioral problems other than those associated with autis-

tic-like features had been observed. Using the Vineland Adaptive Behavior
Scales (VABS; *43*), Dykens and her colleagues examined adaptive behavior
in a small sample of institutionalized adult males with FXS, and found that
they were largely indistinguishable from other males with MR, or those
diagnosed with autism *(44)*. This was confirmed by Kerby and Dawson who
also noted that adaptive behavior levels in adult males with FXS were correlated with their cognitive abilities *(45)*. Institutionalized males with FXS
were compared with noninstitutionalized males. As might be expected,
noninstitutionalized males with FXS functioned at a significantly higher
adaptive behavior level *(46)*. However, both groups of *FRAXA* males manifested unusually high maladaptive behavior levels. Similarly, Kerby and
Dawson examined adult males with FXS and, compared to non-FXS controls, were also observed to be more temperamental, that is, shyer, more
emotional, and more socially withdrawn *(45)*. Cohen et al. had observed
that, compared to Down syndrome controls, age-matched male children with
FXS were more withdrawn socially *(47)*. They did not find any correlation
of social withdrawal with language ability. On the other hand, Wiegers et al.
examined a broad age range of male children, adolescents, and young adults
and found their social adaptability well developed, particularly daily living
skills (DLS) *(48)*. They, however, used a different instrument to evaluate
adaptive behavior which may account for the dissimilarities in their results
compared to previous findings. Strength in DLS in male adults with FXS
had been reported previously *(44)*.

Age-related features of adaptive behavior were also examined by Dykens
et al. *(49)*. Using the VABS, they evaluated children and adolescents with
FXS and found significant interactive effects between test–retest scores and
age. Specifically, younger children exhibited the sharpest increases in age-
equivalent adaptive behavior levels, while adolescents showed modest
decreases. They also found that DLS, which were a relative strength among
young adolescents, decreased on retesting and were not significantly different other adaptive domain scores, that is, Socialization and Communication.
Dykens et al. concluded that the trajectories of adaptive behavior plateau as
children age. In a multicenter retrospective analysis, these results were later
confirmed *(50)*.

To determine whether these findings could be demonstrated prospec-
tively, Fisch and his colleagues began a decade long, prospective longitudinal multicenter study of children and adolescents with the *FRAXA* mutation.
In addition to examining cognitive abilities longitudinally—an issue that
will be addressed shortly—these investigators found that, on retest, adap-

tive behavior composite scores decreased in all but one male and all but three females *(51,52)*. In addition, declines in retest scores were apparent in all behavior domains—Communication, Socialization, and Daily Living Skills—and in all age cohorts examined between ages 4 and 15 years. Decreasing adaptive behavior composites transform into the plateau effect observed by Dykens et al. *(49)*. Recently, Bailey et al. employed a different battery, the Batelle Developmental Inventory (BDI), to evaluate adaptive behavior longitudinally in children ages 2–6 years *(53)*. They also found that adaptive behaviors plateau in younger children, and in all domains in which they were examined: adaptive, cognitive, communication, motor skills, and personal-social.

In an attempt to resolve many discrepant findings reported in emotional–behavioral research, Einfeld et al. *(54)* used the Developmental Behaviour Checklist (DBC) to examine 48 individuals with the fragile X mutation. When compared to MR controls, the prevalence of psychiatric disorders among individuals with fragile X was lower, but not significantly lower, than its prevalence among same age individuals with MR. However, individuals with fragile X were not as antisocial but shyer, manifesting gaze avoidance more frequently than controls. Using the DBC in their follow-up study, Einfeld et al. reexamined individuals assessed earlier and found no significant changes in overall levels of behavioral and emotional disturbance *(55)*. Disruptive behavior, however, declined significantly in both fragile X and control groups, but remained unusually high in the fragile X group. These results are in accord with the findings on maladaptive behavior obtained by Fisch et al. *(56)*. Einfeld et al. also observed an increase in antisocial behavior in both groups *(55)*.

1.3. Neurobehavioral Studies of FXS

Neurobehavioral and neurobiological anomalies, that is, abnormal EEGs, were first reported by Brondum-Nielsen *(11)*. Vieregge and Froster-Iskenius examined 29 cytogenetically positive males with *FRAXA* and noted hypotonia in most individuals *(57)*. Modest hemi- or bilateral pyramidal signs were observed in some cases. Those with no pyramidal signs exhibited a clumsy but not ataxic gait. Several males presented with seizures. EEG studies of 12 males revealed slow background activity in 6. Neuropsychological assessments comparing males with *FRAXA* or Down syndrome showed significant differences in visual–spatial processing *(58)*. Reiss and his colleagues examined males *(59)* and females *(60)* with *FRAXA* and reported significantly lower PV/IC ratios and larger fourth ventricular volumes compared to age- and sex-matched controls. They suggested that neuroanatomical abnormalities in these regions were more likely associated with social and language dysfunction than cognitive impairment.

Using fMRI in concert with a visual–spatial task, Reiss and his colleagues recently examined young females with and without the *FRAXA* mutation *(61)*. Females without the mutation had significantly higher IQ scores. Not unexpectedly, these researchers found that the proportion of correct responses on visual–spatial tasks for the collective group of females studied was strongly and significantly correlated with IQ score. However, females with the *FRAXA* mutation exhibited a significantly lower proportion of correct responses on the more complex of the two visual–spatial procedures (the "2-back") compared to the simpler one ("1-back"). Compared to normal controls, fMRIs taken during visual–spatial tasks revealed significant differences in patterns of voxel activation in the frontal gyrus, parietal lobe, and supramarginal gyrus from those with the *FRAXA* mutation.

1.4. The Heterozygous Female

As might be expected in an X-linked disorder, females with the *FRAXA* mutation tended to be less affected than males. Researchers noted a broad range of IQ scores and milder clinical features *(38,62,63)*, although a few cases in which psychopathology was present were also reported *(64)*. Several early studies of cognitive ability noted significant positive VIQ–PIQ differences *(65,66)*, although later studies by Kemper et al. *(67)* and Wolff et al. *(68)* show as many females with significant negative VIQ-PIQ differences or no differences at all (for a review, *see* Fisch *[69]*). Although their sample was quite small, Mazzocco et al. reported problem-solving deficits in fragile X females consonant with frontal lobe deficiencies *(70)*, and Steyaert et al. found deficits on tests of visual memory *(71)*. Later, using a standardized visual attention task, Steyaert and his colleagues compared female fragile X carriers with controls and found that fragile X females responded significantly more quickly *(72)*.

The suggestion of psychopathology in the heterozygous female was propelled by early anecdotal reports *(62,73,74)*. In their study, Reiss et al. reported significantly greater psychopathology in heterozygous females, particularly schizotypal features in non-retarded females compared to controls *(75)*. On the other hand, Borghgraef et al. *(76)* noted behavioral problems among their nonretarded female carriers the frequency of which was similar to that among controls. Later studies by Freund et al. *(77,78)*, Hull and Hagerman *(79)*, and Sobesky et al. *(80)* also reported higher proportions of mood disorders, particularly major depression, among *FRAXA* female carriers compared to controls. However, the reports by Hull and Hagerman and Sobesky et al. also included females with MR and, as Hagerman and Smith noted earlier *(62)*, individuals with MR are at greater risk to develop psychopathology than individuals with normal range IQ scores. Using the MMPI, Steyaert et al. examined female carriers but found no specific psychopathological profile *(72)* (for a review, *see* Fisch *[69]*).

1.5. Defining the Fragile X Phenotype

Variability in the fragile X phenotype, particularly among heterozygous females, led some investigators to develop screening instruments that utilized clinical features that best exemplify FXS *(18,30)*. Some questionnaires made use of already standardized methods of assessment, for example, Conners Rating Scales to identify behavioral problems such as conduct disorder, hyperactivity, impulsivity, and anxiety *(81)*. Attempts to quantify the clinical phenotype have been modestly successful at best. Using a six-point scale, Reiss et al. found that their screening questionnaire was sensitive in identifying young *FRAXA* males but not older ones *(82)*. Moreover, it did not facilitate identification of young females with *FRAXA*.

1.6. Age-Related Features of the Fragile X Phenotype

Age-related features of adaptive and maladaptive behavior were described earlier. Earliest reports of age-related features in FXS found that cytogenetic frequency of *FRAXA* was inversely correlated with age *(28,83)*, as well as an inverse relationship between age and IQ scores *(28,64)*. Sutherland and Hecht noted lower IQ scores in older *FRAXA* males, but suggested it may have been related to a cohort effect in which older males had been institutionalized but younger males had been placed in intensive training programs *(84)*. However, Hagerman and Smith observed that retest IQ scores were lower than initial test scores in four individual males evaluated *(62)*.

The first systematic examinations of test–retest IQ scores were undertaken by Lachiewicz et al. *(85)* and Borghgraef et al. *(86)*. Unlike Lachiewicz et al., who examined young *FRAXA* males only, Borghgraef et al. compared young *FRAXA* males with age-matched non-*FRAXA* males and found decreasing IQ scores among *FRAXA* males but not among the non-*FRAXA* group. Lachiewicz et al. also found declining IQ scores in the sample of fragile X males they examined. Later, Dykens et al. noted that IQ scores in young males decreased, that is, cognitive development reached plateau, at about the age of 15 years *(87)*. Hagerman et al. also reported declines in IQ scores *(88)*, but unlike Dykens et al., they found decreases in both children and adolescents. In their international retrospective study, Fisch et al. examined test–retest scores of 60 males evaluated with the same IQ test, and also reported significant decreases in most children and adolescents studied *(89)*. Hagerman et al. indicated that decreases may have resulted from the increasing complexity and abstraction associated with subtests for older children *(88)*, whereas Hodapp et al. suggested that other neurobiological factors may have been implicated in the developmental delay *(90)*. Others, for example, Hay *(91)*, suspected that methodological factors may have contributed artifactually to declines in IQ scores. Therefore, Fisch and his colleagues undertook a prospective multicenter study of children and adolescents with the *FRAXA* mutation. Children's ages ranged from 4 to 15 years, and all were tested and retested with the same IQ test, the Stanford–Binet 4th Edition *(92)*. They found that composite IQ scores declined in nearly all males *(51)* and most females tested *(52)*. In addition, Fisch et al. observed that decreases were present in all cognitive areas tested: verbal reasoning, abstract/visual reasoning, quantitative ability, and short-term memory *(51)*.

2. THE *FMR1* GENE: *TRIPLET REPEAT DYNAMICS*

2.1. Genetics and Inheritance Features of Fragile X Syndrome

The report in 1969 by Lubs, who first described the existence of the fragile site at the tip of Xq *(1)*, was confirmed 8 years later by Sutherland *(93)*. Sutherland associated this fragile site with the absence of folic acid in the culture medium and recognized a strong association with an X-linked mental retardation. Cytogenetic testing using folate deficient media became the test of choice and over subsequent years allowed a study of X-linked mental retardation families to be performed worldwide. The prevalence of FXS is now known to be in the order of 1/4000 males and 1/6000 females *(94,95)*. Once families with the fragile X chromosome were identified, genetic linkage studies were launched to locate the gene responsible. It soon became evident that the inheritance of the syndrome was not behaving as an X-linked disease. In classic X-linked disorders, males inheriting the mutated X chromosome develop the trait associated with that mutation. In FXS, early genetic studies showed that the mutation could pass through carrier males without becoming manifest. In addition, these males did not cytogenetically express the fragile X chromosome and so they became known as normal transmitting males.

A large analysis of many fragile X families also revealed another fascinating observation: The risk of a male expressing the phenotype depends on their position within the pedigree, and the risk increases over subsequent generations *(96)*. Opitz denoted the phenomenon "Sherman's paradox" and is now recognized as a form of genetic anticipation. The explanation for these unusual genetics became apparent after the *FMR1* gene and its associated triplet repeat were discovered.

2.2. Molecular Genetics and Cloning of the FMR1 Gene

Application of molecular genetic techniques to the fragile X syndrome in the late 1980s identified several genetic markers in linkage with the locus believed to be disrupted at the fragile X site. In the early 1990s, a complete map spanning the region was determined. The first observations of DNA abnormalities in fragile X individuals came when anomalous methylation was seen in the region believed to include the gene *(97,98)*. Shortly after, the DNA from this methylated region was cloned and the first cases of an unusual form of genetic instability were reported *(99,100)*. Soon afterwards, the *FMR1* gene (standing for Fragile X Mental Retardation) was isolated as being transcribed from the methylated region and encompassing the unstable region *(101)*. This methylation is associated with the loss of *FMR1* mRNA *(102)*.

The first exon of the *FMR1* gene lies within its 5' promoter region. On the normal X chromosome there are between 6 and 52 copies of a CGG repeat (*see* Fig. 1). Typically, these triplets are stably inherited. Almost all (95%) individuals in the normal population have fewer than 40 repeats, and only 1–2% have more than 46. In contrast, in fragile X families, the number of triplets exceeds 55 and, within a family, the number generally increases from one generation to the next, producing progressively longer stretches of the triplet repeat *(103)*.

The process of expansion provides both a molecular explanation for the puzzling genetics of the fragile X syndrome and an assay for its accurate diagnosis. In fragile X families, the *FMR1* $(CGG)_n$ array exists in one of two "states," depending on copy number. Arrays that are longer than 55, but shorter than 200 repeats, are found in carrier females and in the normal transmitting males described earlier. These are termed premutations; they are stable in somatic tissues but are unstable when transmitted to offspring, with most events being expansions. Typically, affected individuals carry an array greater than 200 copies and the *FMR1* gene promoter surrounding the $(CGG)_n$ repeat undergoes an additional change during development and becomes methylated. "Full" mutations of this sort frequently exhibit somatic variation in a cell population, even within the same tissue, resulting in a heterogeneous mixture of alleles.

One other important aspect of transmission of the expanded $(CGG)_n$ in fragile X families is that the conversion from premutation to full mutation occurs exclusively on maternal transmission. The risk of expansion to the full mutation is dependent on the allele length in the mother, such that any

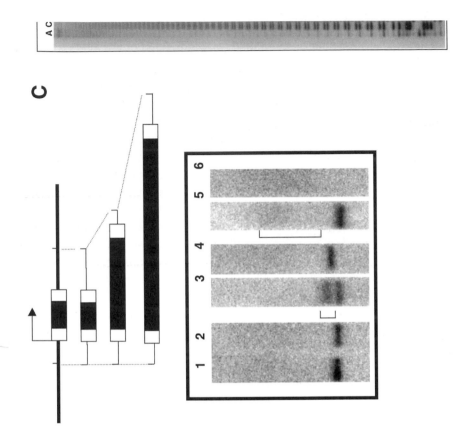

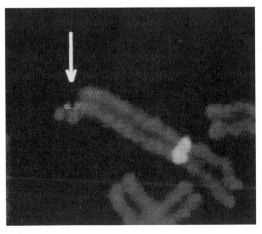

premutation allele above 90 copies has a 100% conversion rate whereas an allele of 70 copies will convert in only 30% of transmissions *(104)*. The progressive expansion coupled with an increased risk of conversion to the full mutation provides a molecular explanation for the Sherman paradox. Daughters of the normal transmitting males, who are always unaffected with FXS and are cytogenetically negative for fragile X expression, only ever inherit a premutation allele from their fathers. Thus an accurate determination of the exact length of the *FMR1* (CGG)$_n$ array in fragile X families is critical to accurate diagnostics within families (reviewed comprehensively in *105*).

The role of the *FMR1* gene in FXS was confirmed by the identification of patients with other types of mutations in individuals who were cytogenetically negative for the fragile X chromosome but who had very similar clinical phenotypes. Most of these carry microdeletions across the *FMR1* promoter and can be explained by the complete absence of *FMR1* gene expression; there are, however, some individuals whose deletions remove larger portions of the gene *(106–114)*. A point mutation converting isoleucine-367 to an asparagine residue was also identified in an individual with severe FXS, a very low IQ *(20)* and extreme macroorchidism syndrome *(115)*. As we will discuss later, this mutation lies within a critical region of the FMR protein and appears to interfere with its function.

2.3. Diagnostics

The length of triplet repeat in the *FMR1* gene is highly indicative of the phenotypic state of the individual and its measurement forms the basis of all

---

Fig. 1. (*Opposite page*) Fragile X diagnostics: from chromosome to DNA to sequence. (**A**) Cytogenetic analysis of the fragile X chromosome induced by folate stress. FISH analysis shows the X chromosome centromere labeled. Arrow highlights the position of fragile site breakage and hybridization of a labeled DNA probe that spans the *FMR1* gene, showing coincident localization. (**B**) Diagnostic DNA analysis by Southern blot hybridization to detect the expanded triplet array (*dark box*) within *FMR1* exon 1 (*open box*). Fragments released by cutting with an enzyme either side of the triplet array releases a fragment that is detected by DNA probe OX1.9. A normal sized fragment is seen in the individuals in *lanes 1* and *2*, whereas progressively larger fragments are seen in the carrier female in *lane 3* and male in *lane 4* (*region highlighted*). Full mutation fragments, seen as a smear of fragments (*region highlighted*) due to heterogeneity between cells is seen in an affected female (*lane 5*) and affected male (*lane 6*). The normal allele is also visible in the female in *lane 5*. (**C**) Sequence analysis of the *FMR1* triplet array from a carrier male with 60 repeats showing the CGG repeat. This type of analysis can be used to determine the AGG interruption profile of intermediate and small premutation arrays.

genetic testing for FXS. Until the triplet expansion was identified, diagnosis had relied almost exclusively on the cytogenetic identification of the fragile X chromosome, an example of which can be seen in Fig. 1a. Apart from the more intensive laboratory procedures involved, one major limitation with the cytogenetic test is that it does not detect carriers. DNA tests are now well established *(105)* and in most laboratories, the length of the $(CGG)_n$ array can be estimated by studying the increase in size of DNA fragments above the normal baseline using Southern blots as shown in Fig. 1b. Genomic DNA is digested with a restriction enzyme and the size of the fragment is estimated after detection with an *FMR1* gene probe. Figure 1b shows an examination of the genomic DNA from peripheral blood lymphocytes of several normal, carrier, and affected fragile X family members. The normal sized DNA fragment is visible as a single 5.2-kb fragment, as seen in lanes 1 and 2. Premutation length expansions can be detected as larger fragments, as seen in lanes 3 and 4, which are a carrier female and male respectively; the female also has a fragment from her normal X chromosome. The full mutation expansion is present as a heterogeneous smear in two individuals in this figure, an affected female (lane 5) and affected male (lane 6). This is due to the extensive heterogeneity described earlier and, as can be seen, can sometimes be difficult to detect, particularly in a female. Only the latter two individuals would be detected as cytogenetically positive.

As mentioned earlier, expanded arrays larger than 200 triplets also undergo methylation and this is associated with the absence of *FMR1* gene transcription. The methylation status of the *FMR1* promoter is routinely tested by combining the simple genomic test with a second enzyme that can test for the presence of methylation. This is a similar assay to that described above but combines a joint detection of both expansion and methylation. Polymerase chain reaction (PCR)-based $(CGG)_n$ amplification tests have also been developed which complement the genomic DNA analysis. Although these can offer a rapid screening test, problems in efficiently amplifying large expansions in the presence of smaller alleles, as occurs in both females and a large number of males who are mosaics of different length arrays, means that verification is usually performed with the more informative genomic tests. In most diagnostics laboratories, PCR tests are used on an exclusion basis to prescreen samples for individuals with normal length arrays.

In addition to the complications of interpreting different length arrays, the degree to which the genotype observed in genomic DNA tests correlates with the phenotype of the individual can be influenced by several other factors. First, as mentioned above, some individuals are mosaic for several classes of $(CGG)_n$ expansion, that is, they carry different lengths of triplet repeat and may well have different levels of *FMR1* methylation in different cells within their body. In these cases, the degree of mental impairment will likely depend on the proportion and distribution of full mutation carrying cells in the brain. Second, random X-inactivation within a female heterozygote means that any phenotype is presumably dependent on the proportion of her brain cells containing the active normal *FMR1* gene. The distribution of these cells within the body will greatly influence the penetrance of the disease.

DNA testing is also used for prenatal diagnosis, where *FMR1* repeat length can be reliably measured *(116–119)*. However, methylation in DNA isolated from CVS tissue does not reflect methylation of the embryo itself, limiting the predictive value of the tests in cases where a small expansion is observed. This is not as problematic with amniocentesis-based tests, in which *FMR1* methylation can be measured more accurately but at a later time in gestation.

As mentioned earlier, the fragile X phenotype results from the lack of the FMRP protein. As we soon discuss, this is determined by both an inhibition of level of gene transcription through *FMR1* promoter methylation and by a direct effect of the triplet repeats on translation. Recently, a direct test for the FMRP protein was been developed and can be used to detect protein levels in blood cells, hair bulbs, CVS cells, and amniocytes *(120–123)*. Levels of FMRP correlate well with the degree of MR seen in fragile patients. In particular, the analysis of hair bulbs is promising as they appear to reflect levels of protein expression in the brain and show a good correlation with female IQ. Direct detection of FMRP is an extremely promising diagnostic test as it resolves many of the issues of mosaicism of methylation and expansion we discussed earlier.

2.4. Genotype–Phenotype Correlations

Among the earliest genotype–phenotype correlations between cytogenetic expression and IQ were observed in heterozygous females *(83)*. Noting an inverse correlation between cytogenetic frequency and IQ in affected males *(28)*, Chudley et al. later confirmed these findings. Fisch et al. *(124)* and Fisch and Fryns *(125)* found that both familial factors and sex contributed to cytogenetic frequency. After the *FMR1* gene was cloned and identified, correlations between mutation size, that is, number of CGG repeats, and cognitive–behavioral features were examined. Staley et al. found IQ scores among premutation females were significantly higher than among females with full mutations *(18)*, while Abrams et al. noted significant inverse correlations between mutation size and IQ among all heterozygous females *(126)*. Staley et al. also reported that males with mosaic full mutations had significantly higher IQ scores that those with full mutations only, although Fisch et al. examined young males with full mutations and, compared to those with mosaics, found no significant differences in IQ scores *(51)*. Based on these and other molecular–cognitive data, Kolehmainen and Karant developed a model to explain the relationship between methylation mosaicism and IQ *(127)*.

2.5. Multiple Molecular Effects of (CGG)$_n$ Expansion: Transcription, Methylation, and Translation

The full mutation *FMR1* (CGG)$_n$ expansion undergoes extensive methylation across the gene promoter and triplet repeat region *(97,98,128)*. In a manner believed to parallel methylation-associated silencing on X-inactivation in female somatic cells, this was predicted to lead to *FMR1* gene silencing through an inhibition of transcription. This was indeed shown to be the case in fragile X families *(129)*, and furthermore, by comparing methylated and unmethylated *FMR1* genes during embryogenesis, gene silencing was shown to correlate directly with methylation *(102)*. In most of these cases, methylation was assessed at only a few sites within the gene promoter. The absence of the encoded FMRP protein in full mutation individuals served to confirm this effect. In addition to methylation, full mutation arrays are associated with other molecular changes to chromatin that include deacetylation of histones, a process that is associated with gene silencing *(130)*.

Methylation across the *FMR1* promoter and the (CGG)$_n$ array has now been studied in more detail using more sensitive techniques that assess multiple sites *(131,132)*. *FMR1* methylation is strikingly variable across the promoter, with some regions more methylated than others, even within areas that are known to be important for transcription factor binding *(131,133)*. The study by Genc et al. found that in mosaic individuals, *FMR1* genes associated with shorter arrays have less methylation *(132)*. The study by Tassone et al. showed that methylation differs according to tissue type *(134)*, supporting earlier observations by Worhle et al. *(135)*. The variable nature of *FMR1* promoter methylation suggests that routinely used diagnostic digests that assess methylation only in a limited area of the promoter cannot be used to infer methylation status across the complete promoter.

In most fragile X individuals, the level of *FMR1* mRNA is not routinely examined as DNA tests designed to assess the expansion/methylation status are sufficiently accurate predictors in most cases. With the development of more quantitative techniques to study gene expression, recent analysis of

FMR1 transcription in both premutation and full mutations individuals has led to a new interpretation of the effects of $(CGG)_n$ expansion on transcription and the role of methylation.

It has become apparent that the relationship between expansion, transcription, and translation is more complex than originally described. Several studies have now shown that cells carrying premutation length *FMR1* $(CGG)_n$ arrays have elevated levels of *FMR1* mRNA *(136–138)*. Longer premutations exhibit increased levels of mRNA as much as fivefold greater than normal length arrays, as shown in Fig. 2a. These elevated levels of *FMR1* mRNA appear to be due to increased transcription, as premutation-containing mRNA did not appear to have an increased stability. This appears to be the case even for small premutation arrays of 55–100 triplets, which can show more than a twofold increase in mRNA levels. This increase in mRNA is not, however, matched by a concomitant increase in FMRP protein expression and FMRP levels are actually decreased in these individuals. An explanation for these observations lies in a report published in 1995 by Feng et al. that suggested that *FMR1* mRNAs carrying longer lengths of $(CGG)_n$ were poorly translated through a direct effect of the CGG triplets on the translation machinery *(139)*. As can be seen in Fig. 2b, the amounts of FMRP decrease directly in proportion to the length of the CGG array within the mRNA such that mRNAs carrying more than 200 triplets are very poorly translated *(138,139)*. Indeed, some individuals with arrays as short as 48 and 55 CGG triplets showed up to a 17% reduction in cellular FMRP. A direct comparison of Figs. 2a and 2b, clearly indicates that as the level of *FMR1* mRNA translation decreases, the cell appears in some way to compensate through a proportionate increase in transcription, suggesting connection between the level of FMRP and its own mRNA. In the fragile X point mutation individual, who produces a nonfunctional FMRP, transcription is at a normal level (from a $[CGG]_{25}$ allele), suggesting that this feedback cannot be based on FMRP function. This effect might therefore be due to a direct *cis* effect of the $(CGG)_n$ array on the promoter.

The elevated *FMR1* mRNA level in premutation individuals and the decreased translation efficiency of *FMR1* mRNAs containing longer $(CGG)_n$ arrays might provide some molecular foundation to support the growing evidence for a clinical phenotype associated with the premutation. It is easy to see how a decreased level of FMRP might contribute to a cellular phenotype through a deficit on cellular protein levels. It is also possible that the presence of an elevated level of *FMR1* mRNA could directly or indirectly interfere with other genes. This has been shown to be the case in DM where the presence of DM mRNA carrying an expanded $(CTG)_n$ repeat binds regu-

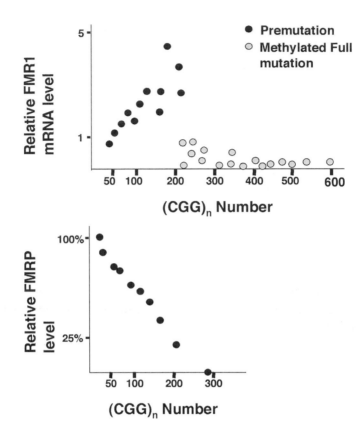

Fig. 2. Effect of $(CGG)_n$ expansion on *FMR1* transcription and translation. The relationship between *FMR1* CGG array length mRNA levels relative to normal (=1) is shown for a range of repeat lengths from normal, intermediate, permutation, and methylated full mutation. This data is a pictorial representation of data presented in refs. *136–138*. As array length increases, the levels of cellular mRNA also increase. In individuals carrying methylated arrays above 200 repeats in length, the levels of mRNAs are dramatically decreased although some expression can be detected at almost normal levels in some males. A similar relationship is shown in the bottom panel between *FMR1* CGG array length and the relative amounts of cellular FMRP. This is a pictorial representation of data showing that as array length increases, the levels of FMRP protein decrease *(138,139)*. Arrays longer than 200 produce little or no FMRP.

latory proteins that play critical roles in the regulation of other genes *(140,141)*. It is the effect on these other genes that gives rise to many of the clinical effects of the expansion in DM. Overall, it is clear that the phenotypic effects of the premutation length arrays in carriers needs to be examined in greater detail. In addition, the observation that some individuals within the high normal/intermediate range have elevated mRNA and decreased FMRP levels suggest that the clinical effects of these arrays should also be reexamined.

The application of these techniques to the analysis of full mutation individuals has also recently found evidence of mRNA production from methylated alleles which were previously considered to be transcriptionally silent (*see* Fig. 2a). Tassone et al. describe a study in which they found *FMR1* mRNA levels approaching those of a normal individual in more than half the sample of 48 full mutation males they examined *(142)*. This is most evident in males with full mutations in the 200–400 repeat range, although arrays as long as 600 triplets do allow some mRNA production, but at a level 0.1% of normal. These males carried methylated full mutation arrays as determined by methylation/expansion diagnostic restriction digests. As mentioned earlier, these diagnostic tests examine only a few areas of the *FMR1* gene promoter and presumably, in these individuals, critical regions of their *FMR1* genes remain unmethylated or with an altered chromatin configuration that allows for at least some mRNA production. No studies have yet been performed to assess the status of chromatin proteins associated with these active genes. However, owing to the suppression of translation which is seen with mRNAs carrying long $(CGG)_n$ arrays (*see* Fig. 2b), these males do not produce any FMRP.

It is clear that the critical determinant of the fragile X clinical phenotype is the level of FMRP present within the cell. This is now known to be dependent on both the repeat length and methylation. Somatic mosaicism of the repeat length and methylation will also play a role as to which cells in the brain contain which length and methylation status of repeat.

2.6. Premature Ovarian Failure and FRAXA

Early studies of premature ovarian failure (POF) found an association between it and mutations at the tip of the long arm of the X chromosome *(143–145)*. In their report of heterozygous females, Cronister et al. found 8 of 61 (13%) of females with the *FRAXA* premutation experienced POF, compared to none of the six females with the full mutation *(146)*. Subsequently, Schwartz et al. examined a larger sample of female *FRAXA* carriers and observed that, among woman older than 40 years, 12 of 49 (25%) of those with the premutation had undergone POF, as opposed to three of eight (38%) carriers with the full mutation *(147)*. Other studies also confirmed findings in which an unusually high proportion of females with the premutation manifested POF *(148,149)*. These early reports led to an international collaborative study by Allingham-Hawkins et al. in which 760 women from *FRAXA* families were evaluated *(150)*. Of those who were older than 40 years, none of the 42 women with the full mutation had undergone POF, whereas 43 of 182 (24%) women with the premutation had. Later, when 106 women who were affected by POF but not previously tested for *FRAXA* were examined, a higher-than-expected proportion (6 of 106, or 6%) were diagnosed with *FRAXA (151)*. Taken together, these findings provide evidence of an association between POF and the *FRAXA* premutation.

The findings also present a conundrum. Previously, women with the *FRAXA* premutation were not thought to exhibit a clinical phenotype, despite a previous report by Sobesky et al. *(152)*. As we discussed, early molecular findings showed no unusual levels of RNA transcription nor in protein expression and a molecular mechanism linking POF with the *FRAXA* premutation was missing. One hypothesis, that the POF gene and *FRAXA* may be in linkage disequilibrium, was presented by Murray et al. *(153)*. In support of their conjecture, Hundschein et al. found evidence that women who inherited the *FRAXA* mutation from their fathers were significantly more likely to manifest POF than those women who inherited the mutation from their mothers *(154)*. These findings, however, were not confirmed by other investigators *(155,156)*. The recent observations discussed in the preceding, that: (1) there are significantly higher mRNA levels in *FRAXA* premutation females compared to either nonmutation controls or females with the full mutation; (2) increased RNA levels are associated with reduced FMRP levels in premutation carriers; and (3) FMRP inhibits many other mRNA levels, provides a possible candidate for investigation of the as yet unknown basis of the *FRAXA*/POF association.

2.7. Triplet Expansion in the FMR1 Gene

2.7.4. The Structure of the FMR1 Triplet Repeat Determines Instability

A detailed analysis of the *FMR1* triplet array in the normal population has shown that it is not a pure $(CGG)_n$ array, but rather that it contains internal interruptions *(103,157–161)*. The majority of normal *FMR1* triplet arrays consist of short tracts of $(CGG)_n$ and single interspersed AGG triplets arranged such that, in most alleles, every 10th triplet is an AGG. Approximately 10–15%, contain portions of $(CGG)_{n>17}$, either as uninterrupted arrays or at the 3' end of compound arrays (*see* Fig. 3). Allelic variation in these normal length arrays is a result of both variation in the $(CGG)_n$ lengths (from 7 to 13, with a modal length of 9 triplets) and the number the $(CGG)_n(AGG)$ blocks present. The most frequent structures of array in the population are 20 and 30 repeat arrays containing either two or three of these interrupted blocks.

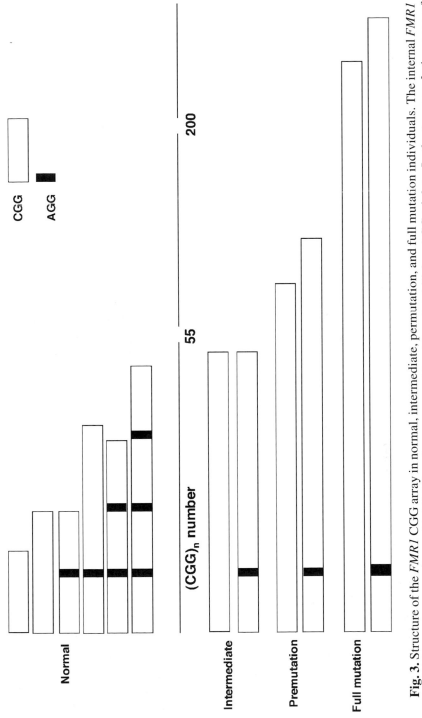

Fig. 3. Structure of the *FMR1* CGG array in normal, intermediate, permutation, and full mutation individuals. The internal *FMR1* (CGG)$_n$ array structure is shown highlighting the pattern and location of stabilising AGG triplets. In the **top panel**, the range of alleles of varying internal structure and length are shown. Note that some alleles carry longer lengths of uninterrupted (CGG)$_n$ at their 3′ end. Shown below are intermediate, permutation, and full mutation length arrays. Note that expansion into this size range due to additional CGG triplets being added within the 3′ uninterrupted portion.

A group of arrays also seen that are longer than normal, but that are not known to be premutations, is also found in the population. These tend to have longer blocks of uninterrupted $(CGG)_n$ at their 3' ends (see Fig. 3). Several have been found to be genetically unstable in family studies. In this class of arrays, the shortest array exhibiting instability has been $(CGG)_{34}$ (162), although an array of $(CGG)_{11}(AGG)(CGG)_{30}$ was also demonstrated as being unstable (159). Thus, uninterrupted repeats as short as $(CGG)_{30}$ were shown to be unstable in some families. More sensitivity can be obtained by analyzing the male germline directly rather than encountering length changes by chance in family studies. A comparison of instability using single-sperm PCR to measure mutation frequency showed that the presence of interrupting AGG triplets has a significant effect on stability (163). In comparing two 39 repeat arrays, the array containing only one AGG triplet showed a more than threefold higher rate of expansion compared to an array containing two AGGs (3% vs <0.9%). Expansions occurred within the 3' uninterrupted portion of the array. An analysis using small pool PCR on sperm DNA reached similar conclusions (164). When an overall comparison is made between $(CGG)_n$ length and genetic instability, the degree of instability correlates well with the increasing length of the uninterrupted $(CGG)_n$ portion. In fragile X families, arrays in which longer uninterrupted 3' $(CGG)_n$ regions are present and expansion occurs within this portion of the array (see Fig. 3), eventually expand to the full mutation length above 200 repeats, wherein methylation arises.

2.7.2. Problems with Intermediate Arrays

Recognition that unstable arrays have longer 3' $(CGG)_n$ blocks raises a question as to whether normal-sized arrays that carry them may be "precursors" that will eventually progress into the premutation range through expansion. Population genetic studies suggest that this may indeed be the case (165–168), as many fragile X chromosomes share common genetic haplotypes with intermediate-sized alleles having longer 3' CGG tracts. As discussed earlier, these intermediate arrays can also exert an effect on FMRP translation but, to date, no study has examined the effects of AGG interruption in longer intermediate arrays on either mRNA levels or on translation. Comparison of a fully interrupted vs uninterrupted array could provide valuable insight into these phenomena.

For diagnostic purposes, difficulties can arise with intermediate length *FMR1* arrays of between 40 and 55 repeats as to whether these are considered potential premutations. We know that array instability is, to a great extent, determined by the pattern of AGG interruption (DNA sequence analysis is shown in Fig. 1c). It would therefore serve a useful purpose in

distinguishing between an uninterrupted array with a higher chance of instability from a fully interrupted array with a lower theoretical risk. At present
the only route for follow up with these borderline arrays is an extended
family analysis as few data are available to provide a quantitative estimate
of instability in the intermediate range. Three factors should, however, be
borne in mind. First, the risk of conversion for any expanded array to a full
mutation is dependent on passage through the female germline; thus, for
alleles transmitted from a male the risk will be zero. Second, arrays within
this intermediate zone of instability are unlikely to carry a significant risk of
conversion to the full mutation in a single generation; one of the smallest
reported arrays that has given rise to a fragile X chromosome contained 56
uninterrupted repeats and expanded over two generations *(162)*. Third, some
intermediate arrays may also give rise to a decreased level of FMRP and the
phenotypic consequences of this are, as yet, unknown.

It should also be noted that one increase in length in a normal length
FMR1 array has been described that resulted in the addition of a complete
AGG-$(CGG)_9$ block of triplet repeat being added to the array *(169)*. This
increases in *FMR1* array length was most likely a result of a genetic
exchange event, rather than through triplet expansion, but could be misin-
terpreted as instability if only the array length was measured. This highlights the importance of examining AGG interruption patterns in cases of
instability to determine if the structure might be considered expansion prone.

2.7.3. The Timing of CGG Triplet Expansion

Examination of repeat length changes in fragile X families shows that, in
general, premutation length arrays are relatively stable. That is, they do not
appear to undergo expansion in the somatic cells within an individual. There
are cases in which expansion has been reported *(170)* and it may be more
common than we currently believe, but the PCR analysis required to examine this is not reliable. In dramatic contrast, premutation arrays that are
somatically stable undergo expansion at some point during germ cell development in the parent or during early embryogenesis in the offspring, or in
both. Key to understanding when expansion occurs, therefore, is the question of what length of repeat is present in the oocyte and sperm of fragile X
carriers. Studies in this area have, unfortunately, been very limited owing to
problems of obtaining suitable material.

Premutation arrays are transmitted by both sexes but expansion to the full
mutation occurs only on transmission from the female. To explain this, it
has been suggested that full mutations are selected against in the male germ
line; cells carrying full mutations would not proliferate and not reach mature
sperm. Supporting evidence came when sperm from full mutation males was

found to contain only premutation length arrays *(171)*. If FMRP is required for proliferation, selection could be due to a selective growth or survival of pregerm cells that have undergone a deletion event to carry premutation length $(CGG)_n$ arrays that would express more FMRP on the strength of having shorter arrays. Using an in vitro cell culture system, Salat et al. have shown that the outgrowth of fibroblasts with reduced $(CGG)_n$ length is associated with increased levels of FMRP *(172)*. It is also possible that the full mutation is selected against on the basis of the triplet repeat itself and its effect on DNA structure, perhaps leading to chromosome breakage and a selective removal of those cells carrying DNA breaks by through cell cycle arrest and apoptosis. This latter hypothesis is supported by the fact that mice that lack FMRP are fertile. Therefore, FMRP is not required for germ cell proliferation, although its presence might still influence cell growth.

As transmission of the full mutation occurs only on female transmission, how much do we know about the mutations lengths here? Two models have been proposed that differ as to the timing of expansion or conversion to the full mutation. The first model assumes that conversion occurs in either germ cell development or meiosis. As a result, the female oocyte would carry a full mutation array that would be inherited and all the somatic tissues of the offspring would carry a full mutation. According to this model, to explain mosaic individuals, some cells must undergo contraction in length. No study has reported a direct examination of oocytes from premutation carrier females, but the study of Malter et al. detected full mutations within oocytes of a full mutation embryo *(173)*. Although this does not provide any direct evidence as to the status of a premutation in the female germline, it does confirm that the full mutation is compatible with oocytes, in apparent contrast to the case in the male germ line, where full mutations remain to be demonstrated.

The alternative model suggests that the expansion to the full mutation occurs during embryogenesis and that the oocytes of a premutation female contain only premutation arrays *(174,175)*. This model suggests that mosaics arise when a small proportion of cells do not undergo conversion to the full mutation, remaining in the somatic cells as premutations. The study of Moutou et al., however, suggests that to explain the frequency of mosaicism that is actually seen in families, the conversion from premutation to full mutation must occur before d 3 after fertilization or before *(176)*. Clearly, we have yet to determine precisely determine when expansion to the full mutation is occurring in FXS.

2.7.4. Triplet Expansion in Other Human Neurological Diseases

Since the identification of the triplet expansion at *FMR1*, expansions of triplet and other simple repeats have now been identified at more than 20 loci (*see* Table 1), many of which are associated with disease. As the process of expansion is generally believed to be similar in these other disorders, comparisons with other expansion diseases might provide valuable insights into the process in FXS. Expansion also influences both the frequency of FXS in the population and also determines the affected status of an individual. As such, understanding the mechanism of expansion might allow for the development of therapeutics to halt or even reverse the process.

In all cases that are associated with clinical disease, the affected status is associated with an increase in repeat length, although the degree of expansion differs among the different diseases. Generally speaking, triplet expansions fall into two categories based on their size: (1) those with large expansions to over 200 repeats of $(CTG)_n$ in myotonic dystrophy or $(GAA)_n$ in Friedreich's ataxia; (2) those with smaller expansions of up to $(CAG)_{130}$ triplets such as occur in Huntington's disease and the spinocerebellar ataxias. Larger expansions are also seen in other simple repeats such as with $(CCTG)_n$ in a second myotonic dystrophy gene, *DM2 (177)*, and $(ATTCT)_n$ in *SCA10 (178)* and in minisatellites associated with some fragile sites (*see* Table 1). Although the effect of expansion at the molecular level on the gene or protein differs among the diseases, the underlying mutational process of triplet expansion is believed shared and insights in one may have major implications for the other diseases.

2.7.5. Somatic Expansion and the Cellular Phenotype

The difference is size of the expansions in the different diseases in Table 1 is also reflected in the occurrence of extensive somatic expansion with longer arrays, a process that can have implications for the disease phenotype. $(CTG)_n$ expansions in myotonic dystrophy (DM) can be extremely large, with continuous somatic expansion of several thousand triplets in a highly tissue specific manner, with muscle cells undergoing extensive expansion in an age-related manner *(179–184)*. The effect of this continued somatic expansion is seen at the cellular level in DM, being directly mediated in proportion to the triplet length through the DM mRNA; cells with longer array lengths have a more severe phenotype. An examination of $(CAG)_n$ arrays in Huntington's disease brains also found evidence for somatic expansion occurring within neuronal cells which show the most degeneration *(185)*. When examined in a mouse model, a localized expansion of more than threefold was found in the effected striatum cell *(186)*. As longer $(CAG)_n$ arrays are believed to result in a more neurotoxic protein, somatic expansion in specific cells presumably leads to a more pronounced cellular phenotype. In most cases, somatic expansion appears to be highly variable between cell types indicating that cell-specific *trans*-acting factors probably play a role. As all expanded triplet repeats are known to expand during germ

Table 1
Repeat Expansions in the Human Genome

Gene or Disorder	Repeat	Location/function	Normal range	Range of expanded alleles
Fragile X syndrome	CGG	5' UTR	6–50	50–2000
FRAXE mental retardation	GCC	5' UTR	6–25	70–2000
FRAXF	CGG	Noncoding	6–29	300–1000
FRA11B	CGG	CBL2 gene, chromosome breakage	11	80–1000
FRA16A	CGG	Unknown	16–49	1000–1900
Friedrich's ataxia	GAA	Intronic	7–22	>200
Myotonic dystrophy	CTG	3' UTR	5–30	>50
Kennedy's disease	CAG	Coding: poly Glu	9–36	38–62
Huntington's disease	CAG	Coding: poly Glu	6–35	36–120
SCA1	CAG	Coding: poly Glu	6–35	40–80
SCA2	CAG	Coding: poly Glu	14–32	33–77
SCA3	CAG	Coding: poly Glu	12–40	67–82
SCA6	CAG	Coding: poly Glu	4–17	20–31
SCA7	CAG	Coding: poly Glu	7–17	38–130
DRPLA	CAG	Coding: poly Glu	3–36	49–88
SCA17	CAG	Coding: poly Glu	29–42	>47
SCA8	CAG	mRNA	16–37	110–250
HDL2	CAG/CTG	mRNA-Alt exon	6–27	>40
DM2	CCTG	Intronic	20–32	100–11000
SCA10	ATTCT	Intronic	10–22	Up to 4500
OPMD	CGG	Coding: poly Ala	6	8–13
EPM1	GC 12mer	Gene promoter	2–3	12–13
FRA10B	AT 42bp	Unknown	Unknown	5–100 kb
FRA16B	AT 33bp	Unknown	Unknown	10–70 kb

line development, this suggests that one common expansion-proficient cellular environment must be present in these stages of development.

The detection of somatic expansion in other triplet expansion associated diseases has been greatly assisted by the ability to analyze the repeat length in detail using PCR. This allows small numbers of cells to be examined by a technique known as small pool PCR. Limitations in the application of PCR to *FMR1* arrays has prohibited the use of this technique in fragile X premutation carriers. In addition, as most DNA testing is performed on peripheral blood lymphocytes, it is possible that this does not accurately reflect the length of CGG in the rest of the somatic tissue. Several reports of somatic instability in premutation length arrays and nonmethylated full mutation length arrays have been reported on Southern blot analysis *(170,187)*, suggesting that it can arise. In addition, somatic instability of nonmethylated full mutations have been observed in postmortem tissues *(188)*.

In most cases of affected fragile X males with more than 200 repeats, the triplet repeat length is highly variable, giving rise to a smear of fragments on a Southern blot (e.g., *see* Fig. 1b, lane 6). This degree of somatic instability is believed established in early development and appears to become stabilized on methylation that occurs about the time of cell differentiation or specialization. One effect of methylation may be to stabilize the arrays. Array stability would lead to similar patterns of somatic variation in length among different tissues *(135,189,190)*, between monozygotic twins *(175)*, and in established fibroblast cell cultures *(174)*.

Somatic expansion of triplet repeats may well play a significant role in the clinical phenotype of some expansion diseases. As levels of FMRP are decreased due to a suppression of translation, somatic expansion may exert a significant effect on the amounts of FMRP within cells throughout the body. Different FMRP levels could contribute to a premutation associated phenotype and almost certainly contribute to the variability of phenotypes in mosaic fragile X individuals.

2.7.6. $(CGG)_n$ Expansion, Methylation, and Fragile Site Expression

Identification of the *FMR1* triplet expansion led to the identification of two other fragile sites in the same chromosomal region, *FRAXE* and *FRAXF* *(191–193)*. Cytogenetically, *FRAXE* and *FRAXF* could not be differentiated from *FRAXA*. However, once a molecular test for FXS was developed, these rare individuals did not exhibit the typical *FMR1* expansion. Similar $(CGG)_n$ expansions were identified at these sites *(194–197)* and subsequently also at several autosomal fragile sites (*see* Table 1). To date, only *FRAXE* appears to be associated with a nonsyndromal phenotype associated with mild learning disabilities *(194,195)*. The association between $(CGG)_n$ expansion and late replication, as predicted by Laird and colleagues *(198,199)* and shown to be the case for *FMR1 (200)*, appears to be a common factor for fragile site expression. Interestingly, repeat amplification of longer repeats has been found at two fragile sites *([201]; see* Table 1). These and other fragile sites, not only those associated with $(CGG)_n$ expansion and methylation, appear to be linked to altered replication patterns and are implicated as sites of chromosome breakage in cancer *(202)*.

2.7.7. Insights into the Process of Triplet Expansion from Model Systems

Despite a decade of research into triplet expansion, we still do not know the exact mechanism by which it occurs. However, the use of model organisms such as mouse, bacteria, and yeast have provided some important clues as to which cellular pathways are involved. As triplet expansion must involve the addition of triplet DNA to the existing array, most experimental systems have focused on errors that could arise during DNA synthesis itself. In most cells, DNA synthesis either is associated with DNA replication and repair that occurs prior to cell division, or is associated with DNA repair in nondividing cells in response to DNA damage. Biochemical and genetic studies of replication in both yeast and bacteria have suggested that the $(CGG)_n$ triplet array, in common with other triplet repeats, has a tendency to form unusual and stable DNA structures during DNA synthesis *(203,204)*. These occur more frequently in the $(CGG)_n$ strand and within arrays that are uninterrupted, observations that correlate well with the fact that, in the *FMR1* array, longer uninterrupted arrays appear to be prone to expansion. Difficulty synthesizing or removing these structures is believed to trigger various pathways of DNA repair.

2.7.7.1. THE FEN1 MODEL OF EXPANSION DURING DNA SYNTHESIS

Evidence for one particular pathway has come from studying human triplet arrays that have been established in yeast, a genetic system that allows knockout studies to be performed very rapidly. Several studies have focused on the FEN1 protein in yeast, which when deleted gives rise to a dramatic level of triplet expansion in yeast *(205,206)*. As most proteins involved in DNA repair and replication are highly conserved in all eukaryotes this system is proving particularly useful in identifying human genes that are involved in the expansion process.

During DNA synthesis associated with replication or DNA repair, DNA polymerase displaces a downstream strand of DNA as it polymerizes from an upstream DNA end. The displaced strand forms a so-called "flap" normally removed by a protein called FEN1. Note that to form these flaps, DNA synthesis continues for a while and, in effect, the DNA displaced is duplicated. The flap is normally removed on FEN1 cleavage and no additional DNA is incorporated. FEN1 cannot process a flap that has formed any secondary structure, however. In the case of the *FMR1* array, it is suggested that structures form within a $(CGG)_n$-containing flap that prevent cleavage from occurring. The structure leads to a stalled or partially replicated array (Fig. 4b). To resolve the discrepancy, one recovery pathway involves formation of a double-stranded DNA break (Fig. 4c) followed by DNA repair by copying from the other array (in replication) or other allele (in repair) (Fig. 4d). In this case, additional DNA is synthesized onto the originally stalled strand. In addition, the displaced flap, which is now extra DNA duplicated during the displacement process, also copies DNA in the same way. The result is the addition of a random number of triplets into the array. This model also explains the length dependency of expansion as this most likely reflects the likelihood that an Okazaki fragment is synthesized within the $(CGG)_n$ array itself during DNA replication, as suggested by Richards and Sutherland *(207)*. Interestingly, several studies reported high rates of sister chromatid exchange in the fragile X region in carriers who might support the notion of DNA repair occurring via this pathway *(208,209)*.

2.7.7.2. MOUSE MODELS OF $(CGG)_N$ TRIPLET EXPANSION

As access to suitable human tissues is limited, the creation of suitable animal models for $(CGG)_n$ expansion is highly desirable. As discussed earlier, access to human germline and embryonic tissues is limited and any suitable model would provide great insights into the process of expansion in these cells. Generally speaking, however, mouse models of expansion have been rather disappointing as the extent of intergenerational expansions has been limited. In the case of $(CAG)_n$ and $(CTG)_n$ triplets, some degree of success has been achieved, although the level of instability which has been seen is considerably less than that seen in humans. Instability has been observed in germ line transmission but larger expansions have been observed in somatic tissues, particularly as a result of aging *(210–212)*.

In the case of transgenic mice carrying $(CGG)_n$ arrays, two approaches have been used: one involves simply inserting, at random, an expanded *FMR1* triplet array into the mouse genome while the second targets the repeat in a site specific manner into the homologous mouse gene. In the case of the fragile X $(CGG)_n$ triplet, little success had been achieved with the first approach; three reports of integrated transgenic $(CGG)_n$ repeats in the human premutation size range all report no instability *(213–215)*. The second approach has proven more successful. A recent report describes the insertion of a $(CGG)_{98}$ human derived triplet array into the mouse *FMR1* gene *(216)*. These mice are the first to show $(CGG)_n$ instability, with array length changes seen in 20% of transmissions and expansions of up to +6 triplets occurring in one generation. Although these changes are small compared to

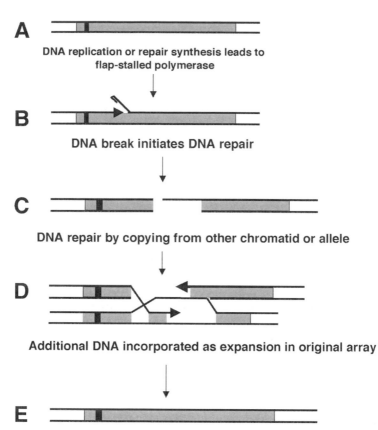

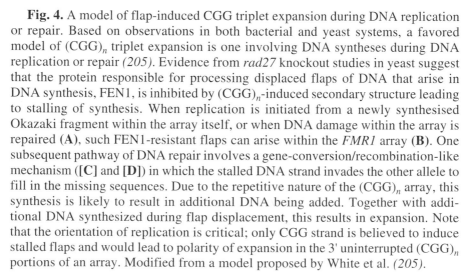

Fig. 4. A model of flap-induced CGG triplet expansion during DNA replication or repair. Based on observations in both bacterial and yeast systems, a favored model of $(CGG)_n$ triplet expansion is one involving DNA syntheses during DNA replication or repair *(205)*. Evidence from *rad27* knockout studies in yeast suggest that the protein responsible for processing displaced flaps of DNA that arise in DNA synthesis, FEN1, is inhibited by $(CGG)_n$-induced secondary structure leading to stalling of synthesis. When replication is initiated from a newly synthesised Okazaki fragment within the array itself, or when DNA damage within the array is repaired (**A**), such FEN1-resistant flaps can arise within the *FMR1* array (**B**). One subsequent pathway of DNA repair involves a gene-conversion/recombination-like mechanism ([**C**] and [**D**]) in which the stalled DNA strand invades the other allele to fill in the missing sequences. Due to the repetitive nature of the $(CGG)_n$ array, this synthesis is likely to result in additional DNA being added. Together with additional DNA synthesized during flap displacement, this results in expansion. Note that the orientation of replication is critical; only CGG strand is believed to induce stalled flaps and would lead to polarity of expansion in the 3' uninterrupted $(CGG)_n$ portions of an array. Modified from a model proposed by White et al. *(205)*.

the sizes of instability seen in the equivalent human premutation, it is hoped that breeding from these mice will eventually lead to a mouse carrying a large expansion array to fully model the fragile X progressive expansion and silencing stages observed in humans.

Studies of $(CTG)_n$ triplet array instability in mice have suggested that proteins involved in the repair of mismatched or mispaired DNA bases can influence levels of somatic instability. By crossing mice carrying $(CTG)_n$ arrays onto various knockout backgrounds it has been shown that somatic instability was prevented in MSH3P-deficient animals but was elevated in MSH6P-deficient animals *(217)*.

3. THE *FMR1* GENE: *FUNCTION*

The coding region of *FMR1* covers 38 kb and consists of 17 exons *(218)*. The gene is highly conserved, having homologues in other primates, mouse, rat, chicken, *Xenopus*, and *Drosophila*. The human gene is expressed predominantly as a 4-kb mRNA that translates into a polypeptide with 614 amino acids and a molecular weight of 69 kDa. Transcripts are found in most tissues including the brain, lung, placenta, kidney, and testes *(219)*. Analysis by *in situ* hybridization in human fetal brain shows *FMR1* is expressed in the proliferating and migrating cells of the nervous system, the retina, and several non-nervous tissues at 8–9 wk, and in nearly all differentiated structures. Expression is highest in cholinergic neurons and pyramidal neurons of the hippocampus at 25 wk *(220)*. Although little is known how many exist, the gene has alternative splice variants that can potentially be used to synthesize many protein isoforms *(221,222)*.

3.1. The FMRP Protein

The FMR protein has been found expressed in virtually every human tissue tested except for skeletal muscle, aorta, and heart, but it is particularly highly expressed in brain and testes, both tissues which are primarily affected in FXS. The protein is predominantly cytoplasmic but certain isoforms have been localized within the nucleus *(223,224)*. In the brain, FMRP is found in all neurons, being concentrated in the cell body, the proximal dendrites, and at synapses, with little present in the axons *(225,226)*. Little expression is seen in non-neuronal cells in the brain. High expression in the testes is found in embryonic primordial germ cells and in adult spematagonia that suggests that FMRP plays an important role in spermatogenesis *(227)*. It also provides some support for the selection hypotheses as to why the male germline does not carry the fragile X full mutation.

A comparison of the amino acid sequence of the FMRP protein with other proteins showed that it contains several predicted important RNA binding domains. One is the KH domain, found in many RNA binding proteins that bind various RNAs including mRNA. The second is an RGG box, found predominantly in nuclear and nucleolar RNA binding proteins. FMRP has been shown to bind RNA *(228)* and is known to selectively bind only a proportion of brain mRNA including its own mRNA *(229,230)*. FMRP has two KH domains, only one of which appears to bind RNA *(231)*. The importance of these domains is highlighted by the observation that the *FMR1* position 304 point mutation occurs in one of the two KH domains present in FMRP. This mutation, however, is within the second KH domain that does not appear to bind RNA but is consistent with the observation that the mutant protein does bind RNA *(230)*. The domain has been shown to have an altered structure *(232,233)* and is clearly critical to FMRP as its presence results in such a severe phenotype. Its precise effect is unknown but it appears to involve the process of protein dimerization. FMRP is known to form homooligomers under normal physiological conditions *(234)*. FMRP containing the point mutation at position 304 does not form dimers and was found not to associate with polyribosomes *(235)*. This suggests that the second KH domain might play a role in the dimerization process or that it is required for interaction with the polyribosome. As mutant FMRP appears to bind mRNA but cannot deliver these to the ribosome it suggests that the mutation might exert its effect through sequestration of couriered mRNAs. Similarly, the complete absence of FMRP, as occurs in FXS, most likely results in an alteration in mRNA delivery to the ribosomes. However, some compensatory mechanism must be in place as the phenotypic effects are not as severe as for the point mutation.

The RGG box is present within the C terminal portion of FMRP. Although the function of these motifs is unclear, they are often found associated with other RNA binding domains and are thought to facilitate the binding of other proteins *(236)*. Darnell et al. *(237)* and Schaeffer et al. *(238)* used the FMRP RGG box to identify target mRNAs and have shown convincingly that the motif binds specifically to mRNAs carrying a structure termed a G quartet. These form in G-rich RNA when two hairpins fold back on themselves and are very stable structures. According to Darnell et al., the specificity of FMRP binding is determined by the RGG box, not the KH domains. Darnell et al. identified 13 specific mRNAs carrying G quartet structures. Six of these are associated with synaptic function and three are involved with neuronal development.

3.1.1. Subcellular Localization and Shuttling Between Nucleus and Cytoplasm

FMRP is found associated with actively translating polyribosomes within the cell, the units of protein production and the association is maintained in an RNA-dependent manner via messenger ribonucleoprotein (mRNP) particles *(224,235)*. As the primary cellular lesion in FXS is within the central nervous system (CNS), the role of FMRP in neurons is of particular interest. In addition to normal cell body based polyribosomes, neurons have additional sites of protein translation at critical sites near synapses, termed synaptosomes. FMRP appears to be an important component of these and thus may play a role in active protein translation near the active site of neuronal connections within the brain *(see* Fig. 5*).*

As mentioned earlier, most cellular FMRP is cytoplasmic, but studies with artificially created isoforms suggested that it must also enter the nucleus. In experiments designed to unravel FMRP function, isoforms that lacked the nuclear export signal present in exon 14 accumulated within the nucleus *(224)*, suggesting that FMRP must normally enter the nucleus. Despite having no obvious homology to known nuclear import signals in other proteins, a region of the protein was found that served to direct FMRP import into the nucleus *(223,239)*. Interestingly, FMRP localized within the nucleus was shown to be phosphorylated, suggesting that this process may be regulated by intracellular signaling. Taken together, FMRP association with mRNA on sites of active translation and the presence of both nuclear import and export signals suggests that it is acting as some form of courier, entering the nucleus on phosphorylation and carrying mRNA from the nucleus to sites of translation. These sites could be within the cell body or possibly to more distant sites in the dendrites *(see* Fig. 5*).* Its exact role within the polyribosome is as yet unknown but recent reports suggest that in some cases it may act as an inhibitor of protein synthesis *(240,241)*.

3.1.2. FMRP and Dendritic Spine Maturation and Processing

Dendrites are the primary areas of synaptic connection between neurons. In response to stimulation, subsets of synapses undergo structural changes in shape and density as well as developing electrophysiological changes. In the dendrite are localized stores of up to 5% of all cellular mRNAs and local translation can occur in response to synaptic stimulation. FMRP has been localized to these polyribosome clusters in dendrites *(226)*, which suggest that it serves to transport mRNA from the nucleus to these sites of local translation. In addition, FMRP appears to be rapidly locally translated in

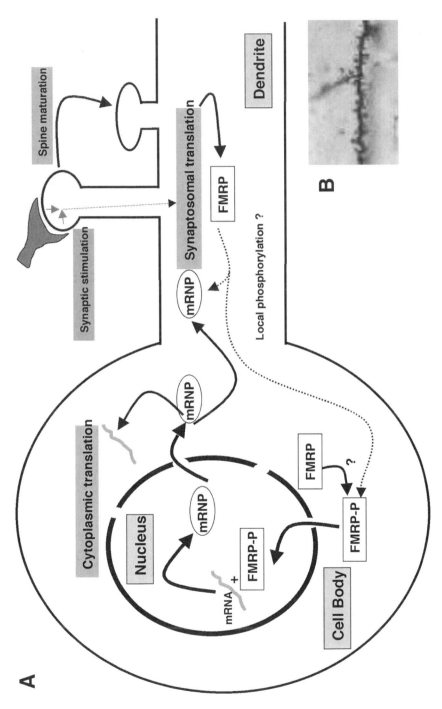

response to metabotrophic glutamate receptor activation *(242)*. It is tempting to speculate therefore that locally synthesized FMRP may return to the nucleus, possibly after local phosphorylation, to replenish local dendritic mRNA supplies *(see* Fig. 5). Clearly FMRP plays an important role in these dendritic polyribosomes and its function may well influence synaptic activity and plasticity. Loss of FMRP is associated with abnormally long and thin dendritic spines in both mouse knockout and human fragile X brain *(243)*. These changes appear to reflect a failure to adopt a mature size and shape, a process known as dendritic pruning. Pruning is a normal part of neuronal development in the brain in which dendrites are eliminated, a process that most likely requires appropriate protein synthesis. This contributes both to the establishment of a less mature neuronal network within the brain and also to a decreased dynamic synaptic response usually made in response to a cognitive task.

3.1.3. FMRP Is Part of a Larger Protein Family

Two *FMR1*-related genes have been identified that have very high amino acid homology with FMRP, FXR1P, and FXR2P *(244,245)*. As might be expected from such a high level of conservation, the proteins also bind RNA and appear to have similar properties to FMRP. They are also found in the mRNP particles and have a very similar pattern of expression to FMRP with high expression in the testis and neurons, although FXR1P is also highly expressed in skeletal muscle *(227,246)*. In testes, a slightly different expression profile is observed for the three proteins. FMRP and FXR1P are highly

---

Fig. 5. (*Opposite page*) Proposed shuttling function of FMRP: intracellular transport of mRNA to sites of translation and local translational regulation. (**A**) FMRP is proposed to act as shuttle protein between the nucleus and cytoplasm, interacting with various proteins and ribonuclear particles during this cycle. Its nuclear localization signal (NLS) allows it to enter the nucleus in the phosphorylated state where it is known to form part of the mRNP particle. Exit from the nucleus is mediated by exportin 1, wherein FMRP is found associated with polyribosomes. In neurons, FMRP is also found at sites of local translation near the base of dendritic spines and is synthesized locally in some spines on stimulation. This suggests that FMRP may act as a shuttle between the nucleus and these sites. FMRP may return to the nucleus, possibly directed by phosphorylation. As FMRP is also known to act as a translation repressor, its loss in FXS, or failure to oligomerize in the I304N FMRP, most likely results in disrupted polyribosome and synaptosome protein synthesis as well as altered mRNA transport. Dendritic spine maturation results in an altered morphology leading to shorter spines, a process that is known to involve microtubules and associated proteins. (**B**) *Inset* is a photograph of dendritic spines on golgi impregnated spiny neurons in chick hyperstriatum (×600). (Courtesy of Michael G. Stewart, Biological Sciences, Open University.)

expressed in fetal primordial germ cells *(227,246)* whereas FXR2P is expressed in interstitial cells. In adults, FMRP is expressed in immature spermatagonia whereas FXR1P is expressed in more advanced cells, suggesting that they might have overlapping but different functions. The presence of nuclear export and import signals suggests that they also shuttle into and out of the nucleus. FXR2P appears to shuttle between the cytoplasm and nucleolus *(247)*. Thus, it may well be that the FMR protein family shuttle into different nuclear compartments, presumably transporting different subsets of RNAs and are found in common only in mRNP complexes.

3.1.4. Interactions with Cellular Components: Clues to FMRP Function

3.1.4.1. CELLULAR mRNAs

As outlined earlier, FMRP has several RNA binding domains and its absence in FXS is predicted to lead to the misregulation or mislocalization of many cellular mRNAs. To identify these downstream targets of FMRP, Brown et al. have used microarrays to identify 432 mRNAs that bind to FMRP in the mouse brain and 251 human mRNAs that have an altered polyribosome profile in human fragile X cells *(248)*. More than 70% of the human mRNA contain G-quartet structures known to interact with the FMRP RGG box. Of these mRNAs, half were found at an elevated level and half were diminished in fragile X cells. Many of these mRNAs appear to have a neuronal function and one in particular, MAP1B appears to play an important role as an FMRP target. The significance of MAP1B became apparent in a study of the *Drosophila melanogaster* FMR1 homolog, *dfxr*. Both the *dfxr* null mutant and an overexpression mutant show synaptic structural defects that are accompanied by altered neurotransmission *(249)*. Studies of the MAP1B homologous gene, Futsch, suggest that *dfxr* is a translational repressor of the MAP1B mRNA *(250)*. The double null mutant for *dfxr* and MAP1B restores normal synaptic function and structure. This indicates that the levels of the microtubule-associated protein MAP1B, are regulated by FMRP binding to its mRNA. In the absence of FMRP, a resultant increased level of translation results in synaptic misfunction that is not seen in the absence of MAP1B.

3.1.4.2. CELLULAR PROTEINS

In addition to interacting with the FXRPs, FMRP also interacts with nucleolin *(251)*. NUFIP1, a nuclear RNA binding protein, as well as two additional proteins cytoplasmic CYFIP1 and CYFIP 2 have also been identified by two hybrid screens as interacting with FMRP *(252,253)*. NUFP1 interacts with the nuclear form of FMRP and CYFIP with the cytoplasmic form. CYFIP1 and CYFIP 2 also colocalize to synaptosomes. CYFIP1 does not interact with either FXR1 or FXR2, whereas CYFIP2 does. Interestingly, CYFIP1 is known to interact with the Rac1 GTPase which is known to play a role in the generation and maintenance of dendritic spines providing a functional link between FMRP and changes in dendritic spines.

The role of FMRP as a negative regulator of translation, as outlined in the case of MAP1B is further substantiated in studies of protein–protein interaction. Y box binding protein 1 (YB1) was identified in mouse as interacting with FMRP and is known to play a role in the regulation of protein translation *(254)*. A similar role for FMRP as a negative regulator of translation was also suggested from direct in vitro observations *(241)*. The failure of the I304N FMRP to act as a translation inhibitor suggests that the process of FMRP homooligomerization is critical in this process. As I304N FMRP is associated with FXS this provides further evidence that translation inhibition plays a central role in the synaptic changes in the disease.

Still outstanding are questions regarding the roles of FXR1P and FXR2P in the phenotype of fragile X individuals as all three proteins can interact with each other and carry mRNA within the cell. Levels of FXRPs in mice lacking FMRP and fragile X patients appear to be normal, which suggests that no gross compensatory up-regulation occurs *(255)*. FXR1 and FXR2, however, do not act as translation inhibitors. It may be that the resultant neuronal changes and deficits that arise in FXS arise only in a subset of cells in which the level of FMRP is critical and that other cells might be protected from the effects of altered mRNA transport by FXR1P and FXR2P.

4. THE *FMR1* KNOCKOUT MOUSE MODEL

4.1. Genetics and Biochemistry

An *fmr1* gene knockout mouse (*fmr1 ko*) was made by the Dutch–Belgian Fragile X Consortium (DBFXC) by a typical homologous recombination knockout strategy wherein all *fmr1* gene expression is destroyed *(256)*. This animal therefore represents a model for development in the complete absence of FMRP and as such would hopefully produce a pronounced phenotype in the animals. In fragile X individuals, some FMRP may be present before methylation silences *FMR1* transcription, depending on the size and concomitant translatability of the mRNA.

A physical analysis of the *fmr1 ko* mice found that macroorchidism was present as the mice aged and that this was associated with an increase in Sertoli cell proliferation *(256,257)*. As described earlier, these KO mice also show abnormal dendritic pruning in neurons in the CNS suggestive of arrested or delayed maturation. At the gross anatomic level, attempts to detect neuroanatomical differences as are seen in human fragile X patients using MRI have been unsuccessful *(258)*. A more detailed description of the cognitive and behavioral studies is described below but of fundamental importance has been the recognition that genetic differences between strains being studied can influence what phenotype is detected *(259)*. It is not known how these differences might also influence the neuroanatomical and biochemical studies that have been performed.

4.2. Cognitive–Behavioral Aspects of the ko Mouse Model

In an examination of various neurological functions and behavioral activities of the *fmr1 ko*, the DBFXC found that mice do not quite manifest the phenotype associated with FXS in humans. *Fmr1 ko* mice exhibit greater exploratory behavior than wild-type *(wt)* littermates and engage in greater motor activity. Using the Morris maze, the DBFXC also examined visual–spatial memory and found that for tasks related to associative processes, that is, latency to find a visible platform, *ko* and *wt* littermates perform equally well. On the other hand, on tasks that involve the use of distal cues, that is, latency to find a hidden platform, *wt* mice showed significantly shorter latencies during the reversal trial condition.

The results of the Morris maze component of the DBFXC study have been essentially replicated by others *(259–261)*. All studies show that both *fmr1 ko* and *wt* littermate controls exhibit significantly improved performances from one block of trials to the next, albeit without significant genotype differences. Even when the Morris maze is modified using an E-shaped configuration, the number of errors produced by *ko* and *wt* controls do not differ significantly *(260)*. Employing another variant of the Morris maze (the "plus" maze) Van Dam et al. examined escape latencies in *fmr1 ko* and *wt* littermate controls and found no significant differences between the two genotypes *(262)*. However, when they examined the proportion of correct trials, they found *fmr1 wt* mice performed significantly better during both the acquisition and reversed trial phases of the experiment.

Demonstration of significant differences in distal visual–spatial learning and memory often involve impairment of long-term potentiation (LTP) in the hippocampus *(263)*. As a result, Godfraind et al. examined LTP in *fmr1 ko* and *wt* mice but found no significant differences in the extracellular postsynaptic potentials between the two groups *(264)*.

Emotional behavior associated with FXS has also been investigated in the *fmr1 ko* mouse. In particular, early studies reported that anxiety and fearfulness were elevated in many individuals with the *FRAXA* mutation *(8,9)*. Paylor et al. demonstrated that conditioned fear is related to amygdala function in the rat *(265)*. Using the conditioned fear paradigm developed by Paylor et al., Paradee et al. examined conditioned fear in the *fmr1 ko* and *wt* littermate controls *(259)*. Curiously, this latter study found significantly lower contextual freezing in the *fmr1 ko* compared to controls. In another study using the same experimental paradigm, however, van Dam et al. also found no significant differences between *fmr1 ko* and *wt* littermate controls *(262)*. This latter study also employed an operant conditioning procedure to produce a conditioned emotional response (CER) in *fmr1 ko* and *wt* littermate controls, finding no significant genotype effects on response rate during the CER phase.

In their attempt to evaluate associative learning and memory in *fmr1 ko* and controls, Fisch et al. performed two experiments *(266)*. The first was used to establish whether ko mice were capable of acquiring and maintaining a bar press response in an operant conditioning environment. The second experiment related to the first examined visual and auditory short-term memory (STM). Moderate-to-severe deficits in both visual and auditory STM are observed in individuals with the *FRAXA* mutation. The second part of this study was designed to elicit how well animals make simple and complex auditory and visual discriminations. The results show that *fmr1 ko* mice acquire auditory and and visual discriminations faster than Fvb controls. Moreover, for the complex discrimination procedure, only *fmr1 ko* mice made the correct discrimination. Fvb controls responded at chance levels only. Since controls were not littermates, it was suggested that genetic strain differences may have played an important role in the outcome. Indeed, in their study, Paradee et al. compared 15th generation E129 *ko* males with E129/C57 *ko* and *wt* male crosses and noted significantly better performances in both *ko* and *wt* E129/C57 crosses compared to E129 *ko* mice *(259)*. Thus, genetic strain is an important factor in determining strengths and weaknesses in Morris maze performance. Strain differences between C57BJ and E129 *fmr1 ko* mice were also demonstrated by Dobkin et al. *(267)*.

To determine whether deficiencies in *fmr1 ko* mice could be rescued, Peier et al. inserted the human *FMR1* gene to a yeast artificial chromosome (YAC), then bred YAC transgenic mice with *FMR1 ko* mice and performed a wide variety of behavioral tests *(268)*. These researchers found that *fmr1 ko* mice show significantly more exploratory behavior than did *wt* littermate controls; and, that YAC *ko* and *wt* mice exhibited significantly less open field activity. As for anxiety-related measures, that is, center-to-total distance, *fmr1 ko* mice showed lower anxiety levels than either *wt* controls or YAC-rescued mice. Fear related startle responses were also lower in *fmr1 ko* mice compared to the other genotypes. In yet another demonstration of learning in the Morris maze, no significant differences in escape latency were observed among the four genotypes.

Taken together, these results suggest that the *fmr1 ko* mouse, at best, exhibits a subtle cognitive–behavioral phenotype. Although it is the case that not all murine knockout models express the genetic disorders associated with their human counterparts, there is evidence to suggest the that the *fmr1 ko* is not a true null mutant. Kosten and colleagues (Kosten, Alsobrook, Nguyen, Aramli, Regan, Lombroso, et al., *unpublished data*) have examined 12 male mice using a delayed matching to sample operant conditioning procedure. After the animals were killed, genotype results indicated eight mice were *kos* and 4 were *wt* littermate controls. However, Western blot analysis revealed that five of the eight knockouts produced FMRP. These results may explain why many researchers have been unable obtain significant differences between the putative genotypes.

A recent report describing a knockout of the mouse *fxr2* gene found no pathological differences in the brain or testis with the normal mouse but did describe a similarity in the *ko* behavioral phenotype that included hyperactivity and a decreased motor and skill learning using a rotarod test *(269)*. In addition the *fxr2 ko* also exhibited other behavioral abnormalities including less contextual conditioned fear and a decreased response to heat stimuli. These observations suggest a role for FXR2P in neuronal function within the CNS.

5. FUTURE RESEARCH AREAS

5.1. Diagnostics

In the last 10 years, thousands of families have been tested using DNA probes for expansions at the *FMR1* gene. Over these years the diagnostic boundaries have been refined and they continue to change. Whereas in previous years, we assumed that the full mutation was due to lack of *FMR1* mRNA, we now know that the lack of FMRP is a product of both methylation inhibition and protein translation suppression. Diagnoses of mosaic individuals will need to measure the amount of FMRP protein present. The FMRP antibody test described earlier will prove especially useful and may eventually replace DNA testing.

5.2. Genetic Treatment: Gene Delivery or Gene Reactivation?

Much interest has been generated by cellular models of gene reactivation. This is based on the observations that the absence of FMRP in fragile X individuals is determined by the lack of *FMR1* mRNA which, in turn, is determined by the methylation induced silencing. Thus, by attempting to reactivate the gene using chemical treatments in cell lines, *FMR1* mRNA production can be increased through the removal of methylation or inhibitory chromatin modifications. The drug 5-azacytidine, which induces gene demethylation by blocking the enzymes responsible for maintaining methylation, increased *FMR1* transcription in full mutation cells *(270)* and acted synergistically with a drug that modified local inhibitory chromatin and resulted in additional transcription *(271)*. However, as has been shown, even in the presence of the full mutation bearing mRNA, the effects of the $(CGG)_n$ repeat on protein translation is dramatic and suggests that gene reactivation would not produce any FMRP for larger full mutation length individuals. There are also questions regarding the toxicity of these drugs, although other drugs are being tested.

Another route for therapy might be to administer FMRP to the cells by gene delivery. Many problems exist with gene therapy based approaches including delivery to all cells in the brain, treating the appropriate developmental window and delivering the appropriate levels of FMRP protein. Evidence from overcorrective FMRP transgenic mice showed that abnormal phenotype can develop if too much FMRP is present *(268)*. In addition, the targeted decrease or increases in downstream targets of FMRP, such as MAP1B, might provide suitable candidate therapies.

REFERENCES

1. Lubs HA. A marker X chromosome. Am J Hum Genet 1969;21:231–44.
2. Martin JP, Bell J. A pedigree of mental defect showing X-linkage. J Neurol Psychiatry 1943;6:154–7.
3. Dunn HG, Renpenning H, Gerrard JW. Mental retardation as a sex-linked trait. Am J Ment Defic 1963;67.
4. Turner G, Till R, Daniel A. Marker X chromosomes, mental retardation and macro-orchidism. N Engl J Med 1978;299:1472.
5. Jacobs PA, Mayer M, Rudak E, et al. More on marker X chromosomes, mental retardation and macro-orchidism. N Engl J Med 1979;300:737–8.
6. Sutherland GR, Ashforth PL. X-linked mental retardation with macro-orchidism and the fragile site at Xq 27 or 28. Hum Genet 1979;48:117–20.
7. Howard-Peebles PN, Stoddard GR. X-linked mental retardation with macro-orchidism and marker X chromosomes. Hum Genet 1979;50:247–51.
8. Opitz JM, Sutherland GR. Conference report: International Workshop on the fragile X and X-linked mental retardation. Am J Med Genet 1984;17:5–94.
9. Hagerman RJ, McBogg PM. The fragile X syndrome: diagnosis, biochemistry, intervention. Denver, CO: Spectra, 1983.

10. Partington MW. The fragile X syndrome II: preliminary data on growth and development in males. Am J Med Genet 1984;17:175–94.
11. Brondum Nielsen K. Diagnosis of the fragile X syndrome (Martin-Bell syndrome). Clinical findings in 27 males with the fragile site at Xq28. J Ment Defic Res 1983;27:211–26.
12. Fryns JP, Jacobs J, Kleczkowska A, van den Berghe H. The psychological profile of the fragile X syndrome. Clin Genet 1984;25:131–4.
13. Thake A, Todd J, Bundey S, Webb T. Is it possible to make a clinical diagnosis of the fragile X syndrome in a boy? Arch Dis Child 1985;60:1001–7.
14. Varley CK, Holm VA, Eren MO. Cognitive and psychiatric variability in three brothers with fragile X syndrome. J Dev Behav Pediatr 1985;6:87–90.
15. Hagerman R, Kemper M, Hudson M. Learning disabilities and attentional problems in boys with the fragile X syndrome. Am J Dis Child 1985;139:674–8.
16. Goldfine PE, McPherson PM, Hardesty VA, Heath GA, Beauregard LJ, Baker AA. Fragile-X chromosome associated with primary learning disability. J Am Acad Child Adolesc Psychiatry 1987;26:589–92.
17. Theobald TM, Hay DA, Judge C. Individual variation and specific cognitive deficits in the fra(X) syndrome. Am J Med Genet 1987;28:1–11.
18. Staley LW, Hull CE, Mazzocco MM, et al. Molecular-clinical correlations in children and adults with fragile X syndrome. Am J Dis Child 1993;147:723–6.
19. Richards BW, Sylvester PE, Brooker C. Fragile X-linked mental retardation: the Martin-Bell syndrome. J Ment Defic Res 1981; 25 Pt 4:253–6.
20. Rhoads FA. Fragile-X syndrome in Hawaii: a summary of clinical experience. Am J Med Genet 1984;17:209–14.
21. Froster-Iskenius U, Schulze A, Schwinger E. Transmission of the marker X syndrome trait by unaffected males: conclusions from studies of large families. Hum Genet 1984;67:419–27.
22. Howard-Peebles PN, Friedman JM. Unaffected carrier males in families with fragile X syndrome. Am J Hum Genet 1985;37:956–64.
23. Madison LS, George C, Moeschler JB. Cognitive functioning in the fragile-X syndrome: a study of intellectual, memory and communication skills. J Ment Defic Res 1986;30:129–48.
24. Veenema H, Carpenter NJ, Bakker E, Hofker MH, Ward AM, Pearson PL. The fragile X syndrome in a large family. III. Investigations on linkage of flanking DNA markers with the fragile site Xq27. J Med Genet 1987; 24:413–21.
25. Curfs LM, Borghgraef M, Wiegers A, Schreppers-Tijdink GA, Fryns JP. Strengths and weaknesses in the cognitive profile of fra(X) patients. Clin Genet 1989;36:405–10.
26. Dykens EM, Hodapp RM, Leckman JF. Strengths and weaknesses in the intellectual functioning of males with fragile X syndrome. Am J Ment Defic 1987;92:234–6.
27. Kemper MB, Hagerman RJ, Altshul-Stark D. Cognitive profiles of boys with the fragile X syndrome. Am J Med Genet 1988;30:191–200.
28. Chudley A, Shepel A, McGgahey E, Knoll J, Gerrard JW. Behavioral phenotype: In Conference report: International Workshop on the Fragile X and X-linked Mental Retardation. Am J Med Genet 1984;17:5–94.

29. Wolff PH, Gardner J, Paccla J, Lappen J. The greeting behavior of fragile X males. Am J Ment Retard 1989;93:406–11.

30. Reiss AL, Freund L. Behavioral phenotype of fragile X syndrome: DSM-III-R autistic behavior in male children. Am J Med Genet 1992;43:35–46.

31. Brown WT, Jenkins EC, Friedman E, et al. Autism is associated with the fragile-X syndrome. J Autism Dev Disord 1982;12:303–8.

32. Meryash DL, Szymanski LS, Gerald PS. Infantile autism associated with the fragile-X syndrome. J Autism Dev Disord 1982;12:295–301.

33. Jorgensen OS, Nielsen KB, Isager T, Mouridsen SE. Fragile X-chromosome among child psychiatric patients with disturbances of language and social relationships. A pilot study. Acta Psychiatr Scand 1984;70:510–4.

34. Venter PA, Op't Hof J, Coetzee DJ. The Martin-Bell syndrome in South Africa. Am J Med Genet 1986;23:597–610.

35. Blomquist HK, Bohman M, Edvinsson SO, et al. Frequency of the fragile X syndrome in infantile autism. A Swedish multicenter study. Clin Genet 1985;27:113–7.

36. Fisch GS. Is autism associated with the fragile X syndrome? Am J Med Genet 1992; 43:47–55.

37. Newall K, Sanborn B, Hagerman R. Speech and language dysfunction in the fragile X syndrome. In: R.J. Hagerman, McBogg PM, eds. The fragile X syndrome. Dillon, CO: Spectra, 1983.

38. Paul R, Leckman J, White B. Report on speech and language in fragile X, International Workshop on the Fragile X and X-linked Mental Retardation, Am J Med Genet 1984;17:5–94.

39. Wolf-Schein EG, Sudhalter V, Cohen IL, et al. Speech-language and the fragile X syndrome: initial findings. ASHA 1987;29:35–8.

40. Sudhalter V, Maranion M, Brooks P. Expressive semantic deficit in the productive language of males with fragile X syndrome. Am J Med Genet 1992;43:65–71.

41. Fisch GS, Holden JJ, Carpenter NJ, et al. Age-related language characteristics of children and adolescents with fragile X syndrome. Am J Med Genet 1999;83:253–6.

42. Roberts JE, Mirrett P, Burchinal M. Receptive and expressive communication development of young males with fragile X syndrome. Am J Ment Retard 2001;106:216–30.

43. Sparrow SS, Balla DA, Cicchetti DV. Vineland Adaptive Behavior Scales. Circle Pines, MN: American Guidance Service, 1984.

44. Dykens E, Leckman J, Paul R, Watson M. Cognitive, behavioral, and adaptive functioning in fragile X and non-fragile X retarded men. J Autism Dev Disord 1988;18:41–52.

45. Kerby DS, Dawson BL. Autistic features, personality, and adaptive behavior in males with the fragile X syndrome and no autism. Am J Ment Retard 1994;98:455–62.

46. Dykens EM, Hodapp RM, Leckman JF. Adaptive and maladaptive functioning of institutionalized and noninstitutionalized fragile X males. J Am Acad Child Adolesc Psychiatry 1989;28:427–30.

47. Cohen IL, Fisch GS, Sudhalter V, et al. Social gaze, social avoidance, and repetitive behavior in fragile X males: a controlled study. Am J Ment Retard 1988;92:436–46.
48. Wiegers AM, Curfs LM, Vermeer EL, Fryns JP. Adaptive behavior in the fragile X syndrome: profile and development. Am J Med Genet 1993;47:216–20.
49. Dykens EM, Hodapp RM, Ort SI, Leckman JF. Trajectory of adaptive behavior in males with fragile X syndrome. J Autism Dev Disord 1993;23:135–45.
50. Dykens E, Ort S, Cohen I, et al. Trajectories and profiles of adaptive behavior in males with fragile X syndrome: multicenter studies. J Autism Dev Disord 1996;26:287–301.
51. Fisch GS, Simensen R, Tarleton J, et al. Longitudinal study of cognitive abilities and adaptive behavior levels in fragile X males: a prospective multicenter analysis. Am J Med Genet 1996;64:356–61.
52. Fisch GS, Carpenter N, Holden JJ, et al. Longitudinal changes in cognitive and adaptive behavior in fragile X females: a prospective multicenter analysis. Am J Med Genet 1999;83:308–12.
53. Bailey DB, Jr., Hatton DD, Skinner M. Early developmental trajectories of males with fragile X syndrome. Am J Ment Retard 1998;103:29–39.
54. Einfeld SL, Tonge BJ, Florio T. Behavioural and emotional disturbance in fragile X syndrome. Am J Med Genet 1994;51:386–91.
55. Einfeld S, Tonge B, Turner G. Longitudinal course of behavioral and emotional problems in fragile X syndrome. Am J Med Genet 1999;87:436–9.
56. Fisch GS, Carpenter NJ, Holden JJ, et al. Longitudinal assessment of adaptive and maladaptive behaviors in fragile X males: growth, development, and profiles. Am J Med Genet 1999;83:257–63.
57. Vieregge P, Froster-Iskenius U. Clinico-neurological investigations in the fra(X) form of mental retardation. J Neurol 1989;236:85–92.
58. Crowe SF, Hay DA. Neuropsychological dimensions of the fragile X syndrome: support for a non-dominant hemisphere dysfunction hypothesis. Neuropsychologia 1990;28:9–16.
59. Reiss AL, Aylward E, Freund LS, Joshi PK, Bryan RN. Neuroanatomy of fragile X syndrome: the posterior fossa. Ann Neurol 1991;29:26–32.
60. Reiss AL, Freund L, Tseng JE, Joshi PK. Neuroanatomy in fragile X females: the posterior fossa. Am J Hum Genet 1991;49:279–88.
61. Kwon H, Menon V, Eliez S, et al. Functional neuroanatomy of visuospatial working memory in fragile X syndrome: relation to behavioral and molecular measures. Am J Psychiatry 2001;158:1040–51.
62. Hagerman R, Smith ACM. The heterozygous female. In: Hagerman RJ, McBogg PM, eds. The fragile X syndrome: diagnosis, biochemistry, intervention. Dillon, CO: Spectra, 1983.
63. Loesch DZ, Hay DA. Clinical features and reproductive patterns in fragile X female heterozygotes. J Med Genet 1988;25:407–14.
64. Hagerman R, Smith ACM, Mariner R. Clinical features of the fragile X syndrome. In: Hagerman RJ, McBogg PM, eds. The fragile X syndrome: diagnosis, biochemistry, intervention. Denver, CO: Spectra, 1983.

65. Miezejeski CM, Jenkins EC, Hill AL, Wisniewski K, Brown WT. Verbal vs. nonverbal ability, fragile X syndrome, and heterozygous carriers. Am J Hum Genet 1984;36:227–9.

66. Miezejeski CM, Jenkins EC, Hill AL, Wisniewski K, French JH, Brown WT. A profile of cognitive deficit in females from fragile X families. Neuropsychologia 1986;24:405–9.

67. Kemper MB, Hagerman RJ, Ahmad RS, Mariner R. Cognitive profiles and the spectrum of clinical manifestations in heterozygous fra (X) females. Am J Med Genet 1986;23:139–56.

68. Wolff PH, Gardner J, Lappen J, Paccia J, Mcryash D. Variable expression of the fragile X syndrome in heterozygous females of normal intelligence. Am J Med Genet 1988;30:213–25.

69. Fisch GS. What is associated with the fragile X syndrome? Am J Med Genet 1993;48:112–21.

70. Mazzocco MM, Hagerman RJ, Cronister-Silverman A, Pennington BF. Specific frontal lobe deficits among women with the fragile X gene. J Am Acad Child Adolesc Psychiatry 1992;31:1141–8.

71. Steyaert J, Borghgraef M, Gaulthier C, Fryns JP, Van den Berghe H. Cognitive profile in adult, normal intelligent female fragile X carriers. Am J Med Genet 1992;43:116–9.

72. Steyaert J, Borghgraef M, Fryns JP. Apparently enhanced visual information processing in female fragile X carriers: preliminary findings. Am J Med Genet 1994;51:374–7.

73. Reiss AL, Feinstein C, Toomey KE, Goldsmith B, Rosenbaum K, Caruso MA. Psychiatric disability associated with the fragile X chromosome. Am J Med Genet 1986;23:393–401.

74. Hagerman RJ, Sobesky WE. Psychopathology in fragile X syndrome. Am J Orthopsychiatry 1989;59:142–52.

75. Reiss AL, Hagerman RJ, Vinogradov S, Abrams M, King RJ. Psychiatric disability in female carriers of the fragile X chromosome. Arch Gen Psychiatry 1988;45:25–30.

76. Borghgraef M, Fryns JP, van den Berghe H. The female and the fragile X syndrome: data on clinical and psychological findings in 7 fra(X) carriers. Clin Genet 1990;37:341–6.

77. Freund LS, Reiss AL, Hagerman R, Vinogradov S. Chromosome fragility and psychopathology in obligate female carriers of the fragile X chromosome. Arch Gen Psychiatry 1992;49:54–60.

78. Freund LS, Reiss AL, Abrams MT. Psychiatric disorders associated with fragile X in the young female. Pediatrics 1993;91:321–9.

79. Hull C, Hagerman RJ. A study of the physical, behavioral, and medical phenotype, including anthropometric measures, of females with fragile X syndrome. Am J Dis Child 1993;147:1236–41.

80. Sobesky WE, Pennington BF, Porter D, Hull CE, Hagerman RJ. Emotional and neurocognitive deficits in fragile X. Am J Med Genet 1994;51:378–85.

81. Lachiewicz AM, Dawson DV. Behavior problems of young girls with fragile X syndrome: factor scores on the Conners' Parent's Questionnaire. Am J Med Genet 1994;51:364–9.

82. Reiss AL, Freund LS, Baumgardner TL, Abrams MT, Denckla MB. Contribution of the FMR1 gene mutation to human intellectual dysfunction. Nat Genet 1995;11:331–4.

83. Jacobs PA, Glover TW, Mayer M, et al. X-linked mental retardation: a study of 7 families. Am J Med Genet 1980;7:471–89.

84. Sutherland GR, Hecht F. Fragile sites on human chromosomes. New York: Oxford University Press, 1985.

85. Lachiewicz AM, Gullion CM, Spiridigliozzi GA, Aylsworth AS. Declining IQs of young males with the fragile X syndrome. Am J Ment Retard 1987;92:272–8.

86. Borghgraef M, Fryns JP, Dielkens A, Pyck K, Van den Berghe H. Fragile (X) syndrome: a study of the psychological profile in 23 prepubertal patients. Clin Genet 1987;32:179–86.

87. Dykens EM, Hodapp RM, Ort S, Finucane B, Shapiro LR, Leckman JF. The trajectory of cognitive development in males with fragile X syndrome. J Am Acad Child Adolesc Psychiatry 1989;28:422–6.

88. Hagerman RJ, Schreiner RA, Kemper MB, Wittenberger MD, Zahn B, Habicht K. Longitudinal IQ changes in fragile X males. Am J Med Genet 1989;33:513–8.

89. Fisch GS, Shapiro LR, Simensen R, et al. Longitudinal changes in IQ among fragile X males: clinical evidence of more than one mutation? Am J Med Genet 1992;43:28–34.

90. Hodapp RM, Dykens EM, Hagerman RJ, Schreiner R, Lachiewicz AM, Leckman JF. Developmental implications of changing trajectories of IQ in males with fragile X syndrome. J Am Acad Child Adolesc Psychiatry 1990;29:214–9.

91. Hay DA. Does IQ decline with age in fragile-X? A methodological critique. Am J Med Genet 1994;51:358–63.

92. Thorndike RL, Hagen EP, Sattler JM. The Stanford-Binet Intelligence Scale. Chicago, IL: Riverside, 1986.

93. Sutherland GR. Fragile sites on human chromosomes: demonstration of their dependence on the type of tissue culture medium. Science 1977;197:265–6.

94. de Vries BB, van den Ouweland AM, Mohkamsing S, et al. Screening and diagnosis for the fragile X syndrome among the mentally retarded: an epidemiological and psychological survey. Collaborative Fragile X Study Group. Am J Hum Genet 1997;61:660–7.

95. Turner G, Webb T, Wake S, Robinson H. Prevalence of fragile X syndrome. Am J Med Genet 1996;64:196–7.

96. Sherman SL, Jacobs PA, Morton NE, et al. Further segregation analysis of the fragile X syndrome with special reference to transmitting males. Hum Genet 1985;69:289–99.

97. Bell MV, Hirst MC, Nakahori Y, et al. Physical mapping across the fragile X: hypermethylation and clinical expression of the fragile X syndrome. Cell 1991; 64:861–6.

98. Vincent A, Heitz D, Petit C, Kretz C, Oberle I, Mandel JL. Abnormal pattern detected in fragile-X patients by pulsed-field gel electrophoresis. Nature 1991;349:624–6.

99. Oberle I, Rousseau F, Heitz D, et al. Instability of a 550-base pair DNA segment and abnormal methylation in fragile X syndrome. Science 1991;252:1097-102.

100. Yu S, Pritchard M, Kremer E, et al. Fragile X genotype characterized by an unstable region of DNA. Science 1991;252:1179–81.

101. Verkerk AJ, Pieretti M, Sutcliffe JS, et al. Identification of a gene (FMR-1) containing a CGG repeat coincident with a breakpoint cluster region exhibiting length variation in fragile X syndrome. Cell 1991;65:905–14.

102. Sutcliffe JS, Nelson DL, Zhang F, et al. DNA methylation represses FMR-1 transcription in fragile X syndrome. Hum Mol Genet 1992;1:397–400.

103. Hirst MC. FMR1 triplet arrays: paying the price for perfection. J Med Genet 1995;32:761–3.

104. Fu YH, Kuhl DP, Pizzuti A, et al. Variation of the CGG repeat at the fragile X site results in genetic instability: resolution of the Sherman paradox. Cell 1991;67:1047–58.

105. Pembrey ME, Barnicoat AJ, Carmichael B, Bobrow M, Turner G. An assessment of screening strategies for fragile X syndrome in the UK. Health Technol Assess 2001;5:1–95.

106. Hirst M, Grewal P, Flannery A, et al. Two new cases of FMR1 deletion associated with mental impairment. Am J Hum Genet 1995;56:67–74.

107. Wohrle D, Kotzot D, Hirst MC, et al. A microdeletion of less than 250 kb, including the proximal part of the FMR-I gene and the fragile-X site, in a male with the clinical phenotype of fragile-X syndrome. Am J Hum Genet 1992;51:299–306.

108. Moore SJ, Strain L, Cole GF, Miedzybrodzka Z, Kelly KF, Dean JC. Fragile X syndrome with FMR1 and FMR2 deletion. J Med Genet 1999;36:565–6.

109. Garcia Arocena D, de Diego Y, Oostra BA, Willemsen R, Mirta Rodriguez M. A fragile X case with an amplification/deletion mosaic pattern. Hum Genet 2000;106:366–9.

110. Tarleton J, Richie R, Schwartz C, Rao K, Aylsworth AS, Lachiewicz A. An extensive de novo deletion removing FMR1 in a patient with mental retardation and the fragile X syndrome phenotype. Hum Mol Genet 1993;2:1973–4.

111. Hammond LS, Macias MM, Tarleton JC, Shashidhar Pai G. Fragile X syndrome and deletions in FMR1: new case and review of the literature. Am J Med Genet 1997;72:430–4.

112. Wiegers AM, Curfs LM, Meijer H, Oostra B, Fryns JP. A deletion of 1.6 Kb proximal to the CGG repeat of the FMR1 gene causes fragile X-like psychological features. Genet Couns 1994;5:377–80.

113. de Graaff E, Rouillard P, Willems PJ, Smits AP, Rousseau F, Oostra BA. Hotspot for deletions in the CGG repeat region of FMR1 in fragile X patients. Hum Mol Genet 1995;4:45–9.

114. Eberhart DE, Warren ST. Nuclease sensitivity of permeabilized cells confirms altered chromatin formation at the fragile X locus. Somat Cell Mol Genet 1996;22:435–41.

115. De Boulle K, Verkerk AJ, Reyniers E, et al. A point mutation in the FMR-1 gene associated with fragile X mental retardation. Nat Genet 1993;3:31–5.

116. Brown WT, Nolin S, Houck G Jr, et al. Prenatal diagnosis and carrier screening for fragile X by PCR. Am J Med Genet 1996;64:191–5.

117. Sutherland GR, Gedeon A, Kornman L, et al. Prenatal diagnosis of fragile X syndrome by direct detection of the unstable DNA sequence. N Engl J Med 1991;325:1720–2.

118. Kallinen J, Heinonen S, Mannermaa A, Ryynanen M. Prenatal diagnosis of fragile X syndrome and the risk of expansion of a premutation. Clin Genet 2000;58:111–5.

119. Hirst. Prenatal diagnosis of fragile X syndrome. Lancet 1991;338:956–8.

120. Willemsen R, Anar B, Otero YD, et al. Noninvasive test for fragile X syndrome, using hair root analysis. Am J Hum Genet 1999;65:98–103.

121. Willemsen R, Smits A, Mohkamsing S, et al. Rapid antibody test for diagnosing fragile X syndrome: a validation of the technique. Hum Genet 1997;99:308–11.

122. Willemsen R, Anar B, De Diego Otero Y, et al. Noninvasive test for fragile X syndrome, using hair root analysis. Am J Hum Genet 1999;65:98–103.

123. Willemsen R, Oostra BA. FMRP detection assay for the diagnosis of the fragile X syndrome. Am J Med Genet 2000;97:183–8.

124. Fisch GS, Silverman W, Jenkins EC. Genetic and other factors that contribute to variability in cytogenetic expression in fragile X males. Am J Med Genet 1991;38:404–7.

125. Fisch GS, Fryns JP. Factors which contribute to cytogenetic frequency of expression in families of fragile X females. Am J Med Genet 1992;43:142–8.

126. Abrams MT, Reiss AL, Freund LS, Baumgardner TL, Chase GA, Denckla MB. Molecular–neurobehavioral associations in females with the fragile X full mutation. Am J Med Genet 1994;51:317–27.

127. Kolehmainen K, Karant Y. Modeling methylation and IQ scores in fragile X females and mosaic males. Am J Med Genet 1994;51:328–38.

128. Hansen RS, Gartler SM, Scott CR, Chen SH, Laird CD. Methylation analysis of CGG sites in the CpG island of the human FMR1 gene. Hum Mol Genet 1992;1:571–8.

129. Pieretti M, Zhang FP, Fu YH, et al. Absence of expression of the FMR-1 gene in fragile X syndrome. Cell 1991;66:817–22.

130. Coffee B, Zhang F, Warren ST, Reines D. Acetylated histones are associated with FMR1 in normal but not fragile X-syndrome cells. Nat Genet 1999;22:98–101.

131. Stoger R, Kajimura TM, Brown WT, Laird CD. Epigenetic variation illustrated by DNA methylation patterns of the fragile-X gene FMR1. Hum Mol Genet 1997;6:1791–801.

132. Genc B, Muller-Hartmann H, Zeschnigk M, et al. Methylation mosaicism of 5'-(CGG)(n)-3' repeats in fragile X, premutation and normal individuals. Nucleic Acids Res 2000;28:2141–52.

133. Schwemmle S, de Graaff E, Deissler H, et al. Characterization of FMR1 promoter elements by in vivo-footprinting analysis. Am J Hum Genet 1997;60:1354–62.

134. Tassone F, Longshore J, Zunich J, Steinbach P, Salat U, Taylor AK. Tissue-specific methylation differences in a fragile X premutation carrier. Clin Genet 1999; 55:346–51.

135. Wohrle D, Hirst MC, Kennerknecht I, Davies KE, Steinbach P. Genotype mosaicism in fragile X fetal tissues. Hum Genet 1992;89:114–6.

136. Tassone F, Hagerman RJ, Taylor AK, Gane LW, Godfrey TE, Hagerman PJ. Elevated levels of FMR1 mRNA in carrier males: a new mechanism of involvement in the fragile-X syndrome. Am J Hum Genet 2000;66:6–15.

137. Tassone F, Hagerman RJ, Loesch DZ, Lachiewicz A, Taylor AK, Hagerman PJ. Fragile X males with unmethylated, full mutation trinucleotide repeat expansions have elevated levels of FMR1 messenger RNA. Am J Med Genet 2000;94:232–6.

138. Kenneson A, Zhang F, Hagedorn CH, Warren ST. Reduced FMRP and increased FMR1 transcription is proportionally associated with CGG repeat number in intermediate-length and premutation carriers. Hum Mol Genet 2001;10:1449–54.

139. Feng Y, Zhang F, Lokey LK, et al. Translational suppression by trinucleotide repeat expansion at FMR1. Science 1995;268:731–4.

140. Mankodi A, Urbinati CR, Yuan QP, et al. Muscleblind localizes to nuclear foci of aberrant RNA in myotonic dystrophy types 1 and 2. Hum Mol Genet 2001;10:2165–70.

141. Savkur RS, Philips AV, Cooper TA. Aberrant regulation of insulin receptor alternative splicing is associated with insulin resistance in myotonic dystrophy. Nat Genet 2001;29:40–7.

142. Tassone F, Hagerman RJ, Taylor AK, Hagerman PJ. A majority of fragile X males with methylated, full mutation alleles have significant levels of FMR1 messenger RNA. J Med Genet 2001;38:453–6.

143. Schwartz C, Fitch N, Phelan MC, Richer CL, Stevenson R. Two sisters with a distal deletion at the Xq26/Xq27 interface: DNA studies indicate that the gene locus for factor IX is present. Hum Genet 1987;76:54–7.

144. Bates A, Howard PJ. Distal long arm deletions of the X chromosome and ovarian failure. J Med Genet 1990;27:722–3.

145. Radhakrishna U, Shah VC, Highland HN, Chinoy NJ, Sheth FJ. A triple-X female with long arm deletion of one of the X-chromosomes associated with primary amenorrhoea: 47,XX, +del(X) (q27.3). Ann Genet 1991;34:40–3.

146. Cronister A, Schreiner R, Wittenberger M, Amiri K, Harris K, Hagerman RJ. Heterozygous fragile X female: historical, physical, cognitive, and cytogenetic features. Am J Med Genet 1991;38:269–74.

147. Schwartz CE, Dean J, Howard-Peebles PN, et al. Obstetrical and gynecological complications in fragile X carriers: a multicenter study. Am J Med Genet 1994;51:400–2.

148. Conway GS, Hettiarachchi S, Murray A, Jacobs PA. Fragile X premutations in familial premature ovarian failure. Lancet 1995;346:309–10.

149. Partington MW, Moore DY, Turner GM. Confirmation of early menopause in fragile X carriers. Am J Med Genet 1996;64:370–2.

150. Allingham-Hawkins DJ, Babul-Hirji R, Chitayat D, et al. Fragile X premutation is a significant risk factor for premature ovarian failure: the International Collaborative POF in Fragile X study—preliminary data. Am J Med Genet 1999;83:322–5.
151. Marozzi A, Vegetti W, Manfredini E, et al. Association between idiopathic premature ovarian failure and fragile X premutation. Hum Reprod 2000;15:197–202.
152. Sobesky WE, Hull CE, Hagerman RJ. Symptoms of schizotypal personality disorder in fragile X women. J Am Acad Child Adolesc Psychiatry 1994; 33:247–55.
153. Murray A, Webb J, Grimley S, Conway G, Jacobs P. Studies of *FRAXA* and FRAXE in women with premature ovarian failure. J Med Genet 1998; 35:637–40.
154. Hundscheid RD, Sistermans EA, Thomas CM, et al. Imprinting effect in premature ovarian failure confined to paternally inherited fragile X premutations. Am J Hum Genet 2000;66:413–8.
155. Murray A, Ennis S, Morton N. No evidence for parent of origin influencing premature ovarian failure in fragile X premutation carriers. Am J Hum Genet 2000;67:253–4; discussion 256–8.
156. Vianna-Morgante AM, Costa SS. Premature ovarian failure is associated with maternally and paternally inherited premutation in Brazilian families with fragile X. Am J Hum Genet 2000;67:254–5; discussion 256–8.
157. Hirst MC, Grewal PK, Davies KE. Precursor arrays for triplet repeat expansion at the fragile X locus. Hum Mol Genet 1994;3:1553–60.
158. Snow K, Doud LK, Hagerman R, Pergolizzi RG, Erster SH, Thibodeau SN. Analysis of a CGG sequence at the FMR-1 locus in fragile X families and in the general population. Am J Hum Genet 1993;53:1217–28.
159. Snow K, Tester DJ, Kruckeberg KE, Schaid DJ, Thibodeau SN. Sequence analysis of the fragile X trinucleotide repeat: implications for the origin of the fragile X mutation. Hum Mol Genet 1994;3:1543–51.
160. Zhong N, Yang W, Dobkin C, Brown WT. Fragile X gene instability: anchoring AGGs and linked microsatellites. Am J Hum Genet 1995;57:351–61.
161. Kunst CB, Warren ST. Cryptic and polar variation of the fragile X repeat could result in predisposing normal alleles. Cell 1994;77:853–61.
162. Eichler EE, Holden JJ, Popovich BW, et al. Length of uninterrupted CGG repeats determines instability in the FMR1 gene. Nat Genet 1994;8:88–94.
163. Kunst CB, Leeflang EP, Iber JC, Arnheim N, Warren ST. The effect of FMR1 CGG repeat interruptions on mutation frequency as measured by sperm typing. J Med Genet 1997;34:627–31.
164. Crawford DC, Wilson B, Sherman SL. Factors involved in the initial mutation of the fragile X CGG repeat as determined by sperm small pool PCR. Hum Mol Genet 2000;9:2909–18.
165. Oudet C, von Koskull H, Nordstrom AM, Peippo M, Mandel JL. Striking founder effect for the fragile X syndrome in Finland. Eur J Hum Genet 1993;1:181–9.

166. Buyle S, Reyniers E, Vits L, et al. Founder effect in a Belgian–Dutch fragile X population. Hum Genet 1993;92:269–72.

167. Hirst MC, Knight SJ, Christodoulou Z, Grewal PK, Fryns JP, Davies KE. Origins of the fragile X syndrome mutation. J Med Genet 1993;30:647–50.

168. Richards RI, Holman K, Kozman H, et al. Fragile X syndrome: genetic localisation by linkage mapping of two microsatellite repeats FRAXAC1 and FRAXAC2 which immediately flank the fragile site. J Med Genet 1991; 28:818–23.

169. Macpherson JN, Curtis G, Crolla JA, et al. Unusual (CGG)n expansion and recombination in a family with fragile X and DiGeorge syndrome. J Med Genet 1995;32:236–9.

170. Wohrle D, Salat U, Glaser D, et al. Unusual mutations in high functioning fragile X males: apparent instability of expanded unmethylated CGG repeats. J Med Genet 1998;35:103–11.

171. Reyniers E, Vits L, De Boulle K, et al. The full mutation in the FMR-1 gene of male fragile X patients is absent in their sperm. Nat Genet 1993;4:143–6.

172. Salat U, Bardoni B, Wohrle D, Steinbach P. Increase of FMRP expression, raised levels of FMR1 mRNA, and clonal selection in proliferating cells with unmethylated fragile X repeat expansions: a clue to the sex bias in the transmission of full mutations? J Med Genet 2000;37:842–50.

173. Malter HE, Iber JC, Willemsen R, et al. Characterization of the full fragile X syndrome mutation in fetal gametes. Nat Genet 1997;15:165–9.

174. Wohrle D, Hennig I, Vogel W, Steinbach P. Mitotic stability of fragile X mutations in differentiated cells indicates early post-conceptional trinucleotide repeat expansion [see comments]. Nat Genet 1993;4:140–2.

175. Devys D, Biancalana V, Rousseau F, Boue J, Mandel JL, Oberle I. Analysis of full fragile X mutations in fetal tissues and monozygotic twins indicate that abnormal methylation and somatic heterogeneity are established early in development. Am J Med Genet 1992;43:208–16.

176. Moutou C, Vincent MC, Biancalana V, Mandel JL. Transition from premutation to full mutation in fragile X syndrome is likely to be prezygotic. Hum Mol Genet 1997;6:971–9.

177. Liquori CL, Ricker K, Moseley ML, et al. Myotonic dystrophy type 2 caused by a CCTG expansion in intron 1 of ZNF9. Science 2001;293:864–7.

178. Matsuura T, Yamagata T, Burgess DL, et al. Large expansion of the ATTCT pentanucleotide repeat in spinocerebellar ataxia type 10. Nat Genet 2000;26:191–4.

179. Ashizawa T, Dubel JR, Harati Y. Somatic instability of CTG repeat in myotonic dystrophy. Neurology 1993;43:2674–8.

180. Thornton CA, Johnson K, Moxley RT, 3rd. Myotonic dystrophy patients have larger CTG expansions in skeletal muscle than in leukocytes. Ann Neurol 1994;35:104–7.

181. Monckton DG, Wong LJ, Ashizawa T, Caskey CT. Somatic mosaicism, germline expansions, germline reversions and intergenerational reductions in myotonic dystrophy males: small pool PCR analyses. Hum Mol Genet 1995;4:1–8.

182. Wong LJ, Ashizawa T, Monckton DG, Caskey CT, Richards CS. Somatic heterogeneity of the CTG repeat in myotonic dystrophy is age and size dependent. Am J Hum Genet 1995;56:114–22.

183. Ohya K, Tachi N, Kon S, Kikuchi K, Chiba S. Somatic cell heterogeneity between DNA extracted from lymphocytes and skeletal muscle in congenital myotonic dystrophy. Jpn J Hum Genet 1995;40:319–26.

184. Peterlin B, Logar N, Zidar J. CTG repeat analysis in lymphocytes, muscles and fibroblasts in patients with myotonic dystrophy. Pflugers Arch 1996; 431:R199–200.

185. De Rooij KE, De Koning Gans PA, Roos RA, Van Ommen GJ, Den Dunnen JT. Somatic expansion of the (CAG)n repeat in Huntington disease brains. Hum Genet 1995;95:270–4.

186. Kennedy L, Shelbourne PF. Dramatic mutation instability in HD mouse striatum: does polyglutamine load contribute to cell-specific vulnerability in Huntington's disease? Hum Mol Genet 2000;9:2539–44.

187. Glaser D, Wohrle D, Salat U, Vogel W, Steinbach P. Mitotic behavior of expanded CGG repeats studied on cultured cells: further evidence for methylation-mediated triplet repeat stability in fragile X syndrome [letter]. Am J Med Genet 1999;84:226–8.

188. Taylor AK, Tassone F, Dyer PN, et al. Tissue heterogeneity of the FMR1 mutation in a high-functioning male with fragile X syndrome. Am J Med Genet 1999;84:233–9.

189. Tassone F, Hagerman RJ, Gane LW, Taylor AK. Strong similarities of the FMR1 mutation in multiple tissues: postmortem studies of a male with a full mutation and a male carrier of a premutation. Am J Med Genet 1999;84:240–4.

190. Reyniers E, Martin JJ, Cras P, et al. Postmortem examination of two fragile X brothers with an FMR1 full mutation. Am J Med Genet 1999;84:245–9.

191. Sutherland GR, Baker E. Characterisation of a new rare fragile site easily confused with the fragile X. Hum Mol Genet 1992;1:111–3.

192. Hirst MC, Barnicoat A, Flynn G, et al. The identification of a third fragile site, FRAXF, in Xq27–q28 distal to both FRAXA and FRAXE. Hum Mol Genet 1993;2:197–200.

193. Flynn GA, Hirst MC, Knight SJ, et al. Identification of the FRAXE fragile site in two families ascertained for X linked mental retardation. J Med Genet 1993;30:97–100.

194. Knight SJ, Flannery AV, Hirst MC, et al. Trinucleotide repeat amplification and hypermethylation of a CpG island in FRAXE mental retardation. Cell 1993;74:127–34.

195. Knight SJ, Voelckel MA, Hirst MC, Flannery AV, Moncla A, Davies KE. Triplet repeat expansion at the FRAXE locus and X-linked mild mental handicap. Am J Hum Genet 1994;55:81–6.

196. Parrish JE, Oostra BA, Verkerk AJ, et al. Isolation of a GCC repeat showing expansion in FRAXF, a fragile site distal to FRAXA and FRAXE [see comments]. Nat Genet 1994;8:229–35.

197. Ritchie RJ, Knight SJ, Hirst MC, et al. The cloning of FRAXF: trinucleotide repeat expansion and methylation at a third fragile site in distal Xqter. Hum Mol Genet 1994;3:2115–21.

198. Laird CD, Lamb MM. Intercalary heterochromatin of *Drosophila* as a potential model for human fragile sites. Am J Med Genet 1988;30:689–91.

199. Laird CD. Proposed mechanism of inheritance and expression of the human fragile-X syndrome of mental retardation. Genetics 1987;117:587–99.

200. Hansen RS, Canfield TK, Lamb MM, Gartler SM, Laird CD. Association of fragile X syndrome with delayed replication of the FMR1 gene. Cell 1993; 73:1403–9.

201. Sutherland GR, Baker E, Richards RI. Fragile sites still breaking. Trends Genet 1998;14:501–6.

202. Richards RI. Fragile and unstable chromosomes in cancer: causes and consequences. Trends Genet 2001;17:339–45.

203. Fry M, Loeb LA. The fragile X syndrome d(CGG)n nucleotide repeats form a stable tetrahelical structure. Proc Natl Acad Sci USA 1994;91:4950–4.

204. Usdin K, Woodford KJ. CGG repeats associated with DNA instability and chromosome fragility form structures that block DNA synthesis in vitro. Nucleic Acids Res 1995;23:4202–9.

205. White PJ, Borts RH, Hirst MC. Stability of the human fragile X (CGG)(n) triplet repeat array in *Saccharomyces cerevisiae* deficient in aspects of DNA metabolism. Mol Cell Biol 1999;19:5675–84.

206. Freudenreich CH, Kantrow SM, Zakian VA. Expansion and length-dependent fragility of CTG repeats in yeast. Science 1998;279:853–6.

207. Sutherland GR, Richards RI. Simple tandem DNA repeats and human genetic disease. Proc Natl Acad Sci USA 1995;92:3636–41.

208. Wenger SL, Hennessey JC, Steele MW. Increased sister chromatid exchange frequency at Xq27 site in affected fragile X males. Am J Med Genet 1987;26:909–14.

209. Branda RF, Arthur DC, Woods WG, Danzl TJ, King RA. Folate metabolism and chromosomal stability in the fragile X syndrome. Am J Med 1984;77: 602–11.

210. Gourdon G, Radvanyi F, Lia AS, et al. Moderate intergenerational and somatic instability of a 55-CTG repeat in transgenic mice [see comments]. Nat Genet 1997;15:190–2.

211. Burright EN, Clark HB, Servadio A, et al. SCA1 transgenic mice: a model for neurodegeneration caused by an expanded CAG trinucleotide repeat. Cell 1995;82:937–48.

212. Mangiarini L, Sathasivam K, Mahal A, Mott R, Seller M, Bates GP. Instability of highly expanded CAG repeats in mice transgenic for the Huntington's disease mutation. Nat Genet 1997;15:197–200.

213. Bontekoe CJ, de Graaff E, Nieuwenhuizen IM, Willemsen R, Oostra BA. FMR1 premutation allele (CGG)81 is stable in mice. Eur J Hum Genet 1997;5:293–8.

214. Lavedan C, Grabczyk E, Usdin K, Nussbaum RL. Long uninterrupted CGG repeats within the first exon of the human FMR1 gene are not intrinsically unstable in transgenic mice. Genomics 1998;50:229–40.

215. Lavedan CN, Garrett L, Nussbaum RL. Trinucleotide repeats (CGG)22TGG (CGG)43TGG(CGG)21 from the fragile X gene remain stable in transgenic mice. Hum Genet 1997;100:407–14.

216. Bontekoe CJ, Bakker CE, Nieuwenhuizen IM, et al. Instability of a (CGG)(98) repeat in the Fmr1 promoter. Hum Mol Genet 2001;10:1693–9.

217. van Den Broek WJ, Nelen MR, Wansink DG, et al. Somatic expansion behaviour of the (CTG)(n) repeat in myotonic dystrophy knock-in mice is differentially affected by Msh3 and Msh6 mismatch-repair proteins. Hum Mol Genet 2002;11:191–8.

218. Eichler EE, Richards S, Gibbs RA, Nelson DL. Fine structure of the human FMR1 gene. Hum Mol Genet 1993;2:1147–53.

219. Hinds HL, Ashley CT, Sutcliffe JS, et al. Tissue specific expression of FMR-1 provides evidence for a functional role in fragile X syndrome [see comments] [published erratum appears in Nat Genet 1993;5:312]. Nat Genet 1993;3:36–43.

220. Agulhon C, Blanchet P, Kobetz A, et al. Expression of FMR1, FXR1, and FXR2 genes in human prenatal tissues. J Neuropathol Exp Neurol 1999;58:867–80.

221. Eberhart DE, Warren ST. The molecular basis of fragile X syndrome. Cold Spring Harb Symp Quant Biol 1996;61:679–87.

222. Verkerk AJ, de Graaff E, De Boulle K, et al. Alternative splicing in the fragile X gene FMR1. Hum Mol Genet 1993;2:1348.

223. Eberhart DE, Malter HE, Feng Y, Warren ST. The fragile X mental retardation protein is a ribonucleoprotein containing both nuclear localization and nuclear export signals. Hum Mol Genet 1996;5:1083–91.

224. Willemsen R, Bontekoe C, Tamanini F, Galjaard H, Hoogeveen A, Oostra B. Association of FMRP with ribosomal precursor particles in the nucleolus. Biochem Biophys Res Commun 1996;225:27–33.

225. Tamanini F, Meijer N, Verheij C, et al. FMRP is associated to the ribosomes via RNA. Hum Mol Genet 1996;5:809–13.

226. Feng Y, Gutekunst CA, Eberhart DE, Yi H, Warren ST, Hersch SM. Fragile X mental retardation protein: nucleocytoplasmic shuttling and association with somatodendritic ribosomes. J Neurosci 1997;17:1539–47.

227. Tamanini F, Willemsen R, van Unen L, et al. Differential expression of FMR1, FXR1 and FXR2 proteins in human brain and testis. Hum Mol Genet 1997;6:1315–22.

228. Siomi H, Siomi MC, Nussbaum RL, Dreyfuss G. The protein product of the fragile X gene, FMR1, has characteristics of an RNA-binding protein. Cell 1993;74:291–8.

229. Ashley CT, Jr., Wilkinson KD, Reines D, Warren ST. FMR1 protein: conserved RNP family domains and selective RNA binding. Science 1993; 262:563–6.

230. Brown V, Small K, Lakkis L, et al. Purified recombinant Fmrp exhibits selective RNA binding as an intrinsic property of the fragile X mental retardation protein. J Biol Chem 1998; 273:15,521–7.

231. Adinolfi S, Bagni C, Musco G, Gibson T, Mazzarella L, Pastore A. Dissecting FMR1, the protein responsible for fragile X syndrome, in its structural and functional domains. RNA 1999; 5:1248–58.

232. Musco G, Kharrat A, Stier G, et al. The solution structure of the first KH domain of FMR1, the protein responsible for the fragile X syndrome [letter]

[published erratum appears in Nat Struct Biol 1997;4:840]. Nat Struct Biol 1997;4:712–6.

233. Musco G, Stier G, Joseph C, et al. Three-dimensional structure and stability of the KH domain: molecular insights into the fragile X syndrome. Cell 1996;85:237–45.

234. Tamanini F, Van Unen L, Bakker C, et al. Oligomerization properties of fragile-X mental-retardation protein (FMRP) and the fragile-X-related proteins FXR1P and FXR2P. Biochem J 1999;343(Pt 3):517–23.

235. Feng Y, Absher D, Eberhart DE, Brown V, Malter HE, Warren ST. FMRP associates with polyribosomes as an mRNP, and the I304N mutation of severe fragile X syndrome abolishes this association. Mol Cell 1997;1:109–18.

236. Kiledjian M, Dreyfuss G. Primary structure and binding activity of the hnRNP U protein: binding RNA through RGG box. EMBO J 1992;11:2655–64.

237. Darnell JC, Jensen KB, Jin P, Brown V, Warren ST, Darnell RB. Fragile X mental retardation protein targets G quartet mRNAs important for neuronal function. Cell 2001;107:489–99.

238. Schaeffer C, Bardoni B, Mandel JL, Ehresmann B, Ehresmann C, Moine H. The fragile X mental retardation protein binds specifically to its mRNA via a purine quartet motif. EMBO J 2001;20:4803–13.

239. Bardoni B, Sittler A, Shen Y, Mandel JL. Analysis of domains affecting intracellular localization of the FMRP protein. Neurobiol Dis 1997;4:329–36.

240. Li Z, Zhang Y, Ku L, Wilkinson KD, Warren ST, Feng Y. The fragile X mental retardation protein inhibits translation via interacting with mRNA. Nucleic Acids Res 2001;29:2276–83.

241. Laggerbauer B, Ostareck D, Keidel E, Ostareck-Lederer A, Fischer U. Evidence that fragile X mental retardation protein is a negative regulator of translation. Hum Mol Genet 2001;10:329–38.

242. Weiler IJ, Irwin SA, Klintsova AY, et al. Fragile X mental retardation protein is translated near synapses in response to neurotransmitter activation. Proc Natl Acad Sci USA 1997;94:5395–400.

243. Irwin SA, Galvez R, Greenough WT. Dendritic spine structural anomalies in fragile-X mental retardation syndrome. Cereb Cortex 2000;10:1038–44.

244. Zhang Y, O'Connor JP, Siomi MC, et al. The fragile X mental retardation syndrome protein interacts with novel homologs FXR1 and FXR2. EMBO J 1995;14:5358–66.

245. Siomi MC, Siomi H, Sauer WH, Srinivasan S, Nussbaum RL, Dreyfuss G. FXR1, an autosomal homolog of the fragile X mental retardation gene. EMBO J 1995;14:2401–8.

246. Khandjian EW, Bardoni B, Corbin F, et al. Novel isoforms of the fragile X related protein FXR1P are expressed during myogenesis. Hum Mol Genet 1998;7:2121–8.

247. Tamanini F, Bontekoe C, Bakker CE, et al. Different targets for the fragile X-related proteins revealed by their distinct nuclear localizations. Hum Mol Genet 1999;8:863–9.

248. Brown V, Jin P, Ceman S, et al. Microarray identification of FMRP-associated brain mRNAs and altered mRNA translational profiles in fragile X syndrome. Cell 2001;107:477–87.

249. Wan L, Dockendorff TC, Jongens TA, Dreyfuss G. Characterization of dFMR1, a *Drosophila melanogaster* homolog of the fragile X mental retardation protein. Mol Cell Biol 2000;20:8536–47.
250. Zhang YQ, Bailey AM, Matthies HJ, et al. *Drosophila* fragile X-related gene regulates the MAP1B homolog futsch to control synaptic structure and function. Cell 2001;107:591–603.
251. Ceman S, Brown V, Warren ST. Isolation of an FMRP-associated messenger ribonucleoprotein particle and identification of nucleolin and the fragile X-related proteins as components of the complex. Mol Cell Biol 1999; 19:7925–32.
252. Schenck A, Bardoni B, Moro A, Bagni C, Mandel JL. A highly conserved protein family interacting with the fragile X mental retardation protein (FMRP) and displaying selective interactions with FMRP-related proteins FXR1P and FXR2P. Proc Natl Acad Sci USA 2001;98:8844–9.
253. Bardoni B, Schenck A, Mandel JL. A novel RNA-binding nuclear protein that interacts with the fragile X mental retardation (FMR1) protein. Hum Mol Genet 1999;8:2557–66.
254. Ceman S, Nelson R, Warren ST. Identification of mouse YB1/p50 as a component of the FMRP-associated mRNP particle. Biochem Biophys Res Commun 2000;279:904–8.
255. Hoogeveen AT, Oostra BA. The fragile X syndrome. J Inherit Metab Dis 1997;20:139–51.
256. DBFXC. Fmr1 knockout mice: a model to study fragile X mental retardation. The Dutch-Belgian Fragile X Consortium. Cell 1994;78:23–33.
257. Slegtenhorst-Eegdeman KE, de Rooij DG, Verhoef-Post M, et al. Macroorchidism in FMR1 knockout mice is caused by increased Sertoli cell proliferation during testicular development. Endocrinology 1998;139:156–62.
258. Kooy RF, Verhoye M, Lemmon V, Van Der Linden A. Brain studies of mouse models for neurogenetic disorders using in vivo magnetic resonance imaging (MRI). Eur J Hum Genet 2001;9:153–9.
259. Paradee W, Melikian HE, Rasmussen DL, Kenneson A, Conn PJ, Warren ST. Fragile X mouse: strain effects of knockout phenotype and evidence suggesting deficient amygdala function. Neuroscience 1999;94:185–92.
260. Kooy RF, D'Hooge R, Reyniers E, et al. Transgenic mouse model for the fragile X syndrome. Am J Med Genet 1996;64:241–5.
261. D'Hooge R, Nagels G, Franck F, et al. Mildly impaired water maze performance in male Fmr1 knockout mice. Neuroscience 1997;76:367–76.
262. Van Dam D, D'Hooge R, Hauben E, et al. Spatial learning, contextual fear conditioning and conditioned emotional response in Fmr1 knockout mice. Behav Brain Res 2000;117:127–36.
263. Morris RG, Anderson E, Lynch GS, Baudry M. Selective impairment of learning and blockade of long-term potentiation by an N-methyl-D-aspartate receptor antagonist, AP5. Nature 1986;319:774–6.
264. Godfraind JM, Reyniers E, De Boulle K, et al. Long-term potentiation in the hippocampus of fragile X knockout mice. Am J Med Genet 1996;64:246–51.

265. Paylor R, Tracy R, Wehner J, Rudy JW. DBA/2 and C57BL/6 mice differ in contextual fear but not auditory fear conditioning. Behav Neurosci 1994; 108:810–7.
266. Fisch GS, Hao HK, Bakker C, Oostra BA. Learning and memory in the FMR1 knockout mouse. Am J Med Genet 1999;84:277–82.
267. Dobkin C, Rabe A, Dumas R, El Idrissi A, Haubenstock H, Brown WT. Fmr1 knockout mouse has a distinctive strain-specific learning impairment. Neuroscience 2000;100:423–9.
268. Peier AM, McIlwain KL, Kenneson A, Warren ST, Paylor R, Nelson DL. (Over)correction of FMR1 deficiency with YAC transgenics: behavioral and physical features. Hum Mol Genet 2000;9:1145–59.
269. Bontekoe CJ, McIlwain KL, Nieuwenhuizen IM, et al. Knockout mouse model for Fxr2: a model for mental retardation. Hum Mol Genet 2002;11:487–98.
270. Chiurazzi P, Pomponi MG, Willemsen R, Oostra BA, Neri G. In vitro reactivation of the FMR1 gene involved in fragile X syndrome. Hum Mol Genet 1998;7:109–13.
271. Chiurazzi P, Pomponi MG, Pietrobono R, Bakker CE, Neri G, Oostra BA. Synergistic effect of histone hyperacetylation and DNA demethylation in the reactivation of the FMR1 gene. Hum Mol Genet 1999;8:2317–23.

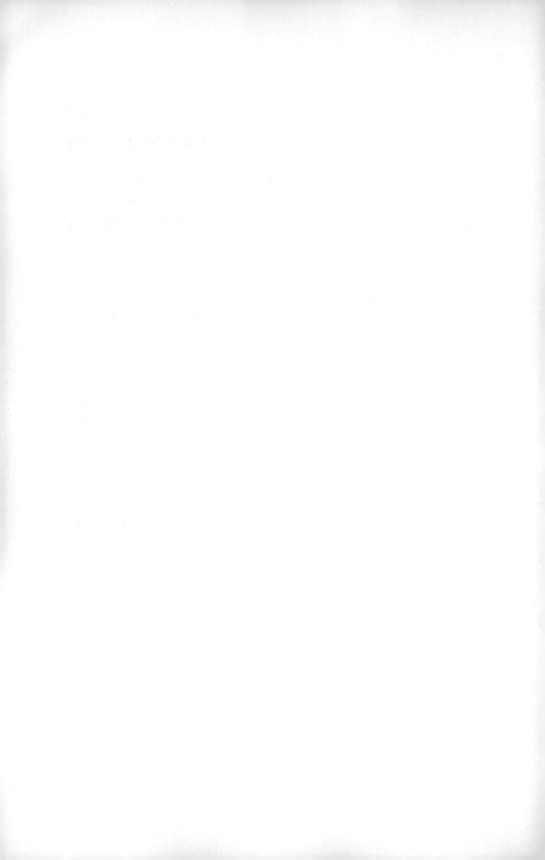

15

Rett Syndrome

Clinical–Molecular Correlates

Alan K. Percy, Joanna Dragich, and N. Carolyn Schanen

1. INTRODUCTION

Rett syndrome (RS) was first recognized in the early 1960s as a developmental disorder affecting young females only. Andreas Rett, a Viennese developmental pediatrician, reported the initial accounts of this unique syndrome, but none was widely circulated *(1)*. Bengt Hagberg identified girls in Sweden with similar clinical features and together with colleagues from France and Portugal presented the first English language publication on RS in 1983 *(2)*. As a result, RS was soon recognized in the United States, Japan, and throughout western Europe *(3–6)*, and has now been reported in all ethnic groups. The prevalence of RS (Table 1) ranges from 1/10,000 in Sweden *(7)* to 1/22,000 in Texas *(8)*. In the United States, more than 3000 females meeting the clinical criteria for RS have been identified. As described in the following paragraphs, mutations in the gene *MECP2*, which encodes methyl-CpG-binding protein 2, have been found in most girls or women (and some boys) with RS. Surprisingly, mutations in this gene can also lead to a wide variety of clinical phenotypes ranging from normal females to fatal encephalopathy in males.

For the purpose of classification, Rett syndrome has been included in DSM-IV and ICD-10 under the general heading of Pervasive Developmental Disorders (PDD), specifically in DSM-IV as 299.80. This category (299.80) includes Asperger syndrome and PDD Not Otherwise Specified. The rationale for placing RS in this category is unclear and has generated lively discussion in the past *(9,10)*. From both clinical and biological perspectives, one cannot imagine a reason to categorize a multisystem disorder *(see* discussion under clinical issues) dominated by neurologic and behavioral aspects in this manner. Particularly in light of the recent molecu-

From: *Contemporary Clinical Neuroscience:*
Genetics and Genomics of Neurobehavioral Disorders
Edited by: G. S. Fisch © Humana Press Inc., Totowa, NJ

Table 1
Rett Syndrome Prevalence Estimates

Location	Year	Number	Prevalence
Western Scotland	1982	19	1/15,000
Switzerland	1982	27	1/24,600
Western Sweden	1982	12	1/13,000
Japan	1988	24	1/25,000
Texas	1990	103	1/22,800
Australia	1995	79	1/22,000
Sweden	1996	69	1/13,000

lar advances in our understanding of RS, it should be classified as a distinct entity, just as fragile X syndrome or Down syndrome.

2. CLINICAL CHARACTERISTICS OF RETT SYNDROME

In its typical clinical presentation, RS is characterized by profound cognitive impairment, communication dysfunction, stereotypic movements, and pervasive growth failure, all of which follow a period of apparently normal development during the first 6–18 mo of life *(11)*. Prior to the identification of a gene for RS, attempts to establish a biologic marker had failed. As such, the diagnosis of RS is based on clinical characteristics. Consensus panels have developed obligate standards (Table 2) for this diagnosis *(12,13)*. These criteria include normal pre- and perinatal periods and developmental progress, which appears normal for the first several months of life, although some delays may be recognized in retrospect. In particular, these children tend to be hypotonic during infancy. Thereafter, purposeful hand skills are lost and psychomotor and communication functions regress, typically occurring as early as 9 mo of age or as late as 2.5 years. During this period, eye contact is poor and socialization and communication skills are severely limited. These features may suggest the diagnosis of autistic spectrum disorder. Also, abnormal sleep patterns and profound irritability without apparent explanation are often noted during this period. The first clinical sign of RS may be a deceleration in the rate of head growth recognizable as early as 3 mo of age. Failure of normal head growth may be profound, leading to microcephaly in some children *(14)*. Stereotypic movements, occurring only during wakefulness, begin between ages 1 and 3 years. These stereotypies consist of hand-washing or hand-wringing movements or hand-clapping/hand-patting movements. Hand stereotypies typically occur at the midline, but may vary to involve one hand in the mouth and another pulling or pick-

Table 2
Rett Syndrome Obligate Clinical Criteria

Criteria	Onset
Normal	—
Apparently normal early development	6–8 mo
Postnatal deceleration of head growth rate	3 mo–4 years
Loss of purposeful hand skills	9 mo–2 1/2 years
Psychomotor regression	9 mo–2 1/2 years
Communication dysfunction	
Autistic features	
Stereotypic movements	1–3 years
Hand washing/wringing	
Hand clapping/patting	
Hand mouthing	
Gait dysfunction	1–4 years
Truncal ataxia	
Absence of	
Organomegaly	
Optic atrophy	
Retinal changes	
Intrauterine growth retardation	

ing at the clothes or hand-patting or hand-wringing behind the back. On occasion, stereotypic movements of orofacial muscles or feet may be noted. Most children with RS are capable of walking. However, between 1 and 4 years, the gait becomes apraxic, that is, has a broad-based, wandering, purposeless character and is often accompanied by truncal ataxia and side-to side rocking while standing. Walking is frequently initiated by first stepping backwards (retropulsion).

The diagnosis of RS requires a thorough history and neurological evaluation to include growth and developmental parameters and implementation of the obligate criteria. The significant overlap in the RS phenotype, as defined by the diagnostic criteria, and that of other neurodevelopmental disorders requires the careful consideration of the relevant differential diagnoses so that the appropriate testing strategies are judiciously employed. During childhood, RS and Angelman syndrome (AS) appear remarkably similar, but may often be distinguished by the absence of regression in most children with AS. Recent data, however, have shown that some children with AS carry mutations in the *MECP2* gene, demonstrating the difficulties in clearly distinguishing these two disorders in the young child *(15)*. For this reason, the initial testing strategy in RS should include mutation analysis on leukocyte DNA for the *MECP2* gene *(16)* in conjunction with the molecular probe for AS and chromosome analysis with high resolution banding. Definitive diagnosis of RS is accomplished by identification of a mutation in the *MECP2* gene combined with a developmental profile that meets the diagnostic criteria. Importantly, up to 20% of individuals with clinically defined RS will not have an identifiable mutation in the coding region of this gene. This does not preclude the diagnosis of RS. The chance of identifying a mutation is lower in atypical RS (<50%) as well as in affected siblings (approx 20%) or in boys (<5%) meeting diagnostic criteria. In a child who has evidence of regression, no mutation in the *MECP2* gene, and normal AS testing, additional testing is warranted, particularly because of overlap with the early stages of infantile or late infantile neuronal ceroid lipofuscinosis and other storage diseases. Ancillary evaluations including audiologic and ophthalmologic assessments and cranial MRI should be considered and specific enzyme testing may be necessary as determined by the presence of retinal or central nervous system (CNS) abnormalities. At this point in our understanding of RS, a broad investigation for inherited metabolic disorders is not warranted unless unusual clinical features are present that would support the need to pursue these diagnostic procedures.

3. CLINICAL STAGING

RS has been characterized in four clinical stages (Table 3), which provide a format for plotting the clinical progression of RS *(17)*. However, the transition from one stage to the next is generally along a continuum rather than an abrupt change. The first stage is the early onset stagnation period, which occurs from age 6 to 18 mo. In most instances, this stage lasts from weeks to months and consists of delay in developmental progress without clear evidence of regression. The second stage is the period of rapid developmental regression with onset ranging from age 1–3 or 4 years. This period is characterized by the loss or regression of previously acquired skills in motor and communication function and by impairment of cognitive performance. This stage may be relatively brief (days to weeks) or last as long as a year. Other diagnoses to consider during this stage include autistic spectrum disorder, infantile neuronal ceroid lipofuscinosis, AS, and an acute toxic or infectious encephalopathy. Infantile neuronal ceroid lipofuscinosis and AS are particularly relevant, as each may resemble the RS phenotype including deceleration in the rate of head growth, seizures, and stereotypic movements. However, the natural histories of these two disorders are quite different from that of RS, and both can now be differentiated from RS by appropriate molecular genetic or biochemical testing.

Table 3
Rett Syndrome Clinical Stages

Stage	Onset	Duration	Clinical features
Early onset stagnation	6–18 mo	Months	Delayed development Hypotonia Slowing of head growth Disinterest in play
Rapid regression	1–3 years	Weeks to months	Psychomotor regression Profound irritability Loss of hand skills Loss of language Hand stereotypies Bruxism Growth decline Seizures Autistic-like interaction
Pseudostationary	2–10 years	Years to decades	Cognitive impairment Improved eye contact Hand stereotypies Breathing irregularities Growth failure Gait apraxia Truncal ataxia Seizures Scoliosis
Late motor deterioration	10–30 years	Years	Loss of gait Progressive scoliosis Improved eye contact Staring gaze Reduced seizures Improved breathing Increasing rigidity or dystonia Muscle wasting Cold, purplish feet

The third stage, the pseudostationary period, may span many years, if not decades. Girls in this stage must have preserved the ability to walk. Communication functions such as socialization and eye contact may improve remarkably during the third stage, but motor function such as walking and the stereotypic hand movements may decline in speed and frequency. Not uncommonly, ambulation may persist into middle age. In this stage, RS must be differentiated from the so-called ataxic static encephalopathies, spinocerebellar degeneration, and neuronal ceroid lipofuscinosis. AS should also be considered as well as idiopathic psychomotor retardation. The fourth stage, late motor deterioration, is defined by absence of the ability to walk, that is, when wheelchair dependency is complete. Despite transition to stage 4, communication functions such as eye contact and socialization may be quite good and continue into adulthood. Girls who never walk transition directly from stage 2 to 4. As such, stage 4 differentiates girls who lose ambulation (4A) from those who never ambulate (4B). Girls in stage 4B are typically severely hypotonic during childhood and then develop progressive motor disability with muscle wasting and skeletal deformities.

4. VARIANT PHENOTYPIC EXPRESSION

Variant phenotypic expressions of RS are well recognized. The most common is the so-called *formes fruste*, which consists of delay in onset of RS features until age 8–10 years *(18)*. Other phenotypes include a preserved speech variant *(19)*, a congenital form lacking any period of developmental progress, and an early onset seizure form *(20)*. The relatively severe epileptic encephalopathy accompanying the early onset seizure form may preclude any semblance of normal early development.

Criteria for delineating the later onset variants *(21)* consist of the following:

- female sex,
- at least 10 years old, and
- fulfilling at least 3 of 6 main criteria and at least 5 of 11 associated features for RS (Table 4).

In a Swedish cohort of 130 females with RS *(11)*, 82% fulfilled the classic criteria, 12% were *formes fruste*, and the remaining 6% were made up by the late regression, preserved speech, or congenital forms. Because of the relative infrequency of males who meet the diagnostic criteria, boys manifesting RS features have also been considered an atypical or variant form. Nonetheless, the RS phenotype has been described in several males, but few have demonstrated mutations in *MECP2* (*see* Subheading 6.). One notable exception has been the identification of classical RS in males with Klinefelter syndrome (47,XXY) *(22–25)*.

5. GENETIC BASIS OF RETT SYNDROME

Since its earliest description, RS was proposed to be a genetic disorder that was transmitted as an X-linked dominant trait with lethality in males,

Table 4
Rett Syndrome Variant Phenotypes Criteria

Inclusion criteria:

> Female
> At least 8–10 years old
> Meet at least 3 of 6 main criteria
> Meet at least 5 of 11 supportive criteria

Six main criteria:

> Loss of finger skills
> Loss of babble/speech
> Loss of communication skills
> Deceleration of head growth
> Hand stereotypies
> RS disease profile

Eleven supportive criteria:

> Irregular breathing
> Teeth grinding
> Scoliosis/kyphosis
> Lower limb amyotrophy
> Laughing/screaming spells
> Cold, purplish feet
> Bloating
> Gait dyspraxia
> RS EEG pattern
> RS eye pointing
> Pain indifference

although no evidence exists of prenatal lethality in males. Prior to the identification of mutations in *MECP2 (16,26,27)*, support for an X-linked transmission of RS followed several lines:

1. RS had been described reliably only in females.
2. Monozygotic twins were consistently concordant, that is, if one twin had RS, the second also had RS, although variability was reported in expression within twin pairs, a common feature of X-linked traits in females.
3. Familial cases were identified in which sisters, half-sisters, or aunt/nieces have RS.
4. Vertical transmission occurred, that is, a woman with RS gave birth to a daughter with RS.
5. Skewed or nonrandom X-chromosome inactivation patterns were noted in obligate carrier females in families with recurrent RS. Skewing of inactivation (i.e., preferential silencing of one copy of the X chromosome in each cell

in females) provides a mechanism that a female carrying a RS mutation could escape its effects.

Mapping the causative gene was not straightforward, however, because RS is largely a sporadic disorder, with much less than 1% representing recurrences within families. In addition, the severe cognitive impairment that accompanies RS makes it unlikely that most affected women would reproduce (i.e., they have reduced reproductive fitness). Efforts to establish linkage to specific regions of the X-chromosome were hampered by the small number of familial cases. Nevertheless, linkage studies eventually focused on Xq28, a very gene rich region *(28–30)*. As a result, mutations were subsequently identified in the gene *MECP2*, which encodes a transcriptional silencer, methyl-CpG-binding protein 2 (MeCP2) *(16)*. MeCP2 is important in the regulation of gene transcription although the target genes have not yet been identified. *MECP2* is expressed ubiquitously in human tissues, but is highly expressed in brain. In girls or women with RS, several different mutations have now been described in *MECP2* although 8 of these mutations account for nearly 70% of those identified to date *(16,25,26,31–44)*. Most of the known mutations are truncating, that is, result in formation of an incomplete form of MeCP2. Missense mutations produce a full-length MeCP2, but one with reduced functional integrity.

At present, mutations in *MECP2* have been identified in 80–85% of females with classic RS. This number is likely to increase as the gene is sequenced more completely. In the case of variant forms of RS, the number with mutations in *MECP2* is considerably lower (<50%). Similarly, *MECP2* mutations have been found in only about 25% of affected sister pairs, which supports the existence of a second, possibly autosomal, locus associated with development of classic RS. Inasmuch as familial recurrences are small, most girls with RS represent new mutations. It had been postulated that mutations in *MECP2* may arise in the paternal germline, leading to an excess of affected females as mutations occurring on the paternal X chromosome would generally lead only to affected daughters. Recent support for this hypothesis has emerged *(45,46)*. However, it is also likely that considerable ascertainment bias exists against the identification of boys with *MECP2* mutations as they may present with a markedly different phenotype.

6. *MECP2* MUTATIONS IN MALES

Although the *MECP2* mutations in RS are dominant acting alleles, a growing number of reports of *MECP2* mutations identified in males have appeared. The initial male phenotype was identified in boys who carry the same *MECP2* mutations that cause classical RS in females. This severe, early onset encephalopathy was first seen in a boy who was found to share the same mutation as his mother, who has a mild learning disability, and his aunt and sister, who have RS *(31,47)*. The features of this phenotype include normal growth parameters at birth, with onset of hypotonia, central apnea, gastroesophageal reflux, and seizures in the first month of life. Similarly, another boy carries the same mutation in *MECP2* as his sister with RS and their mother (a brother died with a similar encephalopathy before mutation testing was available) *(48)*. Recently, this phenotype has also been identified in boys who are not members of RS kindreds, but display similar clinical features in early infancy *(25,49)*. In contrast, typical RS profiles have been identified in at least four boys with Klinefelter syndrome *(22–25)*. Mutations in *MECP2* have been identified in at least two of them *(24,25)*. As a result of X inactivation, the presence of two X chromosomes renders them functionally mosaic for expression of the mutant gene (as in females with RS).

While the very severe phenotype in hemizygous males and the RS-like phenotype of Klinefelter males were somewhat predicted for an X-linked dominant disorder, mutations have been found in karyotypically normal males with various forms of mental retardation. For example, *MECP2* mutations were also found in two 46,XY males with severe cognitive impairment, macrocephaly, chronic diarrhea, and progressive spasticity *(50)*. In this family, both mothers and the two boys share a common mutation in *MECP2*. One mother was normal, but the other had borderline intelligence. In contrast, a more Rett-like phenotype was seen in another boy who lacked stereotypic hand movements *(51)*. Evidence was not presented regarding the presence or absence of deceleration in the rate of head growth. His phenotype is explained by somatic mosaicism for the *MECP2* gene, that is, some of his cells express a mutation in *MECP2*, while other cells have a normal copy of this gene *(51)*. More recent observations of this boy suggest that he now has hand stereotypies and may well fit the criteria for classic RS (Kathy Hunter, International Rett Syndrome Association-[IRSA], personal communication). To add further complexity, recent investigations of this gene as a cause of mental retardation in males led to the identification of mutations in 4 of 185 males with nonspecific mental retardation *(52)*. This frequency suggests that *MECP2* may have a similar frequency as fragile X syndrome among this population and play a major role in the development of mental retardation in males. In the males carrying *MECP2* mutations, regression in skills is not noted generally, however, one common feature has been the absence of language. Importantly, aside from males with Klinefelter syndrome, these other males with *MECP2* mutations do not have the clinical features of RS.

7. PHENOTYPE–GENOTYPE CORRELATIONS

Attempts at providing phenotype–genotype correlations with respect to RS and mutations in *MECP2* have led to mixed results *(25,33,34,53)*. This may be due in part to the multiplicity of mutations associated with RS and the fact that different studies derive their comparisons from a different set of mutations. It may also result from disparate sets of criteria for determining severity of phenotypic features. The factor that appears to have the greatest influence on phenotype is the degree of nonrandom X-chromosome inactivation (XCI) *(53)*. Systematic study of XCI has not been performed, but may vary markedly between tissues. In addition, it is nearly impossible to assay XCI using standard approaches on the relevant cell types, as even studies in brain would assess XCI pattern of very heterogeneous cell populations that include both neuronal and glial lineages. Thus, correlations based on sampling peripheral tissues such as lymphocytes or hair follicles may be misleading.

One lesson to be learned is that comparisons among girls with RS must be based on carefully conducted clinical evaluations using an agreed on set of clinical criteria and clinical severity scales. For example, the clinical criteria for RS and the clinical severity scales differed between the studies of Amir et al. *(53)* and Cheadle et al. *(33)*. As such, direct comparisons between the two studies are not possible. In future, it will be important to base phenotype–genotype correlations on a common clinical severity scale among girls who fulfill the classic criteria or whose deviation from these criteria is clearly indicated. Despite these incongruities, it appears that mutations in the amino-end of the protein lead to more severe clinical features and those toward the carboxy-end result in less severe involvement *(25,33,35,53)*. This is most apparent in the boys with X-linked mental retardation arising from mutations in *MECP2*, which most often show missense mutations in the 3' end of the coding sequence *(52)*. In females, skewed XCI is a significant modifier such that proximal truncating mutations, which would be predicted to produce a more severe clinical picture, may be associated with milder expression if XCI is skewed in favor of the normal X chromosome. Conversely, if XCI were skewed in favor of the XCI bearing the *MECP2* mutation, clinical involvement could be much more severe. Indeed, it might feature a rapidly progressive encephalopathy as already described in males *(31,47,48)*.

8. *MECP2* MUTATIONS EXTENDING BEYOND THE BOUNDARIES OF RETT SYNDROME

The second major outcome from identification of mutations in *MECP2* is the broad spectrum of clinical phenotypes associated with such mutations

Table 5
Rett Syndrome Phenotypes Associated with *MECP2* Mutations

Females

    Rett syndrome
    Formes fruste
    Preserved speech variant
    Delayed onset variant
    Angelman syndrome
    Autistic spectrum disorder
    Mild learning disability
    Normal carriers

Males

    Fatal encephalopathy
    Rett/Klinefelter syndrome
    X-Linked mental retardation/progressive spasticity
    X-Linked mental retardation
    Somatic mosaicism/neurodevelopmental delay

(15,22–25,31,48–52,54). This finding should, however, not be surprising. Similar results have been obtained for a number of inherited disorders. Disease processes associated with mutations in the hexosaminidase A gene (*HEXA*), which is responsible for Tay–Sachs disease, represent the most striking range of clinical expression including dystonia, spinocerebellar degeneration, amyotrophic lateral sclerosis, spinal muscular atrophy, or psychotic depression. Thus, it is hardly surprising that similar variability in clinical presentation should emerge from mutations in *MECP2*. If recent experience is a guide, the span will be broad. The range of disorders associated with *MECP2* mutations now involves both females and males (Table 5). Among females, mutations have been identified in association with RS and its variants, in the Angelman phenotype *(15)*, in autistic spectrum disorder *(25)*, and in normal women as well as those with mild learning disability.

    The array of phenotypes associated with RS is displayed in Fig. 1 as overlapping circles depicting the close relationship between this disorder and individuals with mutations in *MECP2*. Currently, mutations in this gene have not been identified in some girls with RS. Conversely, mutations in *MECP2* have been described in males and females who display features either in common with RS or are completely disparate. The overlap region includes girls with classic and variant forms of RS. This pattern is likely to expand as new associations with *MECP2* mutations are defined. As such, it is neces-

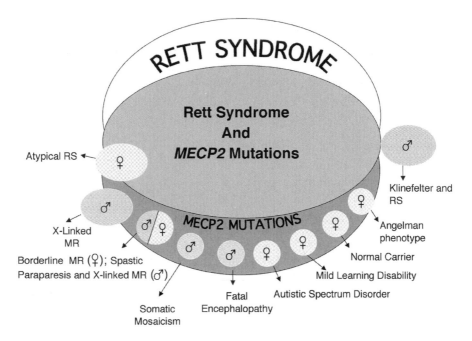

Fig. 1. Overlapping ovals representing individuals with *MECP2* mutations. The upper oval represents females with Rett syndrome, most of whom have mutations in *MECP2*. The lower oval represents females (*lightly shaded ovals*) and males (*darkly shaded ovals*) with mutations in *MECP2* and clinical features distinct from Rett syndrome. The side oval represents males with Klinefelter syndrome, clinical features of Rett syndrome, and mutations in *MECP2*. The oval overlapping the two larger ovals represents females with atypical Rett syndrome and mutations in *MECP2*.

sary to consider how widely to explore other neurodevelopmental disorders with respect to mutations in this gene.

One critical element in advancing our understanding of the role of *MECP2* in neurodevelopmental disabilities is the establishment of firm diagnostic criteria and clinical severity measures that extend over the continuum of clinical involvement for RS and its variant forms. Further, as indicated previously, these tools must be carefully applied. This places the responsibility squarely on the clinician to provide clear and complete descriptions of the clinical presentations for all girls in whom mutations in *MECP2* are identified. One might also ask: How wide should the net be cast in the evaluation of girls or boys with unexplained neurodevelopmental disabilities?

9. PATHOBIOLOGY OF RS

With the identification of mutations in *MECP2* as the principal molecular mechanism underlying RS, it is important to explore the implications of this discovery against the background of available information on the neuropathology of this disorder. Substantial neuropathologic data are available. What remains is to explore the possible relationship of these data with the known neurobiologic properties of the transcriptional repressor, MeCP2.

9.1. Neuropathology

In RS, brain weight is reduced *(55)*, especially with respect to the volume of frontal cortex and deep gray nuclei *(56)*. The brain appears normal to gross inspection, but is small, typically between 60% and 70% of expected weight for age. Although brain weights are uniformly low, no pattern of progressive reduction in size with increasing age, that is, atrophy, is noted. Evidence of disrupted migration is lacking. In addition, melanin deposition in the substantia nigra is markedly reduced. Throughout the brain, neurons are smaller than normal and are too close together, with too few processes as dendritic arborizations are significantly diminished. Golgi studies reveal markedly shortened and relatively primitive dendritic arborizations, resulting in the increase in cell packing density. The absence of any recognizable disease process argues against a neurodegenerative disorder *(55,57–64)*. Thus, RS has the profile of a developmental disorder and not that of a neurodegenerative condition. That is, the fundamental neurobiologic problem appears to be the arrest or interruption of normal neural maturation. This conclusion is based on the substantial neuropathologic evidence noted in the preceding, indicating no progressive neuropathologic features, that is, no evidence of neuronal loss or extensive gliosis. Instead of normal neural maturation, cortical neurons in RS remain small and dendritic connections are reduced, both of which suggest a failure in the proper development or maintenance of synaptic connections.

Although the mechanisms are likely to be very different, several other neurodevelopmental disorders have similar neuropathologic features. These include Down syndrome, in which dendritic branches are significantly reduced after early infancy such that dendritic spines are deficient already by 4 mo of age and remain so into adulthood *(65)*. Decreased dendritic arborizations and dendritic spines are also prominent neuropathologic features of AS *(66)* and fragile X syndrome *(67,68)*. Finally, increased packing density and decreased cell size are noted in autistic spectrum disorder *(69)*.

9.2. Role of MeCP2 in Developmental Neurobiology

The role of MeCP2 in transcriptional silencing and of its subsequent effects on developmental neurobiology is largely unexplored *(70)*. Identification of mutations in this gene in girls with RS has sparked new interest in this area. Methylated CpG residues densely populate heterochromatic regions of chromosomes as well as the promoter regions of many genes. Of the cytosine residues found in CpG nucleotides throughout the mammalian genome, 60–90% are modified by methylation. Germline methylation patterns are erased after fertilization and distinct patterns are reestablished during differentiation *(71)*. Gene silencing through methylation is used in several cellular processes including XCI, imprinting, silencing of endogenous retroviruses, and tissue-specific regulation of transcription. Why neurons are particularly susceptible to dysfunction of epigenetic silencing is still unclear. It is possible that chromatin remodeling may prevent excess transcriptional noise *(70,72)*, allowing postmitotic neurons to function efficiently.

Recently, a clear link between transcriptional repression and histone deacetylation (HDAC) has been uncovered. In yeast and mammals, large protein complexes containing HDACs and various repressor proteins have been shown to inhibit transcription through a mechanism that involves local chromatin remodeling. Histone deacetylation is thought to allow negatively charged DNA to wind more tightly around the histone octamer by revealing positively charged lysine residues on the histone tails *(73)*. Chromatin remodeling has been implicated in gene silencing in several contexts. These include the transcriptional repression of >20 neuron-specific genes in non-neuronal cell types by the neural restrictive silencer factor (NRSF), which associates with the transcriptional repressor Sin3A and HDAC1 *(74,75)*. Treatment of non-neuronal cells with trichostatin A (TSA), a potent inhibitor of HDACs, induces expression of neuron-specific genes silenced by NRSF and provides evidence that HDAC activity is involved in the repression mechanism mediated by NRSF *(76)*. The current model predicts that MeCP2 also mediates gene silencing by attracting HDACs to methylated DNA *(77)*. Similar to NRSF, physical interaction between MeCP2, HDAC1, and HDAC2, and the transcriptional corepressor Sin3A, as well as functional links to the transcriptional apparatus, including the SP1 transcription factor, have been demonstrated *(78–81)*. At present, however, no targets of MeCP2-mediated silencing have been identified nor have chromosomal domains been identified that preferentially associate with MeCP2. Immunofluorescence studies show strong localization of MeCP2 to pericentric heterochromatin in the mouse, while more diffuse staining is seen in the rat *(82)* and human *(83)*. In neurons, MeCP2 is excluded from nucleoli *(84)*, which contain tandemly repeated methylated ribosomal DNA (rDNA) *(85)* and methylated ribosomal RNA (rRNA).

Direct evidence of the effect of mutant MeCP2 indicates that mutations in the methyl-binding domain of this protein interfere with binding to methylated DNA *(86)*. MeCP2 containing the common missense mutations R106W and R133C and a third missense mutation have a 100-fold reduction in affinity for methylated DNA while a third common missense mutation (T158M) has only a twofold reduction in binding affinity.

From our understanding of the neuropathology of RS, *MECP2* would appear to impact fundamental mechanisms in synaptic development *(63,64)*. Fragile X syndrome offers a striking parallel, both in terms of reduced dendritic arborizations *(67,68)* as well as in transcriptional silencing *(70)*. In fragile X syndrome, the responsible gene, *FMR1*, has an expansion of the CGG trinucleotide in the 5'-untranslated region. The effect of this expansion is abnormal methylation of *FMR1* with resultant repression of its transcription through histone deacetylation as described in the preceding *(87–89)*. The FMR1 protein (Fmrp) is found abundantly in neurons where it appears to be critical for protein synthesis *(90,91)*. This impairment of normal protein synthesis in neurons is likely responsible for the clinical and neuropathologic features of fragile X syndrome. In this case, excessive or aberrant transcriptional silencing leads to a loss of function. In RS, the lack of transcriptional silencing appears to lead to a gain of function in that the downstream genes typically influenced by MeCP2 are no longer regulated properly. Whether this is due to a failure to reduce transcriptional noise or altered transcription of brain-specific genes remains to be determined.

As proposed by Michael Johnston (*personal communication*), the hallmark of cellular dysfunction in RS may be the "sick" synapse. This fits well with the known involvement of multiple neurotransmitter systems and abnormalities in dendrite formation and places the timing of cellular dysfunction in the last third of gestation or very early infancy. Evidence that proliferation and migration of neurons proceed appropriately during the first 25 wk of gestation and that deceleration in the rate of head growth is present already by 3 mo of life suggests this temporal boundary *(14)*. Similarly, *MECP2* knockout mouse strains show normal cortical layering, although the brains are smaller than normal. In addition, these mice display delay in onset of abnormalities, suggesting dysfunction of more mature neurons *(92,93)*. The specific neurobiologic events and the downstream genes underlying RS on the one hand and normal neurodevelopment on the other remain to be determined. The unfolding panorama of ongoing investigations including the further elaboration of these mouse models will certainly provide important new insights for both.

10. SPECIFIC CLINICAL ISSUES IN RETT SYNDROME

Considerable variability is now recognized with respect to the functional level of females with RS. Nevertheless, for most of them, a number of specific clinical issues must be addressed over their lifetime. These include cognitive impairment, growth failure, breathing irregularities, seizures, scoliosis, gastrointestinal function, self-abuse, and longevity.

10.1. Cognitive Impairment

Assessment of cognitive function in girls with RS presents unique challenges. Without effective fine motor and communication skills, utilization of standardized tests is often impractical; however, with modification, standardized tests of cognition are considered a necessary part of the evaluation of children with RS and should be integrated into the Individualized Education Program (IEP) evaluations. Available data indicate that cognitive impairment is significant in most children with RS with mental age at the 8–10 mo level and gross motor function ranging from 12–18 mo. Assessments that depend only on visual response also yield cognitive levels in the severely impaired range. Adaptive skills such as feeding, dressing, and toileting functions often fail to develop, although some girls have acquired a degree of function in closely supervised settings. Thus, assistance with these needs must be provided throughout their lives. To maximize their functional levels, girls with RS must receive appropriate educational and habilitation services. These include physical, occupational, and speech therapy with augmentative communication *(94)*.

10.2. Growth Failure

Pervasive growth failure is one of the principal clinical characteristics of RS. The first evidence is often deceleration in the rate of head growth, which appears as early as 3 mo of age *(14,95)*. By age 4–5 years, median head circumference values for girls with RS fall to the second percentile of the normal population. Weight and height growth rates also fail to follow expected patterns and may reflect nutritional difficulties to some extent. For weight, growth rates fall below normal values near the end of the first year of life and median values are less than the 5th percentile about age 7 years. For height or length, growth slows at about 15 mo and median values reach the 5th percentile at age 7 years. Hand and foot growth are affected similarly. Reduction in rate of foot growth is greater and parallels that of height *(96)*. Onset of decline in the rate of hand growth occurs somewhat later and is less significant than that for feet.

10.3. Breathing Irregularities

Irregular breathing during wakefulness is another common feature of RS *(97–99)*. This irregularity may involve hyperventilation or breathholding, and in some girls, may include both. Breathholding may be prolonged, even exceeding 1 min, and may be associated with significant cyanosis. On the other hand, it may be quite subtle and escape recognition by parents and health care providers. In either case, medical intervention is rarely required or even effective. Air swallowing (aerophagia) may be significant, resulting in striking abdominal distension and potentially leading to impaired nutrition. Distension resolves spontaneously, especially during sleep.

Irregular breathing patterns have their onset in early childhood (3–5 years). During the early school-age period (5–10 years), hyperventilation or breathholding may permeate much of the waking activities. After this period, these breathing patterns are less frequent and intense. If irregular breathing is noted during sleep, a search for causes of obstructive apnea should be initiated.

As noted in the preceding, medical management of breathholding or hyperventilation has been rather ineffective. Benefit has been reported with the opiate antagonist, naltrexone, although this response is not reported consistently and could be explained by the sedating properties of this agent *(100)*. In this study, the treatment group demonstrated a greater rate of progression by clinical stage. However, this finding could be explained in part by the greater number of girls in stage II in the treatment group *(7)* than in the placebo group *(3)*. As such, the suggestion of a deleterious effect must be viewed with caution.

10.4. Seizures

Seizure frequency in RS appears to be quite variable with rates ranging from 30% to 80% *(101–104)*. The EEG is abnormal after about age 2 years. The principal EEG features are slow background, absence or reduction of posterior dominant rhythm, and recurrent spike and slow spike and wave activity. Despite the presence of epileptiform EEG changes, the majority of girls with RS may demonstrate few, if any, clinical seizures. Differentiating the often peculiar behavioral patterns from seizures in these girls may be challenging, generally requiring video-EEG monitoring. Seizures typically respond to standard antiepilepsy medications, particularly carbamazepine or sodium valproate, although standard precautions for serious side effects associated with the use of these medications are indicated. Carbamazepine has been tolerated quite well in general, but may produce agitation or self-abusive behavior. Carbamazepine has been associated with significant allergic reactions (Stevens–Johnson syndrome) and neutropenia. Sodium valproate has been associated with thrombocytopenia, pancreatitis, and fulminant liver failure, although these are rare above the age of 2 years and when used as monotherapy. Lamotrigine has also proved effective *(105,106)*, but must be given in slowly increasing dosages to avoid the appearance of skin rash.

10.5. Ambulation

Approximately 80% of girls with RS are able to walk. However, many will lose their ability to walk during or after the period of regression. Overall, about 60% remain ambulatory. For those who are able to walk, ambulation should be encouraged for as long as possible. In addition, weight-bearing strategies are recommended for those who do not walk. This would include the use of standing frames. Bones tend to be undermineralized and weight bearing may aid in improving this problem.

10.6. Scoliosis

Scoliosis is a common feature in RS, increasing in frequency with age. Scoliosis is present in about 8% of preschoolers and in more than 80% of girls over 16 years of age *(107–111)*. The overall incidence is about 50%. Scoliosis usually becomes apparent by 8 years, but earlier diagnosis is possible. Thereafter, it may become clinically significant and require medical or surgical attention. Progression is much more likely in girls who are nonambulatory. Bracing is considered when the curvature reaches 25 degrees although the efficacy of bracing in retarding progression has not been established. When the curvature exceeds 40 degrees, surgery is recommended.

10.7. Gastrointestinal Function

Nutrition can be a major problem in RS, requiring the guidance of a nutritionist to assess the adequacy of dietary intake with respect to caloric content, food consistency, and need for dietary supplementation. Girls with RS appear to have increased protein requirements *(112–114)*. Oral feeding may not be sufficient to maintain proper growth so that gastrostomy feeding may be necessary.

Gastroesophageal reflux and esophagitis may be common in RS. Recent parental reports to IRSA (Kathy Hunter, personal communication) have cited a number of instances of gall bladder disease as the basis for intense and recurring crying episodes and apparent abdominal pain. In some instances, these problems may underlie the unexplained irritability or apparent distress seen in RS. The lack of effective communication makes it quite difficult to interpret signs of distress in RS. As such, referral to a gastroenterologist for evaluation and treatment may be advisable under the circumstances.

Constipation is also a significant problem in RS requiring medical intervention in many instances. Numerous strategies including high-fiber foods, enemas, mineral oil, and milk of magnesia have been employed with variable success. Regular use of enemas is inadvisable due to the possible development of dependency on this mode of treatment. Prolonged use of mineral oil may interfere with proper absorption of the fat-soluble vitamins. Many girls refuse milk of magnesia, even the flavored forms. Miralax (polyethylene glycol) has been utilized recently with apparent efficacy (A. Percy, personal observation). This preparation is more palatable and better tolerated as it is tasteless and odorless and may be dissolved in juice, milk, or water.

10.8. Self-Abuse

Self-abusive behavior such as hair pulling, biting fingers, hands, or other parts of the upper extremities, and hitting themselves about the face or head is a potential problem in RS. Aggressive behavior toward others may also occur. This usually involves hitting, biting, or hair pulling. Care should be taken to exclude other medical problems, particularly gastrointestinal dysfunction as noted previously, or as a side effect of medications already in use before considering pharmacologic intervention. If indicated, risperidone in a low dose (0.25–0.5 mg b.i.d.) may be beneficial for ameliorating these adverse behaviors. The risk for extrapyramidal signs or tardive dyskinesia is minimal at these low dosages. The use of other agents for self-abusive behavior in RS, such as the serotonin reuptake inhibitors, has not been reported.

10.9. Longevity

Survival into adulthood is typical. One systematic, but unpublished study has been conducted, revealing that survival followed that of the general female population to age 10 years. Thereafter, life expectancy was less than expected. For the RS study cohort, survival at age 35 was about 70% compared to 98% for all females, and 27% for individuals with profound cognitive psychomotor impairments. Despite the reduced survival rate, significant issues exist with regard to counseling parents and other caretakers about long-term care and future planning as many of these women may outlive their parents.

Sudden death without apparent explanation has been reported in RS. Concern has been raised recently regarding the possibility of a cardiac basis for sudden death. This concern followed the report of prolonged QT intervals in a significant number of females with RS *(115–117)*. Nevertheless, a cardiac mechanism for sudden death has not been firmly documented.

10.10. Other Associated Features

In addition to the preceding, other features of RS include bruxism (teeth grinding), interrupted sleep patterns, and vasomotor disturbances in the form of cold feet and hands. Bruxism tends to occur more frequently during early childhood and attempts to treat it medically have been ineffective.

Sleep is often disrupted and fragmented *(98)*. Girls with RS may not sleep well for many nights in succession or may be awake during the night, often playing quietly or laughing for no apparent reason. This may result in similar disruptions in the parents' ability to sleep. It may be necessary to employ chloral hydrate, diphenhydramine, or hydroxyzine.

Vasomotor features tend to be more prominent in the lower extremities. These disturbances indicate autonomic nervous system dysfunction for which a precise explanation is lacking. Alteration of biogenic amine metabolites in cerebrospinal fluid *(118,119)* and substance P *(120)* in relevant brain stem nuclei may be involved. Sympathectomy resulting from the surgical management of scoliosis appears to reverse these findings on the operated side. No effective medical treatment has been identified.

11. LONG-TERM MANAGEMENT

In the absence of definitive therapy for RS, long-term management of girls with RS involves physical and occupational therapy, speech therapy, nutritional support, orthopedic intervention, and seizure management *(11,94)*. In particular, emphasis should be placed on establishing optimal communication by accessing the improved social interaction and eye contact, which tend to develop by school age. As noted in the preceding, planning for long-term care needs is essential. The potential for prolonged survival in women with RS mandates that future care needs be considered in light of the possibility that parents may not be able to manage these needs as they themselves age.

12. CONCLUSIONS

To summarize, the recent discovery of mutations in the *MECP2* gene in most females fulfilling the established criteria for RS culminates a decade long search for a genetic explanation for this intriguing disorder *(16)*. Discovery of the gene allows the confirmation of clinical diagnoses and the development of genotype–phenotype correlations. Further, the border zones of clinical involvement for girls who do not meet all diagnostic criteria for RS can now be examined carefully at the molecular genetic level. At present, in our studies and in those of others, the majority of girls fulfilling the criteria for RS have mutations in *MECP2 (25,31–34,37–39,41–44,53)*. The remaining girls may have mutations in as yet unexplored regions of *MECP2* or other genes may produce the disorder.

It is important to note that RS and *MECP2* mutations are not synonymous. The phenotypic spectrum arising from mutations in *MECP2* is remarkable making the decision as to when to pursue molecular analysis in this gene difficult at times. Are we wise enough to determine which individuals and under what circumstances mutational analysis should be requested with a high likelihood of ascertaining a mutation? Recent data suggest that we are not yet able to predict which neurodevelopmental disabilities are likely to be explained by such mutations. Certainly, girls fulfilling some or all criteria for RS should be tested. Based on the variety of clinical phenotypes already described, mutational analysis should also be considered carefully in children with nonsyndromic cognitive impairment, autism with progressive features, unexplained fatal encephalopathy in infancy, and X-linked neurodevelopmental disabilities. It is possible that *MECP2* is one of the more likely suspects involved in various forms of X-linked mental retardation *(52)*.

REFERENCES

1. Rett A. Uber ein eigenartiges hirnatrophisches Syndrom bei Hyperammonamie im Kindesalter. Wien Med Wochenschr 1966;116:723–6.
2. Hagberg B, Aicardi J, Dias K, Ramos O. A progressive syndrome of autism, dementia, ataxia, and loss of purposeful hand use in girls: Rett's syndrome: report of 35 cases. Ann Neurol 1983;14:471–9.
3. Nomura Y, Segawa M, Hasegawa M. Rett syndrome—clinical studies and pathophysiological consideration. Brain Dev 1984;6:475–86.
4. Percy AK, Zoghbi H, Riccardi VM. Rett syndrome: initial experience with an emerging clinical entity. Brain Dev 1985;7:300–4.
5. Holm VA. Rett's syndrome: a progressive developmental disability in girls. Dev Behav Pediatr 1985;6:32–6.

6. Kerr AM, Stephenson JB. A study of the natural history of Rett syndrome in 23 girls. Am J Med Genet 1986;24(Suppl 1):77–83.

7. Hagberg BA. Rett's syndrome: prevalence and impact on progressive severe mental retardation in girls. Acta Paediatr 1985;74:405–8.

8. Kozinetz CA, Skender ML, MacNaughton N, et al. Epidemiology of Rett syndrome: a population-based registry. Pediatrics 1993;91:445–50.

9. Gillberg C. Debate and argument: having Rett syndrome in the ICD-10 PDD category does not make sense (see comments). J Child Psychol Psychiatry Allied Discipl 1994;35:377–8.

10. Rutter M. Debate and argument: there are connections between brain and mind and it is important that Rett syndrome be classified somewhere (comment). J Child Psychol Psychiatry Allied Discipl 1994;35:379–81.

11. Hagberg B. Rett syndrome—clinical & biological aspects. London: MacKeith Press, 1993;1–120.

12. Hagberg B, Goutieres F, Hanefeld F, Rett A, Wilson J. Rett syndrome: criteria for inclusion and exclusion. Brain Dev 1985; 7: 372–3.

13. Anonymous. Diagnostic criteria for Rett syndrome. The Rett Syndrome Diagnostic Criteria Work Group. Ann Neurol 1988; 23: 425–8.

14. Schultz RJ, Glaze DG, Motil KJ, et al. The pattern of growth failure in Rett syndrome. Am J Dis Child 1993; 147: 633–7.

15. Watson P, Black G, Ramsden S, et al. Angelman syndrome phenotype associated with mutations in MECP2, a gene encoding a methyl CpG binding protein. J Med Genet 2001; 38: 224–8.

16. Amir R, Van den Veyver I, Wan M, Tran C, Francke U, Zoghbi H. Rett syndrome is caused by mutations in X-linked MECP2, encoding methyl-CpG-binding protein 2. Nat Genet 1999; 23: 185–8.

17. Hagberg B, Witt-Engerstrom I. Rett syndrome: a suggested staging system for describing impairment profile with increasing age towards adolescence. Am J Med Genet 1986;24(Suppl 1):47–59.

18. Hagberg B, Rasmussen P. "Forme fruste" of Rett syndrome—a case report. Am J Med Genet 1986;24(Suppl 1):175–81.

19. Zappella M. The Rett girls with preserved speech. Brain Dev 1992;14:98–101.

20. Aicardi J. Rett Syndrome. Int Pediatr 1988;3:165–9.

21. Hagberg BA, Skjeldal OH. Rett variants: a suggested model for inclusion criteria. Pediatr Neurol 1994;11:5–11.

22. Vorsanova SG, Demidova IA, Ulas VY, Soloviev IV, Kazantzeva LZ, Yurov YB. Cytogenic and molecular-cytogenic investigation of Rett syndrome: analysis of 31 cases. NeuroReport 1996;8:187–9.

23. Schwartzman JS, Zatz M, dos Reis Vasquez L, et al. Rett syndrome in a boy with a 47,XXY karyotype. Am J Hum Genet 1999;64:1781–5.

24. Leonard H, Silberstein J, Falk R, Houwink-Manville I, Ellaway C, Raffaele LS, Engerstrom IW, Schanen C. Occurrence of Rett syndrome in boys. J Child Neurol 2001;16:333–8.

25. Hoffbuhr K, Devaney JM, LaFleur B, et al. MeCP2 mutations in children with and without the phenotype of Rett syndrome. Neurology 2001;56:1486–95.

26. Dragich J, Houwink-Manville I, Schanen C. Rett syndrome: a surprising result of mutation in MECP2. Hum Mol Genet 2000;9:2365–75.

27. Webb T, Latif F. Rett syndrome and the MECP2 gene. J Med Genet 2001;38:217–23.

28. Schanen C, Dahle E, Capozzoli F, Holm V, Zoghbi H, Francke U. A new Rett syndrome family consistent with X-linked inheritance expands the X chromosome exclusion map. Am J Hum Genet 1997;61:634–41.

29. Sirianni N, Naidu S, Pereira J, Pillotto FR, Hoffman EP. Rett syndrome: confirmation of X-linked dominat inheritance, and localization of the gene in Xq28. Am J Hum Genet 1998;63:1552–8.

30. Schanen NC. Molecular approaches to the Rett syndrome gene. J Child Neurol 1999;14:806–14.

31. Wan M, Lee SS, Zhang X, et al. Rett syndrome and beyond: recurrent spontaneous and familial MECP2 mutations at CpG hotspots. Am J Hum Genet 1999;65:1520–9.

32. Bienvenu T, Carrie A, de Roux N, et al. MECP2 mutations account for most cases of typical forms of Rett syndrome. Hum Mol Genet 2000;9:1377–84.

33. Cheadle J, Gill H, Fleming N, et al. Long-read sequence analysis of the *MECP2* gene in Rett syndrome patients: correlation of disease severity with mutation type and location. Hum Mol Genet 2000;9:1119–29.

34. Huppke P, Laccone F, Kramer N, Engel W, Hanefeld F. Rett syndrome: analysis of MECP2 and clinical characterization of 31 patients. Hum Mol Genet 2000;9:1369–75.

35. Amir R, Zoghbi H. Rett syndrome: methyl-CpG-binding protein 2 mutations and phenotype–genotype correlations. Am J Med Genet 2000;97:147–52.

36. Xiang F, Buervenich S, Nicolao P, Bailey ME, Zhang Z, Anvret M. Mutation screening in Rett syndrome patients. J Med Genet 2000;37:250–5.

37. Amano K, Nomura Y, Segawa M, Yamakawa K. Mutational analysis of the MECP2 gene in Japanese patients with Rett syndrome. J Hum Genet 2000;45:231–6.

38. Buyse IM, Fang P, Hoon KT, Amir RE, Zoghbi HY, Roa BB. Diagnostic testing for Rett syndrome by DHPLC and direct sequencing analysis of the MECP2 gene: identification of several novel mutations and polymorphisms. Am J Hum Genet 2000;67:1428–36.

39. Obata K, Matsuishi T, Yamashita Y, et al. Mutation analysis of the methyl-CpG binding protein 2 gene (MECP2) in patients with Rett syndrome (letter). J Med Genet 2000;37:608–10.

40. Hampson K, Woods CG, Latif F, Webb T. Mutations in the MECP2 gene in a cohort of girls with Rett syndrome. J Med Genet 2000;37:610–2.

41. Bourdon V, Philippe C, Labrune O, Amsallem D, Arnould C, Jonveaux P. A detailed analysis of the MECP2 gene: prevalence of recurrent mutations and gross DNA rearrangements in Rett syndrome patients. Hum Genet 2001; 108:43–50.

42. Nielsen JB, Henriksen KF, Hansen C, Silahtaroglu A, Schwartz M, Tommerup N. MECP2 mutations in Danish patients with Rett syndrome: high frequency

of mutations but no consistent correlations with clinical severity or with the X chromosome inactivation pattern. Eur J Hum Genet 2001;9:178–84.

43. Laccone F, Huppke P, Hanefeld F, Meins M. Mutation spectrum in patients with Rett syndrome in the German population: evidence of hot spot regions. Hum Mutat 2001;17:183–90.
44. Auranen M, Vanhala R, Vosman M, et al. MECP2 gene analysis in classical Rett syndrome and in patients with Rett-like features. Neurology 2001; 56:611–7.
45. Girard M, Couvert P, Carrie A, et al. Parental origin of de novo MECP2 mutations in Rett syndrome. Eur J Hum Genet 2001;9:231–6.
46. Trappe R, Laccone F, Cobilanschi J, et al. MECP2 mutations in sporadic cases of rett syndrome are almost exclusively of paternal origin. Am J Hum Genet 2001;68:1093–101.
47. Schanen NC, Kurczynski TW, Brunelle D, Woodcock M, Dure LS, Percy AK. Neonatal encephalopathy in two boys in families with recurrent Rett syndrome. J Child Neurol 1998;13:229–31.
48. Villard L, Cardoso AK, Chelly PJ, Tardieu PM, Fontes M. Two affected boys in a rett syndrome family: clinical and molecular findings. Neurology 2000;55:1188–93.
49. Imessaoudene B, Bonnefont JP, Royer G, et al. MECP2 mutation in non-fatal, non-progressive encephalopathy in a male. J Med Genet 2001;38:171–4.
50. Meloni I, Bruttini M, Longo I, et al. A mutation in the Rett syndrome gene, *MECP2*, causes X-linked mental retardation and progressive spasticity in males. Am J Hum Genet 2000;67:982–5.
51. Clayton-Smith J, Watson P, Ramsden S, Black G. Somatic mutation in *MECP2* as a non-fatal neurodevelopmental disorder in males. Lancet 2000;356:830–2.
52. Couvert P, Bienvenu T, Aquaviva C, et al. MECP2 is highly mutated in X-linked mental retardation. Hum Mol Genet 2001;10:941–6.
53. Amir R, Van den Veyver I, Schultz R, et al. Influence of mutation type and X chromosome inactivation on Rett syndrome phenotypes. Ann Neurol 2000;47:670–9.
54. De Bona C, Zappella M, Hayek G, et al. Preserved speech variant is allelic of classic Rett syndrome. Eur J Hum Genet 2000;8:325–30.
55. Armstrong D, Dunn K, Schultz R, Herbert D, Glaze D, Motil K. Organ growth in Rett syndrome: a postmortem examination analysis. Pediatr Neurol 1999;20:125–9.
56. Reiss AL, Faruque F, Naidu S, et al. Neuroanatomy of Rett syndrome: a volumetric imaging study. Ann Neurol 1993;34:227–34.
57. Jellinger K, Seitelberger F. Neuropathology of Rett syndrome. Am J Med Genet 1986;24(Suppl 1):259–88.
58. Jellinger K, Armstrong D, Zoghbi HY, Percy AK. Neuropathology of Rett syndrome. Acta Neuropathol 1988;76:142–58.
59. Bauman M, Kemper T. The neuropathology of Rett syndrome is pervasive throughout the brain. Neurology 1991;41(Suppl 1):675P.

60. Armstrong D. The neuropathology of the Rett syndrome. Brain Dev 1992;14:Suppl:S89–98.
61. Bauman ML, Kemper TL, Arin DM. Microscopic observations of the brain in Rett syndrome. Neuropediatrics 1995;26:105–8.
62. Armstrong D. The neuropathology of Rett syndrome—overview 1994. Neuropediatrics 1995;26:100–4.
63. Armstrong D, Dunn J, Antalffy B, Trivedi R. Selective dendritic alterations in the cortex of Rett syndrome. J Neuropathol Exp Neurol 1995;54:195–201.
64. Armstrong D, Dunn K, Antalffy B. Decreased dendritic branching in frontal, motor and limbic cortex in Rett syndrome compared with Trisomy 21. J Neuropathol Exp Neurol 1998;57:1013–7.
65. Takashima S, Ieshima A, Nakamura H, Becker LE. Dendrites, dementia and the Down syndrome. Brain Dev 1989;11:131–3.
66. Jay V, Becker LE, Chan FW, Perry TL, Sr. Puppet-like syndrome of Angelman: a pathologic and neurochemical study. Neurology 1991;41:416–22.
67. Hinton VJ, Brown WT, Wisniewski K, Rudelli RD. Analysis of neocortex in three males with the fragile X syndrome. Am J Med Genet 1991;41:289–94.
68. Comery TA, Harris JB, Willems PJ, et al. Abnormal dendritic spines in fragile X knockout mice: maturation and pruning deficits. Proc Natl Acad Sci USA 1997;94:5401–4.
69. Kemper TL, Bauman M. Neuropathology of infantile autism. J Neuropathol Exp Neurol 1998;57:645–52.
70. Robertson KD, Wolffe AP. DNA methylation in health and disease. Nat Rev Genet 2000;1:11–9.
71. Kafri T, Ariel M, Brandeis M, et al. Developmental pattern of gene-specific DNA methylation in the mouse embryo and germ line. Genes Dev 1992;6:705–14.
72. Bird AP. Gene number, noise reduction and biological complexity. Trends Genet 1995;11:94–100.
73. Ng HH, Bird A. Histone deacetylases: silencers for hire. Trends Biochem Sci 2000;25:121–6.
74. Huang Y, Myers SJ, Dingledine R. Transcriptional repression by REST: recruitment of Sin3A and histone deacetylase to neuronal genes. Nat Neurosci 1999;2:867–72.
75. Naruse Y, Aoki T, Kojima T, Mori N. Neural restrictive silencer factor recruits mSin3 and histone deacetylase complex to repress neuron-specific target genes. Proc Natl Acad Sci USA 1999;96:13,691–6.
76. Chen ZF, Paquette AJ, Anderson DJ. NRSF/REST is required in vivo for repression of multiple neuronal target genes during embryogenesis. Nat Genet 1998;20:136–42.
77. Jones PL, Veenstra GJ, Wade PA, et al. Methylated DNA and MeCP2 recruit histone deacetylase to repress transcription. Nat Genet 1998;19:187–91.
78. Kudo S. Methyl-CpG-binding protein MeCP2 represses Sp1-activated transcription of the human leukosialin gene when the promoter is methylated. Mol Cell Biol 1998;18:5492–9.

79. Nan X, Ng HH, Johnson CA, et al. Transcriptional repression by the methyl-CpG-binding protein MeCP2 involves a histone deacetylase complex. Nature 1998;393:386–9.
80. Chandler SP, Guschin D, Landsberger N, Wolffe AP. The methyl-CpG binding transcriptional repressor MeCP2 stably associates with nucleosomal DNA. Biochemistry 1999;38:7008–18.
81. Kaludov NK, Wolffe AP. MeCP2 driven transcriptional repression in vitro: selectivity for methylated DNA, action at a distance and contacts with the basal transcription machinery. Nucleic Acids Res 2000;28:1921–8.
82. Lewis JD, Meehan RR, Henzel WJ, et al. Purification, sequence, and cellular localization of a novel chromosomal protein that binds to methylated DNA. Cell 1992;69:905–14.
83. Hendrich B, Bird A. Identification and characterization of a family of mammalian methyl-CpG binding proteins. Mol Cell Biol 1998;18:6538–47.
84. Akhmanova A, Verkerk T, Langeveld A, Grosveld F, Galjart N. Characterisation of transcriptionally active and inactive chromatin domains in neurons. J Cell Sci 2000;113 Pt 24:4463–74.
85. Brock GJ, Bird A. Mosaic methylation of the repeat unit of the human ribosomal RNA genes. Hum Mol Genet 1997;6:451–456.
86. Ballestar E, Yusufzai TM, Wolffe AP. Effects of Rett syndrome mutations of the methyl-CpG binding domain of the transcriptional repressor MeCP2 on selectivity for association with methylated DNA. Biochemistry 2000;39:7100–6.
87. Kremer EJ, Pritchard M, Lynch M, et al. Mapping of DNA instability at the fragile X to a trinucleotide repeat sequence p(CCG)n. Science 1991;252:1711–4.
88. Oberle I, Rousseau F, Heitz D, et al. Instability of a 550-base pair DNA segment and abnormal methylation in fragile X syndrome. Science 1991;252:1097–102.
89. Coffee B, Zhang F, Warren ST, Reines D. Acetylated histones are associated with FMR1 in normal but not fragile X-syndrome cells. (erratum appears in Nat Genet 1999 Jun;22[2]:209). Nat Genet 1999;22:98–101.
90. Warren ST, Nelson DL. Trinucleotide repeat expansions in neurological disease. Curr Opin Neurobiol 1993;3:752–9.
91. Feng Y, Absher D, Eberhart DE, Brown V, Malter HE, Warren ST. FMRP associates with polyribosomes as an mRNP, and the I304N mutation of severe fragile X syndrome abolishes this association. Mol Cell 1997;1:109–18.
92. Guy J, Hendrich B, Holmes M, Martin JE, Bird A. A mouse MECP2-null mutation causes neurological symptoms that mimic Rett syndrome. Nat Genet 2001;27:322–6.
93. Chen RZ, Akbarian S, Tudor M, Jaenisch R. Deficiency of methyl-CpG binding protein-2 in CNS neurons results in a Rett-like phenotype in mice. Nat Genet 2001;27:327–31.
94. Budden SS. Rett syndrome: habilitation and management reviewed. Eur Child Adolesc Psychiatry 1997;6:103–7.
95. Stenbom Y, Engerstrom IW, Hagberg G. Gross motor disability and head growth in Rett syndrome—a preliminary report. Neuropediatrics 1995;26:85–6.

96. Schultz R, Glaze D, Motil K, Hebert D, Percy A. Hand and foot growth failure in Rett syndrome. J Child Neurol 1998;13:71–4.

97. Lugaresi E, Cirignotta F, Montagna P. Abnormal breathing in the Rett syndrome. Brain Dev 1985;7:329–33.

98. Glaze D, Frost J, Zoghbi H, Percy A. Rett's syndrome: characterization of respiratory patterns and sleep. Ann Neurol 1987;21:377–82.

99. Southall DP, Kerr AM, Tirosh E, Amos P, Lang MH, Stephenson JB. Hyperventilation in the awake state: potentially treatable component of Rett syndrome. Arch Dis Child 1988;63:1039–48.

100. Percy AK, Glaze DG, Schultz RJ, et al. Rett syndrome: controlled study of an oral opiate antagonist, naltrexone. Ann Neurol 1994;35:464–70.

101. Glaze D, Frost J, Zoghbi H, Percy A. Rett's syndrome: correlation of electroencephalographic characteristics with clinical staging. Arch Neurol 1987;44:1053–6.

102. Hagne I, Witt-Engerstrom I, Hagberg B. EEG development in Rett syndrome. A study of 30 cases. Electroencephalogr Clin Neurophysiol 1989;72:1–6.

103. Glaze D, Schultz R, Frost J. Rett syndrome: characterization of seizures and non-seizures. Electroencephalogr Clin Neurophysiol 1998;106:79–83.

104. Steffenburg U, Hagberg G, Hagberg B. Epilepsy in a representative series of Rett syndrome. Acta Paediatr 2001;90:34–9.

105. Uldall P, Hansen FJ, Tonnby B. Lamotrigine in Rett syndrome. Neuropediatrics 1993;24:339–40.

106. Stenbom Y, Tonnby B, Hagberg B. Lamotrigine in Rett syndrome: treatment experience from a pilot study. Eur Child Adolesc Psychiatry 1998;7:49–52.

107. Holm VA, King HA. Scoliosis in the Rett syndrome. Brain Dev 1990; 12:151–3.

108. Bassett GS, Tolo VT. The incidence and natural history of scoliosis in Rett syndrome. Dev Med Child Neurol 1990;32:963–6.

109. Harrison DJ, Webb PJ. Scoliosis in the Rett syndrome: natural history and treatment. Brain Dev 1990;12:154–6.

110. Guidera KJ, Borrelli J Jr, Raney E, Thompson-Rangel T, Ogden JA. Orthopaedic manifestations of Rett syndrome. J Pediatr Orthop 1991;11:204–8.

111. Lidstrom J, Stokland E, Hagberg B. Scoliosis in Rett syndrome. Clinical and biological aspects. Spine 1994;19:1632–5.

112. Motil KJ, Schultz R, Brown B, Glaze DG, Percy AK. Altered energy balance may account for growth failure in Rett syndrome. J Child Neurol 1994; 9:315–9.

113. Motil K, Shultz R, Wong W, Glaze D. Increased energy expenditure associated with repetitive involuntary movement does not contribute to growth failure in girls with Rett syndrome. J Pediatr 1998;132:228–33.

114. Motil KJ, Schultz RJ, Browning K, Trautwein L, Glaze DG. Oropharyngeal dysfunction and gastroesophageal dysmotility are present in girls and women with Rett syndrome. J Pediatr Gastroenterol Nutr 1999;29:31–7.

115. Sekul EA, Moak JP, Schultz RJ, Glaze DG, Dunn JK, Percy AK. Electrocardiographic findings in Rett syndrome: an explanation for sudden death? J Pediatr 1994;125:80–2.

116. Guideri F, Acampa M, Hayek G, Zappella M, Di Perri T. Reduced heart rate variability in patients affected with Rett syndrome. A possible explanation for sudden death. Neuropediatrics 1999;30:146–8.

117. Guideri F, Acampa M, DiPerri T, Zappella M, Hayek Y. Progressive cardiac dysautonomia observed in patients affected by classic Rett syndrome and not in the preserved speech variant. J Child Neurol 2001;16:370–3.

118. Zoghbi HY, Percy AK, Glaze DG, Butler IJ, Riccardi VM. Reduction of biogenic amine levels in the Rett syndrome. N Engl J Med 1985;313:921–4.

119. Lekman A, Witt-Engerstrom I, Gottfries J, Hagberg BA, Percy AK, Svennerholm L. Rett syndrome: biogenic amines and metabolites in postmortem brain. Pediatr Neurol 1989;5:357–62.

120. Deguchi K, Antalffy B, Twohill L, Chakraborty S, Glaze D, Armstrong D. Substance P immunoreactivity in Rett syndrome. Pediatr Neurol 2000;22:259–66.

Index

From: *Contemporary Clinical Neuroscience:*
Genetics and Genomics of Neurobehavioral Disorders
Edited by: G. S. Fisch © Humana Press Inc., Totowa, NJ

3

T